Satoshi Kuroda
Editor

Moyamoya Disease: Current Knowledge and Future Perspectives

Springer

Foreword

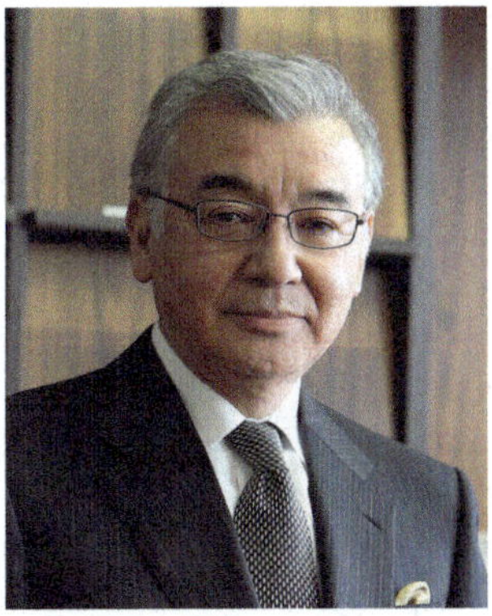

Moyamoya disease is an uncommon cerebrovascular disease characterized by progressive stenosis of the terminal portion of the internal carotid artery and is associated with the dilated, fragile collaterals at the base of the brain. This curious vascular condition was first described by Takeuchi and Shimizu in 1957 as hypoplasia of the bilateral internal carotid arteries. Suzuki and Takaku studied this still-unspecified disease extensively by using cerebral angiography in the relatively early days of the technique and nicely summarized this pathology as "Moyamoya" disease in 1969. Moyamoya means something hazy, like a puff of cigarette smoke in Japanese. This very impressive naming by Suzuki and Takaku must have contributed to spread the idea of the disease worldwide and this evocative name has been used to represent this unique, strange, and mysterious cerebrovascular condition.

Microvascular anastomotic technique has been a potential modality to develop treatment strategy and to enhance the understanding of this pathology. Bypass surgery in patients with Moyamoya disease is one of the finest and most difficult microvascular procedures because the recipient vessels of cortical surface of these patients are exceptionally small and fragile. Surgical bypass from extracranial artery to intracranial artery has been found to be effective with increasing intracranial blood flow but also has found to cause unexpected and unfavorable effects to the patients. To confirm the efficacy of bypass surgery and to reduce complications of bypass surgery, techniques to study cerebral blood flow and metabolism have been accelerated.

Sydney Brenner, a recipient of the 2002 Nobel Prize for discoveries concerning the genetic regulation of organ development and programmed cell death, stated that progress in science depends on new techniques, new discoveries, and new ideas, probably in that order. Although his comments pertained to pure science, they are also applicable to our specialty, including vascular neurosurgery. When we trace the history of the research on diagnosis and treatment of Moyamoya disease, technical advancement came first and such techniques were applied to the patients and many findings were obtained, at least, some of them were not expected, or even not imagined before application of a certain technique. Repeating these processes, we reach to new ideas and such new ideas invite next questions. We are still on such a circuit of resolution.

I know Professor Kuroda personally for many years as a result of his energetic activity in the field of vascular neurosurgery and by collaborating several research works on Moyamoya disease with me. I appreciate very much the enthusiasm, dedication, and energy he has offered to his assignment on this disease. He is a well-trained mountain climber and an outstanding leader of several Alpine clubs in his community. I am sure that there are a lot of similarities between heading for the summit of a high and steep mountain and solving questions and giving answers for the resolution of Moyamoya disease.

This time, he has made a textbook of Moyamoya disease as the editor entitled "*Moyamoya disease—Current Knowledge and Future Perspectives*." This book shows his capacity for organizing researchers and clinicians heading for the top of the mountain, namely for the top of this still challenging disease.

Nobuo Hashimoto
Kyoto University
National Cerebral and Cardiovascular Center
Kyoto, Japan
2020/10/05

Preface

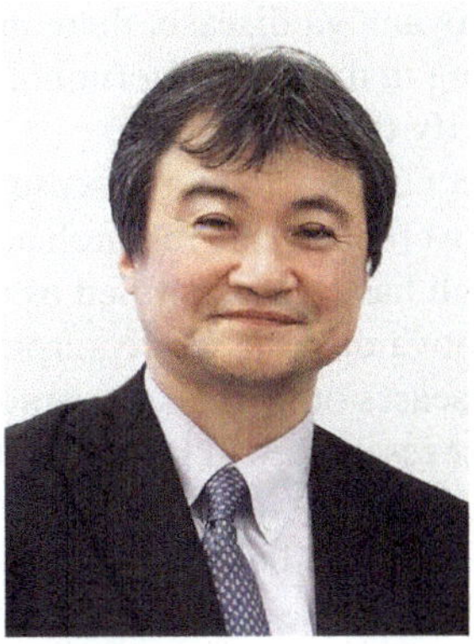

It is with great honor that I can publish this monograph entitled "*Moyamoya Disease—Current Knowledge and Future Perspectives*" with Springer as my own editor, and I feel a tremendous amount of responsibility. My first encounter with moyamoya disease was in the summer of 1985, when I was a medical student rotating in the Department of Neurosurgery during my clinical internship. A young child with multiple cerebral infarcts, resulting in cognitive dysfunction, and the brilliant bypass surgery performed by a still-young Prof. Hiroyasu Kamiyama, are still etched in my eyelids. In the spring of 1986, I could finally become a neurosurgeon and chose the hard path of cerebrovascular neurosurgeon to save as many patients with moyamoya disease as possible. Although I have treated a lot of patients and conducted a lot of research in the past 35 years, I have to say that there are still a lot of issues to be solved for moyamoya disease.

This disease, which still retains many mysterious elements, was discovered in Japan in the 1950s and then sparked a lot of debate in the 1960s in Japan and elsewhere over its etiology and pathology. Exactly 50 years have passed since Prof. Jiro Suzuki and Prof. Akira Takaku first proposed the name moyamoya disease and established the concept of the disease in an English-language medical journal in 1969, but the debate is still going on in a shape-shifting fashion. With this 50-year milestone, I wanted to publish a monograph that explores recent advances in the science and medicine of moyamoya disease, with an emphasis on the new insights gained in the last decade, and to serve as a beacon for the future. For this publication, I would like to express my deepest gratitude and respect to the leading neurosurgeons and researchers from Japan, Korea, China, the United States, and Europe, with whom I have become friends through academic activities such as scientific conferences, for agreeing to the purpose of this monograph and for putting their best efforts into writing the manuscript, despite their busy lives.

In this monograph, we will begin with a review of the evolution of the history, concept, and diagnostic criteria of moyamoya disease under the title of "Part I: Concept of moyamoya Disease." As the diagnostic criteria for moyamoya disease are revised every decade or so, the concept of the disease is by no means settled, and disagreements about the diagnosis are still not so rare. In the case of moyamoya syndrome and unilateral moyamoya disease, there are differences in interpretation among researchers, including in the field of terminology, even now and I wanted to take this opportunity to clarify the situation.

In "Part II: Genetic Aspect of moyamoya Disease," we asked the top researchers to write about one of the most remarkable research achievements of the last decade: the RNF213 mutation, which has been identified as a major susceptibility gene for the development of moyamoya disease. More surprisingly, RNF213 mutation has been identified in several diseases other than moyamoya disease. In the next decade, we are confident that further research will be conducted in this field.

"Part III: Pathophysiology of moyamoya Disease" begins with thorough discussion on the pathophysiology of TIA, headache, and ischemic stroke as old and new topics. moyamoya disease is a unique disorder in that hyperventilation such as eating hot noodles and crying induces TIA and that a migraine-like headache attack occurs upon waking. Although many studies have been conducted to elucidate the pathogenesis of this disease in the 1980s and the 1990s, many questions remain unanswered. I would be very happy if this monograph would serve as an opportunity for young readers to consider future research. The randomized clinical trial, Japan Adult Moyamoya (JAM) trial, has provided us novel knowledge and concept on adult hemorrhagic-type moyamoya disease over the past 10 years. In recent years, it has become clear that moyamoya disease causes cognitive dysfunction in adults as well as in children, and in this chapter, an on-going multi-centered cohort study conducted in Japan will be discussed. The pathophysiology and natural course of asymptomatic moyamoya disease, which is recognized more common than thought before, is still unknown. Therefore, no treatment guidelines have been established yet. An on-going multi-center cohort study, Asymptomatic Moyamoya Registry (AMORE) study in Japan, will be introduced in this chapter.

While many specific pathophysiology and imaging findings of moyamoya disease have been reported in the past, novel findings have been further obtained in the past decade. Therefore, "Part IV: Update on Neuroradiology in moyamoya Disease" was arranged. The results of a series of studies by the JAM Trial Group have reorganized the anatomy and pathophysiological functions of bleeding-prone moyamoya vessels and newly defined as "dangerous periventricular anastomosis." For the past 50 years, morphological information on the lumen of the affected arteries has been the only clue for the diagnosis of moyamoya disease; however, recent MR studies have shown that moyamoya disease causes specific shrinkage of the affected arteries, and thus the concept of the disease and diagnostic criteria may change significantly in near future. Although the disease progression was previously believed very rare in adults, recent longitudinal studies have found that it is not uncommon in adults. There is increasing evidence that hyperperfusion occurs after surgical revascularization at a very high rate in moyamoya disease. Although the pathogenesis is still far from being fully understood, the postoperative management of moyamoya disease has undergone a major renovation over the past decade. Recently, the transient development of high signal intensity in the brain surface on FLAIR images has been widely recognized. Although the pathogenesis is still unknown, the findings are thought almost unique to moyamoya disease, and further studies are awaited.

In recent years, surgical revascularization has been accepted to significantly reduce the recurrence of TIA, ischemic stroke as well as hemorrhagic stroke. However, given that many patients with moyamoya disease are children and young adults, I believe that it is incumbent on us neurosurgeons to clarify the long-term clinical prognosis more than ever before. Therefore, in "Part V: Real World of Surgical Revascularization for Moyamoya Disease," I first outlined about it and wrote about the real world in Japan. Then, prominent neurosurgeons from Asia, the United States, and Europe have also been asked to review in detail the long-term prognosis after surgery in their respective regions. This monograph is not intended to be a detailed discussion of surgical techniques. I have decided to add the detailed descriptions of the issues that should still be familiar to us in performing surgical revascularization for patients with moyamoya disease.

In summary, I have described the background and aims of the chapters of this monograph. As an editor, it is my distinct pleasure if this monograph will be useful to you as you can learn about the fundamentals of moyamoya disease, the advances in basic and clinical research, and the prospects for future research.

Wishing all patients suffering from Moyamoya disease to live their peaceful daily life of mind.

Toyama, Japan
December 1, 2020

Satoshi Kuroda

Part I

Concept of Moyamoya Disease

History of Disease Entity and Diagnosis Criteria

1

Satoshi Kuroda

Abstract

This chapter reviews the history of this mysterious moyamoya disease. Since the 1950s, this rare disease has been discovered in Japan and gradually gaining recognition around the world. It has been just 50 years since Suzuki and Takaku first published the term "moyamoya disease" in an English language journal in 1969. Looking back over the past 50 years, the author would like to review the state of affairs at the time when the causes and concepts of this disease were hotly debated. It may be helpful to us in the future when new diseases appear in front of us. It is no secret, however, that it is nearly impossible to write a history that will satisfy everyone. Therefore, the author appreciates it if the readers would kindly understand that this historical review is only from the author's point of view and they would forgive him.

In this chapter, the author describes the evolution of the diagnostic criteria for moyamoya disease. Since the diagnostic criteria for moyamoya disease were first established in 1979 by a Japanese research group, they have been revised approximately every 10 years in 1988, 1995, 2009, and 2018. The author would like to look back at that history and explore the background with the readers. Finally, the challenges of the diagnostic criteria and the prospects for the future will be discussed.

S. Kuroda (✉)
Department of Neurosurgery, Graduate School of Medicine and Pharmaceutical Science, University of Toyama, Toyama, Japan
e-mail: skuroda@med.u-toyama.ac.jp

S. Kuroda (ed.), *Moyamoya Disease: Current Knowledge and Future Perspectives*, https://doi.org/10.1007/978-981-33-6404-2_1

Keywords

Moyamoya disease · History · Diagnosis criteria

1.1 Introduction

Moyamoya disease is a very specific disease characterized by progressive stenosis of the terminal portion of the internal carotid artery and the formation of an abnormal network of dilated, fragile perforators around the basal ganglia, thalamus, and lateral ventricles. Moyamoya disease was first reported in Japan in the 1950s and has widely been recognized over the world. It occurs in children and adults, and presents with a variety of symptoms, including headache, TIA, ischemic stroke, intracranial bleeding, and involuntary movements. Initially, there was no effective treatment for the disease; however, since the late 1960s, surgical revascularization was found to be an effective treatment.

In this chapter, the author reviews the history of moyamoya disease and describes in detail the historical transition of the diagnosis criteria for moyamoya disease. The issues and future perspectives of the diagnosis criteria are also discussed.

1.2 History of Moyamoya Disease

The history of moyamoya disease has recently been described in the monographs written in English [1, 2]. In writing this chapter, however, the author tried to revisit the history of the moyamoya disease by reading the monographs, proceedings, and review articles from the 1960s. Based on previous review articles, Takeuchi and Shimizu reported a case of bilateral internal carotid arteries in 1955 and published it as a case report in 1957, which is believed as probably the first case of moyamoya disease on cerebral angiography that has appeared in the literature [3]. Since then, a significant number of similar cases were reported from Western countries as well as from Japan in the 1960s and 1970s. Interestingly, the first three cases reported from California were all Japanese Americans [4, 5].

At that time, various theories have been raised as to the cause of this peculiar cerebral angiography seen in moyamoya disease, including carotid artery hypoplasia [3], hypoplasia of the circle of Willis [6], cerebral juxta-basal telangiectasia [7], carotid artery occlusion [8], a network-like vascular anomaly of internal carotid artery [9], and angiomatous malformation [10, 11]. In addition to the papers cited here, many other reports were made in Japan at the time, which strongly suggests that Japanese neurologists and neurosurgeons were engaged in heated discussions about this novel, mysterious disease discovered in Japan in the 1960s and 1970s. However, many of these records are from the annual scientific meetings and their proceedings in Japan and are written in Japanese, and so the author must say that he only quotes original articles written in Japanese or English without citing them in this book, which is likely to be read by readers in countries other than Japan. These valuable records are described in detail in a proceeding by Prof. Tatsuyuki Kudo from Keio University, Tokyo (1967) [12], a review article by Prof. Akira Nishimoto from Okayama University, Okayama (1979) [13] and a monograph by Prof. Jiro Suzuki from Tohoku University, Sendai (1983) [14]. So, the author would like to recommend to the readers who are interested in this topic to read them. Especially, the monograph edited by Prof. Suzuki has been translated and published in English, which will be of great help to the non-Japanese readers (Fig. 1.1).

In 1963, Suzuki et al. performed a detailed review of the findings on cerebral angiography in six cases of moyamoya disease, and concluded that these abnormal net-like vessels at the base of the brain are collateral blood vessels in response to the acquired and gradual narrowing of the terminal portion of the internal carotid artery at the 22nd Annual Meeting of the Japan Neurosurgical Society. At the same time, they also speculated that this group of cases belonged to a single, novel clinical entity. In fact, on the front page of the monograph mentioned above, he put his own words, "Moyamoya vessels are collateral pathways of the brain (1963)" along with the words by Dr. John Hunter in 1785, "Blood goes where it is needed." [14].

Around this time, Prof. Suzuki's concept began to be recognized by many neurologists and neurosurgeons, but the names of the disease still varied widely among them, including spontaneous occlusion of the circle of Willis [15, 16], cerebral arterial rete [17], Nishimoto disease, and Nishimoto-Takeuchi-Kudo disease [18–22]. In 1966, Suzuki and co-workers first proposed the term "moyamoya" disease in a Japanese written medical journal [23]. He described how he arrived at this naming in his monograph as follows: *"Moyamoya" was thought to be appropriate since the abnormal net-like vessels at the base of the brain, as seen in angiograms, are hazy in appearance – like a puff of cigarette smoke drifting in the air, which is commonly described as moyamoya by native speakers of Japanese. As described below,*

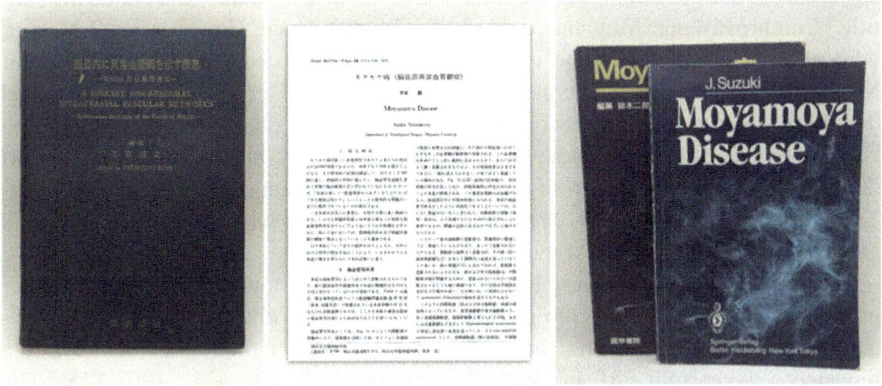

Fig. 1.1 History of moyamoya disease. (*Left*) a proceeding by Prof. Tatsuyuki Kudo from Keio University, Tokyo (1967) [12], (*Middle*) a review article by Prof. Akira Nishimoto from Okayama University, Okayama (1979) [13], and (*Right*) Japanese- and English-written monographs by Prof. Jiro Suzuki from Tohoku University, Sendai (1983) [14]

moreover, in follow-up angiograms of this disease in young patients, the sequential changes – from an initially thick "cloud", to a gradually thinning and shrinking "fog", to the eventual disappearance of the net-like vessels around the internal carotid artery – are also reminiscent of the misty "moyamoya" changes in cigarette smoke. He further stated as follow: *Certainly, moyamoya is an unusual word to enter into medical terminology, but it is appropriate for a number of reasons. It expresses the fact that its etiology is as hazy as the pattern of the abnormal vessels itself. Moreover, the disease was first reported in Japan and continues to show a high incidence there. Usage of a Japanese word emphasize these facts and has thus far been well received in the West as well as in Japan* [14]. Subsequently, Suzuki and Takaku published the first English written article entitled, "Cerebrovascular moyamoya disease, Disease showing abnormal net-like vessels in base of brain," using their new term "moyamoya." Since then, the term "moyamoya" is rapidly recognized worldwide because of its ease of use and euphony [24]. One of the authors, Prof. Akira Takaku was appointed to the University of Toyama as a professor and moved from Sendai to Toyama in 1980. Much later on, the author also moved to the same University of Toyama as a professor in 2012, and had the chance to ask Prof. Takaku about the backgrounds of the naming of moyamoya disease in the 1960s. The following is the narrative by Prof. Takaku: At that time, Prof. Suzuki was concerned that the term "moyamoya" was a Japanese term that was somehow familiar but not international and inappropriate as an academic term. However, he thought that since the disease was discovered in Japan, it would be appropriate to describe it in Japanese. He also thought that if he could properly explain why he named it as moyamoya disease, people overseas might understand it. He also considered that the rhythmic rhyming word "moyamoya" would be easy for foreigners to pronounce. Anyway, Prof. Suzuki was wondering if and how the four syllable words "moyamoya" would be received by foreigners. When Prof. Suzuki and Prof. Takaku submitted their paper to the *Archives of Neurology* journal, they initially chose the main title of their article as "Diseases showing abnormal net like vessels in base of brain," and added the subtitle "Cerebrovascular Moyamoya disease" with diffidence. However, Prof. Merritt, who was a chief editor of the journal at the time, insisted that "Cerebrovascular Moyamoya disease" should be the main title of the article. Prof. Takaku still believed that Prof. Merritt's wise decision was a major turning point in making the name "moyamoya disease" widely known throughout the world (cited from Annual Report 2013 of Department of Neurosurgery, University of Toyama). Very regretfully, Prof. Takaku passed away in 2015, so the author would like to write down Prof. Takaku's narrative here by translating it into English.

According to a review article by Nishimoto [13], however, there were other groups in Japan that called the disease as "chiri-chiri" disease rather than "moyamoya" disease at the same time. Nishimoto described that Maki and Nakada reported a 1-year-old girl and named it "chiri-chiri" disease in 1967 [25]. The Japanese term "chiri-chiri" means "curly" or "wrinkled," e.g., curly hair is called as "chiri-chiri hair" in Japanese; the people may have imagined that the blood vessels within the abnormal vascular networks were comparable to hair, rather than to cigarette smoke. So, in the late 1960s, there was a moyamoya—chiri-chiri controversy in Japan. In fact, when the author started his residency program at the Department of Neurosurgery, Hokkaido University Hospital, Sapporo in 1986, he heard the same story from senior colleagues many times.

1.3 Diagnosis Criteria of Moyamoya Disease

In the 1970s, the Japanese Ministry of Health and Welfare organized a research group to investigate the causes of moyamoya disease and to establish treatment and prevention methods for the disease. First, the Research Committee on Vascular Abnormality in the Brain and Spinal Cord (headed by Prof. Katsutoshi Kitamura) was organized in 1974, and 189 cases of moyamoya disease were registered from all over Japan during the 2 years from 1974 to 1975. Then, in 1977, the research committee was reorganized and given a new name. Thus, the Research Committee on Spontaneous Occlusion of the Circle of Willis ("Moyamoya Disease"), headed by Prof. Fumio Gotoh, was newly established for the same purpose [13]. This research group first established the guideline for the diagnosis of spontaneous occlusion of the circle of Willis (moyamoya disease) in 1978 and published it in their annual report in 1979 [26]. This guideline consisted of the following structure: (1) a general description of moyamoya disease, (2) indispensable angiographic findings, (3) unknown cause and no special underlying diseases, and (4) pathological findings for diagnostic reference. The guidelines clearly stated that cerebral angiography is mandatory for diagnosis and that at least the findings shown in Table 1.1 must be present on cerebral angiography (Table 1.1). In this guideline, ***definite case*** must fulfill all three findings on cerebral angiography, plus other special underlying diseases must not be presented. On the other hand, ***probable case*** should fulfill two findings on cerebral angiography (2-a and 2-b), plus other special underlying diseases must not be presented. In other words, a definite case was defined as having bilateral lesions and a probable case was defined as having unilateral lesions. Since then, moyamoya disease has been diagnosed on the basis of morphological findings of the lumen of the affected arteries on cerebral angiography, which has been maintained to date.

This guideline was revised by the Research Committee, headed by Prof. Hajime Handa, in 1988 [27]. In the revised version, the possibility of familial occurrence of moyamoya disease was first noted in the general description. Specific examples of

Table 1.1 Cerebral angiographic findings to be presented for diagnosis moyamoya disease (An excerpt from the Guideline 1978) Ref. [13]. *English translation by the author*

Cerebral angiography is mandatory for diagnosis and at least the following findings must be present on cerebral angiography
a. Stenosis or occlusion at the terminal portion of the internal carotid artery and at the proximal portion of the anterior and the middle cerebral arteries.
b. Abnormal vascular networks in the vicinity of the occlusive or stenotic lesion on the arterial phase.
c. These findings should present bilaterally.

causative comorbidities that should be excluded when diagnosing moyamoya disease were presented. They included atherosclerosis, meningitis, brain tumor, Down syndrome, von Recklinghausen's disease, head trauma, and irradiation. In addition, pediatric cases with typical angiographic findings on one side and an apparent stenosis of the terminal portion of the contralateral internal carotid artery were classified into ***definite cases***, because these patients usually develop moyamoya vessels thereafter [28].

The guidelines for the diagnosis and treatment of spontaneous occlusion of the circle of Willis ("Moyamoya" disease) have been extensively revised in 1995 [29], and was published in English in 1997 by the Research Committee headed by Prof. Masashi Fukui [30]. The guideline consisted of (1) guidelines for the diagnosis, (2) general information, (3) treatment, and (4) guidelines for making a diagnosis using MRI and MRA. The most significant change in the diagnosis of moyamoya disease at that time was the emergence of MR angiography. Although cerebral angiography had been considered essential for the diagnosis of moyamoya disease until then, noninvasive MR angiography has been reported to be useful for the diagnosis of moyamoya disease since the early 1990s [31–33]. Yamada et al. (1992) reported that MR angiography can accurately detect occlusive lesions at the terminal portion of the internal carotid artery and associated moyamoya vessels, although some occlusive lesions were overestimated because of a flow-related artifact on MR [33]. Houkin et al. (1994) also analyzed the findings on MR angiography in 39 patients with moyamoya disease and found good correlations between cerebral angiography and MR angiography when detecting the stenotic lesions at the carotid fork and moyamoya vessels [32]. Numerous studies to date have recognized that MR angiography is an extremely useful modality not only for the diagnosis of moyamoya disease, but also for determining the stage of the disease and for observing the progression of the disease and collateral formation after surgical revascularization due to its noninvasive nature [34–39]. As a result, the 1997 revision of the guidelines for the diagnosis of moyamoya disease stated for the first time that the diagnosis of moyamoya disease can be made without cerebral angiography only if the findings on MR angiography meet certain criteria (Table 1.2). At the same time, the guidelines for making a diagnosis using MRI and MRA were also presented (Table 1.3) [30]. In addition, autoimmune disease was added as a comorbidity that should be ruled out when diagnosing moyamoya disease of unknown etiology [30].

Subsequently, the guidelines for diagnosis and treatment of moyamoya disease (spontaneous occlusion of the circle of Willis) were revised by the Research Committee on the Pathology and Treatment of Spontaneous Occlusion of the Circle of Willis, headed by Prof. Nobuo Hashimoto, in 2009 [40] and its English version was published in 2012 [41]. From this revised guideline, the world's preferred name of the disease, moyamoya disease, has been used as the official name of the disease, whereas the previous guideline used spontaneous occlusion of the circle of Willis as the official name of the disease, with moyamoya disease written in parentheses. The guideline consisted of eight chapters, including (1) concepts of the disease, (2) epidemiology, (3) pathology/etiology, (4) symptoms, (5) similar conditions, (6) diagnosis, (7) treatment, and (8) prognosis. Although the diagnostic criteria were not

Table 1.2 Guideline 1995 for the diagnosis of moyamoya disease (Fukui et al. 1997) Ref. [30]

1.1. Diagnosis criteria

(A) Cerebral angiography is indispensable for the diagnosis, and should present at least the following findings:

1. Stenosis or occlusion at the terminal portion of the internal carotid artery and/or at the proximal portion of the anterior and/or the middle cerebral arteries.
2. Abnormal vascular networks in the vicinity of the occlusive or stenotic lesions in the arterial phase.
3. These findings should present bilaterally.

(B) When magnetic resonance imaging (MRI) and magnetic resonance angiography (MRA) clearly demonstrate all the below-described findings, conventional cerebral angiography is not mandatory.

1. Stenosis or occlusion at the terminal portion of the internal carotid artery and at the proximal portion of the anterior and middle cerebral arteries on MRA.
2. An abnormal vascular network in the basal ganglia on MRA.

Note: An abnormal vascular network can be diagnosed when more than two apparent flow voids are seen in one side of the basal ganglia on MRI.

3. (1) and (2) are seen bilaterally (refer to the image diagnostic guideline by MRI and MRA).

(C) Because the etiology of this disease is unknown, cerebrovascular disease with the following basic diseases or conditions should thus be eliminated:

1. Atherosclerosis
2. Autoimmune disease
3. Meningitis
4. Brain neoplasm
5. Down syndrome
6. Recklinghausen's disease
7. Head trauma
8. Irradiation to the head
9. Others

(D) Instructive pathological findings:

1. Intimal thickening and the resulting stenosis or occlusion of the lumen are observed in and around the terminal portion of the internal carotid artery usually on both sides. Lipid deposits are occasionally seen in the proliferating intima.
2. Arteries constituting the circle of Willis such as the anterior and the middle cerebral and the posterior communicating arteries often show stenosis of various degrees of occlusion associated with fibrocellular thickening of the intima, a waving of the internal elastic lamina, and an attenuation of the media.
3. Numerous small vascular channels (perforators and anastomotic branches) are observed around the circle of Willis.
4. Reticular conglomerates of small vessels are often seen in the pia mater.

1.2. Diagnosis

In reference to 1.1 mentioned above, the diagnostic criteria are classified as follows: Autopsy case not undergoing cerebral angiography should be investigated separately while referring to (D).

1. ***Definite case***:

One which fulfills either (A) or (B) and (C). In children, however, a case which fulfills (A) (1) and (2) or (B) (1) and (2) on one side and with remarkable stenosis at the terminal portion of the internal carotid artery on the opposite side is also included.

2. ***Probable case***:

One which fulfills either (A) (1) and (2) or (B) (1) and (2) and (C) (unilateral involvement).

Table 1.3 Guideline 1995 for the usage of MRI and MRA to make a diagnosis of moyamoya disease (Fukui et al. 1997) Ref. [30]

Guidelines for making a diagnosis using MRI and MRA

(A) When magnetic resonance imaging (MRI) and magnetic resonance angiography (MRA) clearly demonstrate all the findings described below, conventional cerebral angiography:

1. Stenosis or occlusion at the terminal portion of the internal carotid artery and at the proximal portion of the anterior and middle cerebral arteries on MRA.
2. An abnormal vascular network in the basal ganglia.
3. (1) and (2) are seen bilaterally.

(B) Imaging methods and judgment

1. More than a 1.0-tesla magnetic field strength is recommended.
2. There are no restrictions regarding the MRA imaging method.
3. The imaging parameters, such as the magnetic field strength, the imaging methods and the use of contrast medium, should be clearly documented.
4. An abnormal vascular network can be diagnosed when more than two apparent flow voids are seen on one side of the basal ganglia on MRI.
5. Either an over- or underestimation of the lesion could be made according to the imaging conditions. To avoid a false-positive diagnosis, only definite cases should thus be diagnosed based on the MRI and MRA findings.

(C) Because similar vascular lesions secondary to other disorders are sometimes indistinguishable from this disease in adults, a diagnosis of MRI and MRA without conventional angiography is thus only recommended in childhood cases.

Table 1.4 Suzuki's angiographical stage Ref. [24]

Stage	Cerebral angiographic findings
I	Narrowing of the carotid fork
II	Initiation of the moyamoya (dilated major cerebral artery and a slight moyamoya vessel network)
III	Intensification of the moyamoya (disappearance of the middle and anterior cerebral arteries, and thick and distinct moyamoya vessels)
IV	Minimization of the moyamoya (disappearance of the posterior cerebral artery, and narrowing of individual moyamoya vessels)
V	Reduction of the moyamoya (disappearance of all the main cerebral arteries arising from the internal carotid artery system, further minimization of the moyamoya vessels, and an increase in the collateral pathways from the external carotid artery system)
VI	Disappearance of the moyamoya (disappearance of the moyamoya vessels, with cerebral blood flow derived only from the external carotid artery and the vertebrobasilar artery systems)

revised, Suzuki's angiographic stage (Table 1.4) [24] and MRA-based disease stage (Table 1.5) [36] were described for the first time in Chap. 6 "Diagnosis." In Chap. 7 "Treatment," the recommendation grade and evidence level are first described for each treatment in accordance with the development and spread of evidence-based medicine (EBM) in the medical community over the world, although the author will skip it here [41].

The most recent guideline was established in 2015 by The Research Committee on Spontaneous Occlusion of the Circle of Willis ("Moyamoya Disease"), headed by Prof. Kiyohiro Houkin and was published in Japanese in 2018 [42]. An English

Table 1.5 Houkin's MRA stage Ref. [36]

MRA findings	Score
(1) Internal carotid artery	
Normal	0
Stenosis of C1	1
Discontinuity of the C1 signal	2
Invisible	3
(2) Middle cerebral artery	
Normal	0
Stenosis of M1	1
Discontinuity of the M1 signal	2
Invisible	3
(3) Anterior cerebral artery	
Normal A2 and its distal	0
A2 and its distal signal decrease	1
Invisible	2
(4) Posterior cerebral artery	
Normal P2 and its distal	0
P2 and its distal signal decrease	1
Invisible	2
MRA total score	MRA stage
0–1	1
2–4	2
5–7	3
8–10	4

version has not been published officially. Its structure remains the same as the 2009 version, but there have been major revisions to the diagnosis criteria. First, the site of an occlusion or stenotic lesion was previously defined as "the terminal portion of the internal carotid artery and the proximal portion of the anterior and middle cerebral arteries," but the 2015 revision changed it to "*the arteries centered on the terminal portion of the intracranial internal carotid artery*." It is because there have been several reports of cases with occlusion or severe stenosis of the proximal portion of the middle cerebral artery associated with typical moyamoya vessels, but without obvious stenotic lesions at the terminal portion of the internal carotid artery. Previously, such cases were not diagnosed as moyamoya disease because they were not considered to meet the diagnostic criteria for moyamoya disease. However, Kim et al. (2016) collected 81 cases with an isolated middle cerebral artery stenosis or occlusion. All of them were younger than 60 years. According to the findings on high-resolution MRI (see Chap. 14), they were classified into atherosclerosis group (n = 45) and non-atherosclerosis group (n = 36). The latter was characterized by younger age, smaller number of vascular risk factors, thinner intima-media thickness, and more frequent mutation at *RNF213*, a susceptibility gene for moyamoya disease. More interestingly, Choi et al. (2012) reported a 25-year-old female with chronic headache due to an isolated middle cerebral artery stenosis on the right side. She was conservatively followed up and repeated cerebral angiography revealed the isolated middle cerebral artery stenosis progressed to typical moyamoya disease [43]. These observations strongly suggest that stenotic lesions may start to develop at the proximal portion of the middle cerebral artery, but not at the terminal portion of the internal carotid artery in moyamoya disease. Based on these considerations, the pathogenesis of these cases is now thought very similar to that of moyamoya disease, but a significant number of such cases have not been diagnosed as moyamoya disease according to previous diagnostic criteria. Therefore, the Research Committee decided to revise the diagnosis criteria as written above in 2015.

Second, the 2015 edition eliminated the distinction between definite and probable cases. In the past, cases with bilateral stenotic lesions at the terminal part of the internal carotid artery and its branches were classified as ***definite*** cases and cases with unilateral stenotic lesions were classified as ***probable*** cases, but all cases are simply defined as moyamoya disease without distinction between definite cases and probable cases since 2015 [42]. It is based on increasing evidence that a significant number of unilateral moyamoya disease progress to bilateral moyamoya disease, especially in pediatric patients. They also share a similar genetic background (see Chap. 3) [44–46]. Therefore, the pathophysiology and genetics are recognized as very similar between bilateral and unilateral moyamoya disease, and the distinction between bilateral and unilateral cases has gradually become less significant.

Although different from the diagnostic criteria, this 2015 version of the diagnostic and treatment guidelines for moyamoya disease is notable for incorporating new findings throughout, including the revision to the treatment guidelines for hemorrhagic-type adult moyamoya disease in view of the recent series of studies of the Japan Adult Moyamoya (JAM) Trial. However, this 2018 edition has been published in Japanese only [42], while the English written version has not yet been officially released. Therefore, there is an urgent need to publish an English written version that should serve as the basis for discussions on the future development of a unified international moyamoya disease concept and diagnostic criteria over the world.

Finally, the author will also discuss future issues. As pointed out earlier, moyamoya disease is diagnosed based on the findings on cerebral angiography or MR angiography, i.e., the diagnosis completely depends on morphological information about the lumen of the affected arteries. Therefore, when encountering a patient with stenosis or occlusion of an intracranial artery due to other causes, it is not infrequently difficult to distinguish them from moyamoya disease. Particularly in patients older than 50 years, it is not uncommon to meet with difficulty in accurately diagnosing whether the stenotic lesion is caused by moyamoya disease or by atherosclerosis. This obscures the debate over whether *RNF213* mutants are involved in intracranial artery stenosis lesions other than moyamoya disease or not. Therefore, we need to further improve the accuracy of the diagnosis of moyamoya disease in the next revision.

Acknowledgment This work was partly supported by a grant from the Research Committee on Moyamoya Disease, the Japanese Ministry of Health, Labour and Welfare.

References

1. Tominaga T. Overview. Moyamoya disease update. Tokyo: Springer; 2010.
2. Yoshimoto T, Numagami Y, Shirane R. History and dedicated researchers. Moyamoya disease. Rolling Meadows: American Association of Neurological Surgeons; 2001.
3. Takeuchi K, Shimizu K. Hypoplasia of the bilateral internal carotid arteries. No To Shinkei. 1957;9:37–43.
4. Leeds NE, Abbott KH. Collateral circulation in cerebrovascular disease in childhood via rete mirabile and perforating branches of anterior choroidal and posterior cerebral arteries. Radiology. 1965;85:628–34.
5. Weidner W, Hanafeewmarkham CH. Intracranial collateral circulation via leptomeningeal and rete mirabile anastomoses. Neurology. 1965;15:39–48.
6. Kudo T, Takayama R, Mikawakuchi K, Ishimori S, Otake S, KNakagawa K. Occlusion of internal carotid artery. Brain Nerve (Tokyo). 1957;9:757.
7. Sano K. Cerebral juxta-basal telangiectasia. Brain Nerve (Tokyo). 1965;17:748–50.
8. Takeuchi K, Kobayashi S. Arterial occlusion at the base of brain in children. No To Shinkei 1965;17:779–80.
9. Moriyasu N, Nishio S. FIve cases of network like vascular anomaly of internal carotid artery. Brain Nerve (Tokyo). 1965;17:761–3.
10. Maki Y, Nakada Y. Autopsy cases showing angiomatous anomaly of carotid artery at the base of the brain. Brain Nerve (Tokyo). 1965;17:764–6.
11. Nishimoto A, Sugiu R, Takeuchi S. Hemangiomatous malformation of bilateral internal carotid artery at the base of brain. Brain Nerve (Tokyo). 1966;17:750–2.
12. Kudo T. Historical overview. In: Kudo T, editor. 25th congress of Japan neurosurgical society, vol. 1966. Tokyo: Igaku Shoin; 1967. p. 12–22.
13. Nishimoto A. Moyamoya disease(author's transl). Neurol Med Chir (Tokyo). 1979;19:221–8.
14. Suzuki J. Moyamoya disease. Berlin Heidelberg: Springer; 1983.
15. Kudo T. Occlusion of the circle of Willis with special reference to its developmental process. No To Shinkei. 1966;18:889–96.
16. Kudo T. Spontaneous occlusion of the circle of Willis. A disease apparently confined to Japanese. Neurology. 1968;18:485–96.
17. Handa H, Tani E, Kajikawa H, Sato K, Yamashita J. Autopsy case of the so-called cerebral arterial rete in an adult. No To Shinkei. 1969;21:181–91.
18. Klaus E, Farkova H, Urbanek K. Case of "Moyamoya disease" (Nishimoto-Takeuchi-Kudo syndrome). Fortschr Geb Rontgenstr Nuklearmed. 1970;113:603–8.
19. Nishimoto A, Takeuchi S. Abnormal cerebrovascular network related to the internal cartoid arteries. J Neurosurg. 1968;29:255–60.
20. Simon J, Sabouraud O, Guy G, Turpin J. A case of Nishimoto's disease. Apropos of a rare and bilateral disease of the internal carotid. Rev Neurol (Paris). 1968;119:376–83.
21. Urbanek K, Farkova H, Klaus E. Nishimoto-Takeuchi-Kudo disease: case report. J Neurol Neurosurg Psychiatry. 1970;33:671–3.
22. Vuia O, Alexianu M, Gabor S. Hypoplasia and obstruction of the circle of Willis in a case of atypical cerebral hemorrhage and its relationship to Nishimoto's disease. Neurology. 1970;20:361–7.
23. Suzuki J, Takaku A, Asahi M. Evaluation of a group of disorders showing an abnormal vascular network at the base of the brain with a high incidence among the Japanese. 2. Follow-up studies by cerebral angiography. No To Shinkei. 1966;18:897–908.
24. Suzuki J, Takaku A. Cerebrovascular "moyamoya" disease. Disease showing abnormal net-like vessels in base of brain. Arch Neurol. 1969;20:288–99.
25. Maki Y, Nakada Y. So-called "Chiri-Chiri" disease. J Chiba Medical Soc. 1976;43:667.
26. The Research Committee on Spontaneous Occlusion of the Circle of Willis ("Moyamoya Disease") (1979) The diagnostic guide of the "spontaneous occlusion of the circle of Willis".

Annual Report 1978 of The Research Committee on Spontaneous Occlusion of the Circle of Willis ("Moyamoya Disease") of the Ministry of Health and Welfare, Japan.
27. Kitamura K (1988) Revision of the diagnostic guide of the spontaneous occlusion of the circle of Willis. Annual Report 1987 of the Research Committee on the Pathology and Treatment of Spontaneous Occlusion of the Circle of Willis ("Moyamoya Disease") of the Ministry of Health and Welfare, Japan.
28. Ikezaki K, Fukui M. Definition (guidelines). In: Moyamoya disease. Rolling Meadows: American Association of Neurological Surgeons; 2001.
29. The Research Committee on Spontaneous Occlusion of the Circle of Willis ("Moyamoya Disease") (1996) The diagnostic guideline of the "spontaneous occlusion of the circle of Willis" (new diagnostic criteria). Annual Report 1995 of the Research Committee on Spontaneous Occlusion of the Circle of Willis ("Moyamoya Disease") of the Ministry of Health and Welfare, Japan.
30. Fukui M. Guidelines for the diagnosis and treatment of spontaneous occlusion of the circle of Willis ('moyamoya' disease). Research Committee on Spontaneous Occlusion of the Circle of Willis (Moyamoya disease) of the Ministry of Health and Welfare, Japan. Clin Neurol Neurosurg. 1997;99(Suppl 2):S238–40.
31. Hasuo K, Yasumori K, Yoshida K, Hirakata R, Kuroiwa T, Mizushima A, Matsushima T, Fukui M, Masuda K. Magnetic resonance imaging compared with computed tomography and angiography in moyamoya disease. Acta Radiol. 1990;31:191–5.
32. Houkin K, Aoki T, Takahashi A, Abe H. Diagnosis of moyamoya disease with magnetic resonance angiography. Stroke. 1994;25:2159–64.
33. Yamada I, Matsushima Y, Suzuki S. Moyamoya disease: diagnosis with three-dimensional time-of-flight MR angiography. Radiology. 1992;184:773–8.
34. Houkin K, Kuroda S, Ishikawa T, Abe H. Neovascularization (angiogenesis) after revascularization in moyamoya disease. Which technique is most useful for moyamoya disease? Acta Neurochir. 2000;142:269–76.
35. Houkin K, Nakayama N, Kuroda S, Ishikawa T, Nonaka T. How does angiogenesis develop in pediatric moyamoya disease after surgery? A prospective study with MR angiography. Childs Nerv Syst. 2004;20:734–41.
36. Houkin K, Nakayama N, Kuroda S, Nonaka T, Shonai T, Yoshimoto T. Novel magnetic resonance angiography stage grading for moyamoya disease. Cerebrovasc Dis. 2005;20:347–54.
37. Kuroda S, Ishikawa T, Houkin K, Nanba R, Hokari M, Iwasaki Y. Incidence and clinical features of disease progression in adult moyamoya disease. Stroke. 2005;36:2148–53.
38. Smith ER, Scott RM. Progression of disease in unilateral moyamoya syndrome. Neurosurg Focus. 2008;24:E17.
39. Yoon HK, Shin HJ, Lee M, Byun HS, Na DG, Han BK. MR angiography of moyamoya disease before and after encephaloduroarteriosynangiosis. AJR Am J Roentgenol. 2000;174:195–200.
40. Research Committee on intractable diseases of the Ministry of Health LaWJ. Recommendations for the management og moyamoya disease. A statement from Research Committee on Spontaneous Occlusion of the Circle of Willis (Moyamoya disease) surgery for cerebral. Stroke. 2009;37:321–37.
41. The Research Committee on the Pathology and Treatment of Spontaneous Occlusion of the Circle of Willis. Guidelines for diagnosis and treatment of moyamoya disease (spontaneous occlusion of the circle of Willis). Neurol Med Chir (Tokyo). 2012;52:245–66.
42. Tominaga T, Suzuki N, Miyamoto S, Koizumi A, Kuroda S, Takahashi JC, Fujimura M, Houkin K. Recommendations for the management of moyamoya disease: a statement from Research Committee on Spontaneous Occlusion of the Circle of Willis (Moyamoya disease) [2nd edition]. Surg Cerebr Stroke. 2018;46:1–24.
43. Choi HY, Lee JE, Jung YH, Cho HJ, Kim DJ, Heo JH. Progression of isolated middle cerebral artery stenosis into moyamoya disease. Neurology. 2007;68:954.

44. Inoue T, Murakami N, Sakadume S, Kido Y, Kikuchi A, Ichinoi N, Suzuki K, Kure S, Sakuta R. Differing phenotypes of Moyamoya disease in a familial case involving heterozygous c.14429G > A variant in RNF213. Pediatr Int. 2015;57:798–801.
45. Mineharu Y, Takagi Y, Takahashi JC, Hashikata H, Liu W, Hitomi T, Kobayashi H, Koizumi A, Miyamoto S. Rapid progression of unilateral moyamoya disease in a patient with a family history and an RNF213 risk variant. Cerebrovasc Dis. 2013;36:155–7.
46. Miyawaki S, Imai H, Shimizu M, Yagi S, Ono H, Mukasa A, Nakatomi H, Shimizu T, Saito N. Genetic variant RNF213 c.14576G>A in various phenotypes of intracranial major artery stenosis/occlusion. Stroke. 2013;44:2894–7.

Moyamoya Syndrome

2

Kristin Lucia, Güliz Acker, and Peter Vajkoczy

Abstract

Moyamoya syndrome refers to the presence of an underlying condition in addition to the angiographic findings of moyamoya disease. The diseases which may accompany moyamoya disease and therefore classify a patient as suffering from moyamoya syndrome are wide-ranging and are not uniformly recognized in international comparison. This chapter will focus on the epidemiology in Asia, Europe, and North America. The most frequent underlying conditions reported in patients with moyamoya syndrome will be discussed, as well as their possible pathophysiological links to moyamoya disease. Finally, an overview of long-term outcomes following surgical intervention as well as new perspectives in patient care will be given.

Keywords

Moyamoya syndrome · Quasi-moyamoya disease · Epidemiology · Surgical revascularization · Outcome

---

K. Lucia · G. Acker · P. Vajkoczy (✉)
Department of Neurosurgery, Charité–Universitätsmedizin Berlin (corporate member of Freie Universität Berlin, Humboldt–Universität zu Berlin, and Berlin Institute of Health), Berlin, Germany
e-mail: kristin-elizabeth.lucia@charite.de; gueliz.acker@charite.de; peter.vajkoczy@charite.de

S. Kuroda (ed.), *Moyamoya Disease: Current Knowledge and Future Perspectives*, https://doi.org/10.1007/978-981-33-6404-2_2

2.1 Terminology

Moyamoya disease (MMD) constitutes the spontaneous bilateral stenosis or occlusion of the terminal portions of the internal carotid artery or proximal middle cerebral artery resulting in the formation of dilated, net-like collateral vessels at the base of the brain [1, 2]. According to the current international guidelines, moyamoya syndrome (termed quasi-moyamoya) "refers to the presence of stenosis or occlusion of the terminal portion of the internal carotid artery or proximal portion of the anterior and/or middle cerebral arteries accompanied by an abnormal vascular network detected in association with an underlying disease. Even in cases with unilateral lesions, if an underlying disease is present, the condition is considered as quasi-moyamoya disease" [2]. This chapter will focus on this moyamoya variant disease in regard to epidemiology, underlying conditions, and future perspectives in diagnosis and patient care.

2.2 Epidemiology

Similar to MMD, the prevalence of MMS is reported to be highest in Asian countries [2]. In Japan, the annual incidence of MMD is 1.13/100.000, which is approximately tenfold higher than the annual reported incidence of MMS at 0.11/100.000 [3, 4].

Regardless of ethnicity, MMS patients have been found to have a strong female predominance of approximately 3:1 and present more commonly with ischemia than hemorrhagic events. MMS patients also tend to present at a younger age than those with MMD [3, 5–9].

Differences in epidemiological analysis arise between international series based mainly on the scope of underlying medical conditions recognized as being associated with angiographic MMD. These conditions will be further detailed in chap. 2.3. In particular, inclusion of cardiovascular risk factors such as atherosclerosis have proven controversial in regard to the pathophysiology of MMD. Asian studies include atherosclerosis as an associated condition for classification as MMS, whereas European and North American studies regard atherosclerosis as a separate pathophysiological entity and consider it a risk factor for stroke [9]. The classification of patients with unilateral disease as MMS also remains variable in the literature [5, 7]. Table 2.1 provides an overview of the major international epidemiological studies on MMS and individual contributions will be discussed in detail below.

2.2.1 Japan

In the Japanese cohort surveyed by Hayashi et al., 109 MMS patients were identified (42 males, 66 females). These patients were observed to be younger (mean age at onset of 30.6 years) than MMD patients and included 7% familial cases, which presumably can be accounted for by the congenital nature of several underlying

Table 2.1 Epidemiological studies on MMS

Study	Country	Adult/ Pediatric cohort	MMS/MMD (% MMS)	Number of males/ females	Mean age at onset (years)	Ischemic/ hemorrhagic stroke	Unilateral/ Bilateral	Familial	Associated conditions
Hayashi et al. (2014)	Japan	Adult Pediatric	108 (MMS only)	42/66	30.6	40%/7%	46%/54%	7%	Atherosclerosis: 29% Down syndrome: 15% NF-1: 14%
Wei et al. (2014)	Taiwan	Adult Pediatric	37/90 (45%)	13/24	35.9	73%/11%	Unilateral excluded	–	Atherosclerosis: 32% Graves' disease: 19% Homocystinuria: 8%
Zhao et al. (2017)	China	Adult Pediatric	64/693 (9%) 10 pediatric 54 adult	33/31	31.5	71%/22%	50%/50%	3.1%	Atherosclerosis: 50% Hyperthyroidism: 19% Hx of tumor/radiation: 8%
Gross, Du (2013)	USA	Adult	6/41 (15%)	0/6	31.2	74%/17%	Unilateral excluded	–	Sickle cell disease: 50% Connective tissue disease: 16% NF-1:16% Hyperthyroidism: 16%
Guzman et al. (2009)	USA	Adult Pediatric	23/329 (7%) 16 pediatric 7 adult	–	–	78%/4.8%	14%/86%	–	NF-1: 31% pediatric, 43% adult Down syndrome: 19% pediatric, 43% adult Primordial dwarfism: 19% pediatric, 14% adult
Acker et al. (2016)	Germany	Adult Pediatric	61 (MMS only) 21 pediatric 40 adult	Adult: 11/29 Pediatric: 5/16	30	Adult: 84%/8% Pediatric: 20%/65%	Adult: 7.3%/85% Pediatric	0%	Down syndrome: 14.8% (pediatric), 30% (adult) Hyperthyroidism: 12% (adult) NF-1: 10% (pediatric)
Kraemer et al. (2019)	Germany	Adult	17/200	3:14	32.4	Ischemic: 88% Hemorrhagic: 6%	Unilateral excluded	6.8%	n.a

Where available, data is reported for pediatric and adult populations. The three most common accompanying conditions as reported in the individual studies are listed. Data not reported in the study are indicated by "–"

conditions that are used to define MMS. A separate examination of MMS cases with and without atherosclerosis revealed that the mean age of atherosclerotic patients was higher (53.5 years).

MMS patients presented less commonly with hemorrhagic stroke than MMD patients (7% vs. 40%, respectively). Focal neurological deficits (TIA/Stroke) were observed in over 50% of cases. Atherosclerosis was reported as the most frequently associated condition (29%), followed by Down syndrome (15.1%), NF-1 (14%), history of cranial irradiation or brain tumor (7.5%), and hyperthyroidism (7.5%). Other conditions found included a history of meningitis, leukemia, renal hypertension, and aortic coarctation.

Angiographic findings of MMS patients at diagnosis revealed unilateral disease in 46% of cases with stenoocclusion of the ICA found in 62% (left side) and 65% (right side) followed by MCA stenoocclusion in 13–14%. The majority of patients (60%) showed a disease severity of Suzuki III° at diagnosis. Signs of ischemia were found on MRI in approximately 64% of the patients, hemorrhage in 7%, and no signs of ischemia or hemorrhage were found on MRI in approximately 27%. Surgical treatment analogous to definite MMD was performed in 60% of MMS patients.

Overall, the Japanese population of MMS patients differs from MMD primarily in regard to unilaterality, younger age at diagnosis, and lower incidence of hemorrhage versus ischemia [3, 4, 10].

2.2.2 Taiwan

A single-center Taiwanese series examining 90 MMD patients found 41% of patients had accompanying medical conditions to be considered as MMS [5]. The mean age at onset in this population was 35.9 years. Similar to the Japanese cohorts, atherosclerosis was included as a concurrent condition when classifying for MMS. Importantly, this study examined only patients with bilateral stenoocclusive disease. Overall, 28 patients with unilateral disease were excluded from the original series of 118 cases. Whereas 81.1% of patients had one underlying condition, up to 18.9% had two or more accompanying diseases. The most common accompanying diagnosis in this cohort was atherosclerosis (32%) followed by thyroid disease (29% total, of which 18% were Graves' Disease). Interestingly, no cases of Down syndrome were reported in this series.

Patients with MMS presented more often with ischemia than did MMD patients (73% vs. 64%, respectively). Accordingly, more hemorrhage was observed in MMD than MMS patients (26% vs. 10%, respectively). MMS patients were more commonly treated with antiplatelet therapy than MMD patients, which may also be attributed to the frequency of atherosclerosis and dyslipidemia found in MMS patients. The surgical strategies employed in MMS patients did not differ from those for MMD patients with approximately 24% of MMS and 30% of MMD patients receiving revascularization surgery.

2.2.3 China

In a single-center review of 693 MMD patients 64 (9%) were classified as MMS (including atherosclerosis). The mean age of patients at diagnosis was similar to the Japanese and Taiwanese cohorts at 31.5 years. Interestingly the gender distribution among this Chinese cohort was nearly equal between men and women (33 men, 31 women). Hemorrhage was found to be less frequent at presentation than ischemia (21.9% vs. 70.3%). Atherosclerosis was the most common associated disorder in MMS patients (50%), followed by hyperthyroidism (18.8%), anemia (7.8%), and history of cranial radiation therapy or brain tumor (7.8%). No cases of Neurofibromatosis 1 or Down syndrome were reported.

Disease severity according to Suzuki grading was slightly higher than the Japanese cohort with a majority of patients showing Suzuki III° and IV° (20.3% and 42.2%). In this series, 50% of patients were found to have unilateral vasculopathy with stenoocclusion of the ICA most commonly observed, followed by the middle cerebral artery. No data was provided on stenoocclusion of the posterior circulation. Analysis of the natural course of MMS patients in this series revealed the history of previous ischemia or hemorrhage as predictive of future adverse events as has been reported in Japanese and Chinese MMD patients [11, 12].

2.2.4 Korea

Epidemiological reports on a single-center series of 296 angiographically confirmed MMD patients in Korea found four cases of MMS with underlying conditions included fibromuscular dysplasia, thyrotoxicosis, and cerebral palsy [13]. In this series, atherosclerosis was not used to classify MMS and no further subgroup analysis was performed. Further national reports to date have excluded MMS from analysis [14, 15].

2.2.5 United States of America

Data on North American MMS patients is available from three retrospective analyses. Gross and Du report in a single-center review of 41 adult MMD patients in which six were identified as MMS after excluding unilateral cases [7]. All MMS patients were females, whereas MMD patients showed the standard gender distribution of a 3:1 female to male ratio. MMS patients were younger than MMD patients at diagnosis (mean age 31 vs. 40 years old). Four (67%) MMS patients had presented with ischemia and two with hemorrhagic events (33%). Patients diagnosed with MMD also presented more commonly with ischemia (74%) than hemorrhagic insults (17%). Disease severity as determined by mean Suzuki grading among MMS and MMD patients in this cohort were similar (2.8 vs. 2.5, respectively). Among the concurrent diagnoses of these MMS patients, sickle cell disease was found in three cases with one case each of connective tissue disease, NF-1, and hyperthyroidism.

A further retrospective analysis conducted in the western United States surveyed 298 patients over 10 years [16]. Patients with MMS were not separately addressed in this study; however, 4.4% of cases had concurrent diagnoses of sickle cell disease, 48% of which were African Americans. Down syndrome was reported in 3% of patients and NF-1 in 2.3%.

Guzman et al. reviewed a series of 329 surgically treated patients with MMD and found 23 (16 pediatric and 7 adults) to have MMS [8]. The overall cohort of patients in this study showed a female predominance of 3:1 in adult cases with an 1:1 distribution in the first decade of life. This study also included cases of unilateral disease which was found in 15% of MMS patients. The most common accompanying diagnosis was found to be NF-1 (31% of children, 43% of adults) followed by Down syndrome (19% of children, 43% of adults) and primordial dwarfism in 19% of children and 14% of adults MMS patients. Of the patients presenting with unilateral MMS, 37.5% had NF-1 as a concurrent diagnosis. Patients presented mainly with ischemic stroke (78.2%) with hemorrhagic events occurring much less frequently (4.8%). Ischemic stroke was more common among pediatric MMS patients than pediatric MMD patients (78 vs. 51%). In this study patients with MMS were found to have an increased risk of postoperative stroke (OR 4.16, $p = 0.09$) compared to those with MMD as well as higher surgical morbidity (8.7% vs 3.5%).

2.2.6 Germany

In the largest European analysis of MMS, Acker et al. retrospectively identified 61 cases of MMS from a single center [9]. When examining patients for criteria of MMS, this study performed in our institute did not include atherosclerosis as a concurrent diagnosis associated with MMS as we consider atherosclerosis to be a separate disease entity not associated with the vasculopathic changes observed in MMD. All patients were of Caucasian descent. The gender distribution of pediatric and adult patients was similar with an approximately 3:1 female to male ratio. This European Caucasian cohort showed a predominance of adult presentation in contrast to the pediatric peak found in Asian MMS populations. Pediatric patients comprised approximately one-third of the cohort, of which no cases presented with hemorrhagic events. Among adult patients, 12.2% presented with hemorrhage and 82.7% presented with ischemic events. Thirty percent of all patients showed no sign of ischemic lesions on MRI. The average age of onset in adult patients was 38.2 years and in pediatric patients 5.4 years. The most common underlying condition in both pediatric and adult populations was Down syndrome (14.8% and 30%, respectively), followed by hyperthyroidism in adults (12.2%) and NF-1 in children (10%). Angiographic analysis of this cohort showed 79% of patients with bilateral disease. The rate of unilateral MMS is therefore much lower than previously reported Asian cohorts (11% vs. 46%) [3]. The mean Suzuki grade of all patients was 3. The pattern of stenoocclusive lesions in this cohort showed predominant involvement of the ICA alone or with the MCA/ACA in 89% of patients. The posterior circulation was found to be affected in 40% of pediatric and 27% of adult patients. Surgical treatment was provided for 92% of patients with combined revascularization being performed most often.

A further German series from Kraemer et al. reporting on 200 patients with moyamoya vasculopathy included only 17 cases which were classified as MMS (8.5%) [17]. However, the authors also defined several patients with underlying conditions as MMD in this series. Further details on the underlying conditions for MMS were not available. Gender distribution (82% female, 18% male), mean age at onset (32.4), and rate of ischemic versus hemorrhagic stroke (88% vs. 6%, respectively) were similar to the population described by Acker et al. In this cohort, 6.8% of MMS cases were determined to be familial and no affection of the posterior circulation were described on angiographic examination.

2.3 Associated Conditions

The Guidelines for Diagnosis and Treatment of Moyamoya Disease present an extensive overview of the underlying conditions that are recognized in association with MMD and therefore define the categorization of MMS:

"Atherosclerosis, autoimmune disease (systemic lupus erythematosus, antiphospholipid antibody syndrome, periarteritis nodosa and Sjörgen's syndrome), meningitis, von Recklinghausen's disease, brain tumors, Down's syndrome, head injury, irradiation, hyperthyroidism, stenocephaly, Turner's syndrome, Alagille's syndrome, William's syndrome, Noonan's syndrome, Marfan's syndrome, tuberous sclerosis, Hirschprung's disease, glycogen storage disease type I, Prader-Willi syndrome, Wilms tumor, primary oxalosis, sickle cell disease, Fanconi's anemia, spherocytosis, eosinophilic granuloma, type II plasminogen deficiency, leptospirosis, pyruvate kinase deficiency, protein someone deficiency, protein C deficiency, fibromuscular hyperplasia, osteogenesis imperfecta, polycystic kidney, oral contraceptives, and drug poisoning (cocaine, etc.)" [2].

An overview of the literature available on the most common underlying conditions in MMS can be found in Table 2.2.

2.3.1 Neurofibromatosis Type 1 (von Recklinghausen's Disease)

Neurofibromatosis type 1 (NF-1) or von Recklinghausen's disease is an autosomal dominant condition resulting from loss of function mutations in the NF-1 (neurofibromin) gene leading to overactivation of the RAS pathway and promoting uncontrolled proliferation [23]. Disease prevalence is found to be approximately 1 in 4000–5000 with an equal male to female distribution [18]. Patients can present with visible lesions such as café au lait patches, neurofibromas, lisch nodules, and bony dysplasia. Although the increased RAS activation promoting cellular proliferation may be presumed to affect smooth muscle cells of the tunica intima as may be seen in moyamoya vessels [19], a definite pathophysiological link between NF-1 and MMD has yet to be determined.

Table 2.2 Overview of selected MMS associated conditions

Condition	Pathogenesis	Comment	Proposed pathophysiological links to MMD
NF-1 (Morbus Recklinghausen)	Autosomal dominant loss of function mutation of Neurofibromin and constitutive activation of the RAS pathway	– Predominantly unilateral MMD [18–21] – NF-1 increases the risk of radiation-associated MMD by 7% [22]	RAS-mediated proliferation of smooth muscle cells of the tunica intima [23]
Down syndrome	Aneupleudic triplication of chromosome 21	– Progressive hypertension may preclude ischemic insult in patients with Down Syndrome MMS [24]	Proliferation of the alpha-chain of collagen type VI located on chromosome 21 (29)
Grave's disease	Autoimmune disorder of thyroid-stimulating antibodies targeting TSH receptors	– Primary treatment involving strict pharmacological control of hyperthyroidism. – Thyrotoxic state can increase the risk of infarction [25–27].	– Autoimmune-mediated vascular remodelling [28–30] – Sympathetic induction of vascular wall remodeling [25, 31] – Vasculitis-induced reaction to thyrostatic drugs [32]
Sickle cell disease	Autosomal recessive point mutation of β-globin gene	– Male predominance reported [33]. – Higher rates of unilateral disease in European patients with SCD [34, 35].	n.a
History of radiation	Acquired	– Patients with concurrent NF-1 may have an increased risk of MMD following radiation [36]. – Manifestation of MMD ranges between 2 and 5 years after skull base radiation [21, 37].	– Radiation-induced ischemic necrosis followed by vascular remodeling [38]

Selected underlying conditions in MMS for which the greatest amount of evidence in the current literature exists. Case reports have therefore not been included in this overview

Studies in North American and European children with NF-1 have found that between 2.5 and 6.4% of all cases also display cerebral vasculopathy in the sense of MMD [20–22, 39]. These studies also found predominantly unilateral stenoocclusion with the median age of diagnosis of MMS being between 5 and 12 years of age. Patients with optic glioma associated with NF-1 were found to be at higher risk of having cerebral vasculopathy [21, 39]. Furthermore, MMD was found in 3.5% of patients receiving radiation for primary brain tumors and the presence of NF-1 additionally increased rates of MMD threefold with each 100 cGy increase in radiation dose causing an increased rate of MMD by 7% [40].

A North American pediatric series of 2543 MMD patients observed 29 (6.4%) cases of concurrent NF-1 [41]. Up to 43% of adult MMS cases were found to have an underlying NF-1 diagnosis in a North American cohort of 329 patients. In a Japanese cohort of adult MMD patients, NF-1 was found to occur in 14% of cases [3] and in a German series of 61 MMS cases 10% of pediatric patients were also diagnosed with NF-1 [9]. Results from a single-center North American series of 39 children with MMD and NF-1 found that two-thirds of these patients displayed symptoms of ischemic insult and 56% of these children showed radiographic evidence of stroke [42]. Surgical treatment was performed in 32/39 patients all using pial synangiosis. In 48% of patients, radiographic evidence of disease progression was observed, although 95% of patients remained clinically stable. Due to the recognized association with cerebral vasculopathy and MMD with increased risk of stroke, neuroimaging is considered an optional screening tool at baseline following initial diagnosis of NF-1 in asymptomatic patients but is mandatory in those with neurological symptoms [43].

2.3.2 Down Syndrome (Trisomy 21)

Down Syndrome is an aneuploidy disorder causing triplication of chromosome 21 affecting multiple organ systems and which is associated with increasing maternal age at conception. An increased coincidence of MMD with Down syndrome has been observed, although the pathophysiological basis remains unclear. A possible mechanism has been postulated to involve increased expression of collagen type VI due to the location of its alpha-chains on chromosome 21 which promotes intimal thickening in the cerebral vessels of MMD patients [44].

Reports of underlying Down syndrome in MMD patients are primarily found in North American and European populations. In a North American pediatric series of 2545 MMD patients 8.6% were found to have underlying Down Syndrome [41]. A further North American series of 509 patients found that 3.8% of those admitted to hospital for moyamoya disease had Down syndrome. This study estimated a 26-fold greater prevalence of Down syndrome in Patients with MMD versus the prevalence of Down syndrome among live births [45]. These patients with coincidental MMD and Down syndrome presented more frequently with ischemic events than hemorrhagic insults (15.3% vs. 2.7%), and bilateral involvement was found in all patients with Down syndrome and MMD (16 of 181 cases) in a North American cohort [46]. In this series 16 of 18 patients received surgical revascularization, 15 or which were indirect via pial synangiosis and in one case direct revascularization through STA-MCA bypass was performed. Furthermore, Down syndrome was found to be the most common underlying condition in both pediatric and adult populations (14.8% and 30%, respectively) in a German patient cohort [9]. In contrast to the North

American and European data, rates of Down syndrome in MMD patients is much lower (1:532) in the Japanese population [24] and the current Korean and Chinese reports on MMS describe no coincidental cases of Down syndrome [5, 14].

Interestingly, a North American series of 30 patients with Down syndrome and MMD compared to 116 Down syndrome patients without MMD found that a significant rise in blood pressure was observed in MMD patients over 24 months preceding presentation with clinical symptoms of ischemia [28] indicating a possible clinical parameter which can be used to screen for incipient disease progression.

2.3.3 Thyroid Disease

Thyroid disease, particularly hyperthyroidism due to Grave's disease represents a heterogenous group of underlying conditions in MMD patients. Elevated thyroid autoantibodies have been reported in stroke patients with MMD compared to those without MMD and up 29% of MMS patients in a Chinese series were found to suffer from Grave's disease [5, 29]. Patients with Grave's disease and MMD were found to be older than those with underlying Down syndrome or NF-1, and most patients with Grave's disease and MMD were found to be in a thyrotoxic state at the time of an ischemic event [30].

Several hypotheses regarding the pathophysiology connecting MMD with thyroid disease have been proposed. Similar to the T-cell-mediated autoimmune targeting of TSH receptors in Grave's disease, it has been postulated that an autoimmune reaction may also occur in the vascular walls of MMD patients, although a target of such reactions has not yet been identified [25, 31, 32]. Thyroid hormones may sensitize to the sympathetic nervous system and induce changes in vascular walls [47, 48].

Further mechanisms involving vasculitis-induced alterations due to antithyroid drugs [26] or cerebrovascular changes induced by thyrotoxicosis have been proposed [27, 49], however, the exact mechanism of action remains unclear.

Treatment of patients with MMD and thyroid disease primarily involves strict pharmacological management of hyperthyroidism although surgical revascularization has been recommended in patients with evidence of reduced cerebrovascular reserve capacity due to the increased infarction risk during thyrotoxic states [47, 50, 51]. Patients undergoing revascularization surgery should be kept in a euthyroid state. Surgical strategies used in MMD patients with hyperthyroidism include indirect techniques (EDAS, pial synangiosis) as well as combined revascularization (STA-MCA plus EMS) [33–35].

2.3.4 Sickle Cell Disease

Sickle cell disease (SCD) is an autosomal recessive condition caused by a point mutation in the HBB gene on Chromosome 11 coding for beta-globin causing recurring small vessel occlusion. Retrospective analysis of a North American series of SCD patients who suffered ischemic stroke revealed that 19 of 44 patients (43%)

displayed angiographic MMD. In this series, the average age at the time of ischemic insult was 17 years old, and in contrast to the overall female predominance in MMS, 68% of these patients were male [52]. Pediatric SCD patients with MMD were also shown to be more than twice as likely to suffer an ischemic insult than those without MMD [52]. In a European series of 25 adult SCD with MMD, 32% of these patients showed a unilateral disease pattern which is higher than the 21% described in a cohort of MMS cases with diverse accompanying diseases described in a previous European series [9, 53]. Pediatric SCD patients with MMV have been successfully treated with surgical revascularization via pial synangiosis effectively reducing the rate of ischemic stroke over two years of follow-up [54].

2.3.5 Others

In addition to the aforementioned conditions that have been confirmed to coincide with MMD in several international series, further case reports have illustrated the presence of additional disorders that may accompany MMD. Rheumatic conditions such as systemic lupus erythematodes and Sjörgen's syndrome have been found to coincide with cases of unilateral MMD with affection of the posterior circulation [55]. Antiphospholipid syndrome and thrombophilia (Protein S and Protein C deficiency) have been described in pediatric patients with MMD [56, 57]. Pediatric case reports have also shown coincidence of inherited metabolic syndromes, Fanconi's anemia, phakomatosis, and ulcerative colitis [36, 37, 58–60].

2.3.6 Acquired Conditions

In addition to inherited disease patterns, several acquired conditions are associated with MMD. Of these, the history of cranial radiation has been most intensively studied. Here, radiation induces ischemic necrosis and promotes pathological vascular remodeling [38]. Patients receiving radiation for tumors of the skull base such as craniopharyngioma, optic glioma, or germ cell tumors are at increased risk of developing MMD [61]. The time point at which MMD can be observed following radiation can range between 2 and 5 years, however, this can vary greatly [40, 62]. A case series of 54 pediatric patients receiving radiotherapy in the parasellar region revealed that up to 95% of children developed MMD within 12 years of initial radiation [63]. Development of MMD has also been reported in patients receiving proton beam therapy [64]. Additional case reports have confirmed postinfectious cases of MMD particularly in children and adolescents after bacterial meningitis [65, 66].

2.4 Surgical Revascularization and Outcome

To date, surgical revascularization remains the primary treatment for MMD as it aims at restoring perfusion in order to stabilize cerebrovascular hemodynamics and reduce hemorrhagic and ischemic events [12, 67]. Both direct and indirect revascularization techniques have been successfully employed in MMS patients [68]. Among indirect revascularization techniques, pial synangiosis and EDAS are most commonly reported in the literature, particularly in pediatric patients [69, 70]. In a retrospective single-center analysis of surgical revascularization performed on MMS versus MMD patients, MMS patients were found to have an increased risk of postoperative stroke (OR 4.16, $p = 0.09$) compared to those with MMD as well as higher surgical morbidity (8.7% vs. 3.5%) [8]. It may be hypothesized that the presence of accompanying disease per se increases the risk of surgical morbidity, although this has not yet been thoroughly examined in larger case-control studies.

Long-term follow up of MMS patients following surgical treatment have shown that while approximately 30% of unilateral cases had progressed to bilateral disease over a mean time of 2.2 years [69], no significant increase in ischemia or hemorrhage was observed [70]. Factors associated with progression include contralateral abnormalities on initial angiography, a previous history of congenital cardiac anomaly, history of cranial irradiation, Asian ancestry, and familial MMS [69]. Patients diagnosed with MMS at a younger age were found to progress more rapidly than were those diagnosed later in life [69].

In the largest European Caucasian series of MMS patients, a study performed in our institute reports that 92% of patients received surgical treatment [9]. Combined revascularization techniques (STA-MCA bypass plus EDS and or EMS) were used most commonly in this cohort. Long-term follow up in these patients (mean 51 months) showed that 88% of patients had no new symptoms, whereas four patients (18%) reported persisting TIA symptoms which were not associated with new ischemic lesions on MRI scans. Bypass patency was found to be present in 89% of cases at long-term follow up controls. Four patients underwent revision bypass surgery using intermediate- and high-flow bypasses as well as STA-MCA with the use of the frontal STA branch.

2.5 Future Perspectives in Diagnosis and Patient Care

Recognition of MMS as a disease variant of MMD is established in the current international guidelines for diagnosis and treatment of moyamoya disease. Despite an extensive list of underlying conditions that constitute MMS in these guidelines there is great variation of how MMS is defined in clinical practice and research. Standardization of terminology as well as underlying conditions could simplify international collaboration when dealing with this rare condition.

With increasing integration of next generation sequencing technologies in the clinical routine, there is great potential for expanding our current knowledge of the etiology and pathophysiological mechanisms connecting the underlying conditions discussed in this chapter with MMD. Although linkage studies performed in families with MMD have introduced five potential candidate genes associated with the development of the MMD phenotype, no clear susceptibility gene has yet been identified [71]. In regard to MMS, an autosomal recessive homozygous mutation of the GUCY1A3 gene (coding for the α-subunit of a major NO receptor) has been identified as causing abnormal vascular remodeling in patients with Achalasia and MMS [72]. Furthermore, X-linked deletions on Xq28 leading to loss of the MTCP1/MTCP1NP and BRCC3 genes have been found in three unrelated families to cause a phenotype with short stature, facial dysmorphism, and hypergonadotropic hypogonadism in addition to MMD [73].

Insights into the genetic links between MMD and the accompanying diseases found in MMS could provide a means of screening for patients at risk of developing ischemic or hemorrhagic stroke and guide the timing of possible surgical treatment to improve long-term outcome in this heterogenous group.

References

1. Suzuki J, Takaku A. Cerebrovascular "moyamoya" disease. Disease showing abnormal net-like vessels in base of brain. Arch Neurol. 1969;20(3):288–99.
2. Guidelines for diagnosis and treatment of moyamoya disease (spontaneous occlusion of the circle of Willis). Neurol Med Chir (Tokyo). 2012;52(5):245–66.
3. Hayashi K, Horie N, Izumo T, Nagata I. Nationwide survey on quasi-moyamoya disease in Japan. Acta Neurochir. 2014;156(5):935–40.
4. Hayashi K, Horie N, Suyama K, Nagata I. An epidemiological survey of moyamoya disease, unilateral moyamoya disease and quasi-moyamoya disease in Japan. Clin Neurol Neurosurg. 2013;115(7):930–3.
5. Wei Y-C, Liu C-H, Chang T-Y, Chin S-C, Chang C-H, Huang K-L, et al. Coexisting diseases of moyamoya vasculopathy. J Stroke Cerebrovasc Dis. 2014;23(6):1344–50.
6. Zhao M, Lin Z, Deng X, Zhang Q, Zhang D, Zhang Y, et al. Clinical characteristics and natural history of quasi-moyamoya disease. J Stroke Cerebrovasc Dis. 2017;26(5):1088–97.
7. Gross BA, Du R. The natural history of moyamoya in a North American adult cohort. J Clin Neurosci. 2013;20(1):44–8.
8. Guzman R, Lee M, Achrol A, Bell-Stephens T, Kelly M, Do HM, et al. Clinical outcome after 450 revascularization procedures for moyamoya disease. J Neurosurg. 2009;111:927–35. (Clinical article)
9. Acker G, Goerdes S, Schmiedek P, Czabanka M, Vajkoczy P. Characterization of clinical and radiological features of quasi-moyamoya disease among European Caucasians including surgical treatment and outcome. Cerebrovasc Dis. 2016;42(5–6):464–75.
10. Baba T, Houkin K, Kuroda S. Novel epidemiological features of moyamoya disease. J Neurol Neurosurg Psychiatry. 2008;79(8):900–4.
11. Duan L, Bao XY, Yang WZ, Shi WC, Li DS, Zhang ZS, et al. Moyamoya disease in China: its clinical features and outcomes. Stroke. 2012;43(1):56–60.
12. Kuroda S, Hashimoto N, Yoshimoto T, Iwasaki Y. Radiological findings, clinical course, and outcome in asymptomatic moyamoya disease: results of multicenter survey in Japan. Stroke. 2007;38(5):1430–5.
13. Ikezaki K, Han DH, Kawano T, Inamura T, Fukui M. Epidemiological survey of moyamoya disease in Korea. Clin Neurol Neurosurg. 1997;99(Suppl 2):S6–10.
14. Ahn IM, Park DH, Hann HJ, Kim KH, Kim HJ, Ahn HS. Incidence, prevalence, and survival of moyamoya disease in Korea: a nationwide, population-based study. Stroke. 2014;45(4):1090–5.
15. Kim T, Lee H, Bang JS, Kwon OK, Hwang G. Oh CW. Epidemiology of moyamoya disease in Korea: based on National Health Insurance Service data. J Korean Neurosurg Soc. 2015;57(6):390–5.
16. Uchino K, Johnston SC, Becker KJ, Tirschwell DL. Moyamoya disease in Washington state and California. Neurology. 2005;65(6):956–8.

17. Kraemer M, Schwitalla JC, Diesner F, Aktas O, Hartung HP, Berlit P. Clinical presentation of moyamoya angiopathy in Europeans: experiences from Germany with 200 patients. J Neurol. 2019;266(6):1421–8.
18. Ferner RE. Neurofibromatosis 1. Eur J Hum Genet. 2007;15(2):131–8.
19. Masuda J, Ogata J, Yutani C. Smooth muscle cell proliferation and localization of macrophages and T cells in the occlusive intracranial major arteries in moyamoya disease. Stroke. 1993;24(12):1960–7.
20. Cairns AG, North KN. Cerebrovascular dysplasia in neurofibromatosis type 1. J Neurol Neurosurg Psychiatry. 2008;79(10):1165–70.
21. Ghosh PS, Rothner AD, Emch TM, Friedman NR, Moodley M. Cerebral vasculopathy in children with neurofibromatosis type 1. J Child Neurol. 2013;28(1):95–101.
22. Rosser TL, Vezina G, Packer RJ. Cerebrovascular abnormalities in a population of children with neurofibromatosis type 1. Neurology. 2005;64(3):553–5.
23. Bajaj A, Li QF, Zheng Q, Pumiglia K. Loss of NF1 expression in human endothelial cells promotes autonomous proliferation and altered vascular morphogenesis. PLoS One. 2012;7(11):e49222.
24. Fukushima Y, Kondo Y, Kuroki Y, Miyake S, Iwamoto H, Sekido K, et al. Are down syndrome patients predisposed to moyamoya disease? Eur J Pediatr. 1986;144(5):516–7.
25. Panegyres PK, Morris JG, O'Neill PJ, Balleine R. Moyamoya like disease with inflammation. Eur Neurol. 1993;33(3):260–3.
26. Chastain MA, Russo GG, Boh EE, Chastain JB, Falabella A, Millikan LE. Propylthiouracil hypersensitivity: report of two patients with vasculitis and review of the literature. J Am Acad Dermatol. 1999;41(5 Pt 1):757–64.
27. Colleran KM, Ratliff DM, Burge MR. Potential association of thyrotoxicosis with vitamin B and folate deficiencies, resulting in risk for hyperhomocysteinemia and subsequent thromboembolic events. Endocr Pract. 2003;9(4):290–5.
28. Santoro JD, Lee S, Mlynash M, Nguyen T, Lazzareschi DV, Kraler LD, et al. Blood pressure elevation and risk of moyamoya syndrome in patients with trisomy 21. Pediatrics. 2018;142(4):e20180840.
29. Kim SJ, Heo KG, Shin HY, Bang OY, Kim GM, Chung CS, et al. Association of thyroid autoantibodies with moyamoya-type cerebrovascular disease: a prospective study. Stroke. 2010;41(1):173–6.
30. Ohba S, Nakagawa T, Murakami H. Concurrent Graves' disease and intracranial arterial stenosis/occlusion: special considerations regarding the state of thyroid function, etiology, and treatment. Neurosurg Rev. 2011;34(3):297–304. discussion
31. Weng L, Cao X, Han L, Zhao H, Qiu S, Yan Y, et al. Association of increased Treg and Th17 with pathogenesis of moyamoya disease. Sci Rep. 2017;7(1):3071.
32. Soliman M, Kaplan E, Yanagawa T, Hidaka Y, Fisfalen ME, De Groot LJ. T-cells recognize multiple epitopes in the human thyrotropin receptor extracellular domain. J Clin Endocrinol Metab. 1995;80(3):905–14.
33. Nakamura K, Yanaka K, Ihara S, Nose T. Multiple intracranial arterial stenoses around the circle of Willis in association with Graves' disease: report of two cases. Neurosurgery. 2003;53(5):1210–4. discussion 4–5
34. Im SH, Oh CW, Kwon OK, Kim JE, Han DH. Moyamoya disease associated with Graves' disease: special considerations regarding clinical significance and management. J Neurosurg. 2005;102(6):1013–7.
35. Golomb MR, Biller J, Smith JL, Edwards-Brown M, Sanchez JC, Nebesio TD, et al. A 10-year-old girl with coexistent moyamoya disease and Graves' disease. J Child Neurol. 2005;20(7):620–4.
36. Cohen N, Berant M, Simon J. Moyamoya and Fanconi's anemia. Pediatrics. 1980;65(4):804–5.
37. Tsuruta D, Fukai K, Seto M, Fujitani K, Shindo K, Hamada T, et al. Phakomatosis pigmentovascularis type IIIb associated with moyamoya disease. Pediatr Dermatol. 1999;16(1):35–8.
38. Murphy ES, Xie H, Merchant TE, Yu JS, Chao ST, Suh JH. Review of cranial radiotherapy-induced vasculopathy. J Neuro-Oncol. 2015;122(3):421–9.

39. Rea D, Brandsema JF, Armstrong D, Parkin PC, deVeber G, MacGregor D, et al. Cerebral arteriopathy in children with neurofibromatosis type 1. Pediatrics. 2009;124(3):e476–83.
40. Ullrich NJ, Robertson R, Kinnamon DD, Scott RM, Kieran MW, Turner CD, et al. Moyamoya following cranial irradiation for primary brain tumors in children. Neurology. 2007;68(12):932–8.
41. Titsworth WL, Scott RM, Smith ER. National Analysis of 2454 pediatric moyamoya admissions and the effect of hospital volume on outcomes. Stroke. 2016;47(5):1303–11.
42. Koss M, Scott RM, Irons MB, Smith ER, Ullrich NJ. Moyamoya syndrome associated with neurofibromatosis type 1: perioperative and long-term outcome after surgical revascularization. J Neurosurg Pediatr. 2013;11(4):417–25.
43. Miller DT, Freedenberg D, Schorry E, Ullrich NJ, Viskochil D, Korf BR. Health supervision for children with neurofibromatosis type 1. Pediatrics. 2019;143(5):e20190660.
44. Karousou E, Stachtea X, Moretto P, Viola M, Vigetti D, D'Angelo ML, et al. New insights into the pathobiology of down syndrome--hyaluronan synthase-2 overexpression is regulated by collagen VI α2 chain. FEBS J. 2013;280(10):2418–30.
45. Kainth DS, Chaudhry SA, Kainth HS, Suri FK, Qureshi AI. Prevalence and characteristics of concurrent down syndrome in patients with moyamoya disease. Neurosurgery. 2013;72(2):210–5. discussion 5
46. Jea A, Smith ER, Robertson R, Scott RM. Moyamoya syndrome associated with Down syndrome: outcome after surgical revascularization. Pediatrics. 2005;116(5):e694–701.
47. Liu JS, Juo SH, Chen WH, Chang YY, Chen SS. A case of graves' diseases associated with intracranial moyamoya vessels and tubular stenosis of extracranial internal carotid arteries. J Formos Med Assoc. 1994;93(9):806–9.
48. Morita S, Ueda Y, Eguchi K. Anti-thyroid drug-induced ANCA-associated vasculitis: a case report and review of the literature. Endocr J. 2000;47(4):467–70.
49. Iso H, Moriyama Y, Sato S, Kitamura A, Tanigawa T, Yamagishi K, et al. Serum total homocysteine concentrations and risk of stroke and its subtypes in Japanese. Circulation. 2004;109(22):2766–72.
50. Kushima K, Satoh Y, Ban Y, Taniyama M, Ito K, Sugita K. Graves' thyrotoxicosis and moyamoya disease. Can J Neurol Sci. 1991;18(2):140–2.
51. Tendler BE, Shoukri K, Malchoff C, MacGillivray D, Duckrow R, Talmadge T, et al. Concurrence of Graves' disease and dysplastic cerebral blood vessels of the moyamoya variety. Thyroid. 1997;7(4):625–9.
52. Dobson SR, Holden KR, Nietert PJ, Cure JK, Laver JH, Disco D, et al. Moyamoya syndrome in childhood sickle cell disease: a predictive factor for recurrent cerebrovascular events. Blood. 2002;99(9):3144–50.
53. Kauv P, Gaudré N, Hodel J, Tuilier T, Habibi A, Oppenheim C, et al. Characteristics of moyamoya syndrome in sickle-cell disease by magnetic resonance angiography: an adult-cohort study. Front Neurol. 2019;10:15.
54. Kennedy BC, McDowell MM, Yang PH, Wilson CM, Li S, Hankinson TC, et al. Pial synangiosis for moyamoya syndrome in children with sickle cell anemia: a comprehensive review of reported cases. Neurosurg Focus. 2014;36(1):E12.
55. Matsuki Y, Kawakami M, Ishizuka T, Kawaguchi Y, Hidaka T, Suzuki K, et al. SLE and Sjögren's syndrome associated with unilateral moyamoya vessels in cerebral arteries. Scand J Rheumatol. 1997;26(5):392–4.
56. Tsuda H, Hattori S, Tanabe S, Nishioka S, Matsushima T, Ikezaki K, et al. Thrombophilia found in patients with moyamoya disease. Clin Neurol Neurosurg. 1997;99(Suppl 2):S229–33.
57. Booth F, Yanofsky R, Ross IB, Lawrence P, Oen K. Primary Antiphospholipid syndrome with Moyamoya-like vascular changes. Pediatr Neurosurg. 1999;31(1):45–8.
58. Shanahan P, Hutchinson M, Bohan A, O'Donoghue D, Sheahan K, Owens A. Hemichorea, Moya-Moya, and ulcerative colitis. Mov Disord. 2001;16(3):570–2.
59. Kotagal S, Peterson PL, Martens ME, Lee CP, Nigro M, Archer CR. Impaired NADH-CoQ reductase activity in a child with moyamoya syndrome. Pediatr Neurol. 1988;4(4):241–4.

60. van Diemen-Steenvoorde R, van Nieuwenhuizen O, de Klerk JB, Duran M. Quasi-moyamoya disease and heterozygosity for homocystinuria in a five-year-old girl. Neuropediatrics. 1990;21(2):110–2.
61. Keene DL, Johnston DL, Grimard L, Michaud J, Vassilyadi M, Ventureyra E. Vascular complications of cranial radiation. Childs Nerv Syst. 2006;22(6):547–55.
62. Morris B, Partap S, Yeom K, Gibbs IC, Fisher PG, King AA. Cerebrovascular disease in childhood cancer survivors: a children's oncology group report. Neurology. 2009;73(22):1906–13.
63. Desai SS, Paulino AC, Mai WY, Teh BS. Radiation-induced moyamoya syndrome. Int J Radiat Oncol Biol Phys. 2006;65(4):1222–7.
64. Reynolds MR, Haydon DH, Caird J, Leonard JR. Radiation-induced moyamoya syndrome after proton beam therapy in the pediatric patient: a case series. Pediatr Neurosurg. 2016;51(6):297–301.
65. Czartoski T, Hallam D, Lacy JM, Chun MR, Becker K. Postinfectious vasculopathy with evolution to moyamoya syndrome. J Neurol Neurosurg Psychiatry. 2005;76(2):256–9.
66. Dhawan SR, Sahu JK, Vyas S, Singhi SC, Singhi PD. Pyogenic meningitis complicated with extensive central nervous system vasculitis and moyamoya vasculopathy. J Pediatr Neurosci. 2018;13(3):343–5.
67. Jeon JP, Kim JE, Cho WS, Bang JS, Son YJ, Oh CW. Meta-analysis of the surgical outcomes of symptomatic moyamoya disease in adults. J Neurosurg. 2018;128(3):793–9.
68. Horn P, Pfister S, Bueltmann E, Vajkoczy P, Schmiedek P. Moyamoya-like vasculopathy (moyamoya syndrome) in children. Childs Nerv Syst. 2004;20(6):382–91.
69. Smith ER, Scott RM. Progression of disease in unilateral moyamoya syndrome. Neurosurg Focus. 2008;24(2):E17.
70. Fryer RH, Anderson RC, Chiriboga CA, Feldstein NA. Sickle cell anemia with moyamoya disease: outcomes after EDAS procedure. Pediatr Neurol. 2003;29(2):124–30.
71. Kamada F, Aoki Y, Narisawa A, Abe Y, Komatsuzaki S, Kikuchi A, et al. A genome-wide association study identifies RNF213 as the first moyamoya disease gene. J Hum Genet. 2011;56(1):34–40.
72. Hervé D, Philippi A, Belbouab R, Zerah M, Chabrier S, Collardeau-Frachon S, et al. Loss of $\alpha 1\beta 1$ soluble guanylate cyclase, the major nitric oxide receptor, leads to moyamoya and achalasia. Am J Hum Genet. 2014;94(3):385–94.
73. Miskinyte S, Butler MG, Hervé D, Sarret C, Nicolino M, Petralia JD, et al. Loss of BRCC3 deubiquitinating enzyme leads to abnormal angiogenesis and is associated with syndromic moyamoya. Am J Hum Genet. 2011;88(6):718–28.

Unilateral Moyamoya Disease: A Distinct Entity?

3

Yohei Mineharu and Susumu Miyamoto

Abstract

The clinical features of unilateral moyamoya disease differ from those of bilateral moyamoya disease, e.g., cerebral blood flow pattern and age distribution, and it remains to be determined whether unilateral moyamoya disease belongs to the same clinical entity as moyamoya disease or constitutes a distinct entity. However, both share many common features, e.g., both are chronically progressive. Moreover, bypass surgery is effective in preventing stroke. The R4810K mutation in *RNF213* contributes greatly to the disease risk in East Asian countries. Considering that prevention of the disease progression is the main therapeutic strategy for moyamoya disease, clarification of the mechanisms of disease progression is very important. In this context, unilateral moyamoya disease would serve as a model for disease progression because the unaffected side allows observation of the phenotypes of progression from a very early stage. In this chapter, we summarize the diagnostic criteria and clinical and radiological features of unilateral moyamoya disease and discuss current topics, including the differential diagnosis from transient cerebral arteriopathy, biomarkers of unilateral moyamoya disease, contralateral progression, and posterior cerebral artery involvement. Knowledge on the characteristics of unilateral moyamoya disease is important for understanding the pathophysiology of moyamoya disease.

Keywords

Unilateral · Moyamoya · *RNF213* · Contralateral progression · Focal cerebral arteriopathy · Pediatric · Stroke

Y. Mineharu · S. Miyamoto (✉)
Department of Neurosurgery, Kyoto University Graduate School of Medicine, Kyoto, Japan
e-mail: mineharu@kuhp.kyoto-u.ac.jp; miy@kuhp.kyoto-u.ac.jp

S. Kuroda (ed.), *Moyamoya Disease: Current Knowledge and Future Perspectives*, https://doi.org/10.1007/978-981-33-6404-2_3

3.1 Introduction

Unilateral moyamoya disease was formerly considered a distinct clinical entity and has been regarded as "probable" moyamoya disease. The diagnostic criteria of moyamoya disease are gradually changing with growing understanding of the genetics and pathophysiology of the disease, and currently, both bilateral and unilateral lesions are regarded as "definite" moyamoya disease. Unilateral moyamoya disease constitutes 10%–20% of all cases of moyamoya disease. Although the rate of contralateral progression varies among studies, it occurs in both children and adults. Considering that unilateral and bilateral moyamoya disease are classified under a single family and share common genetic factors, i.e., *RNF213* mutations [1, 2], they are safely considered to share a common pathological background. However, some reports have shown that the progression pattern or cerebral blood flow (CBF) pattern differs between unilateral and bilateral moyamoya disease, and thus, whether they are the same clinical entity remains to be determined. It is also possible that the contribution of nongenetic factors is different between unilateral and bilateral moyamoya disease.

Regardless of whether unilateral and bilateral moyamoya disease are identical, they share common features that are useful in understanding the pathophysiology of the disease. The distinguishing characteristics of both unilateral and bilateral moyamoya disease are progressive stenosis around the terminal region of the internal carotid artery (ICA) and the development of fine collaterals. Understanding the mechanism of disease progression will improve the management of patients. Although it is possible that the process of progression may differ between unilateral and bilateral moyamoya disease, it is advantageous to be able to observe the progressive changes from a very early stage (Suzuki stage 0–1) in cases of contralateral progression in unilateral moyamoya disease. Therefore, it is necessary to review the characteristics of unilateral moyamoya disease in association with bilateral moyamoya disease and other unilateral arteriopathies such as focal cerebral arteriopathy (FCA) to better understand the pathophysiology of moyamoya disease.

3.2 Definition of Unilateral Moyamoya Disease

Unilateral moyamoya disease was formerly regarded as a distinct clinical entity and has been regarded as "probable" moyamoya disease. In 2012, childhood-onset unilateral moyamoya disease with stenotic changes on the contralateral side was regarded as "definite" moyamoya disease [3]. According to the current guidelines of the Research Committee on Spontaneous Occlusion of Circle of Willis (moyamoya disease) [4], both bilateral and unilateral lesions are regarded as "definite" moyamoya disease when patients are diagnosed by conventional angiography, although when diagnosis is performed with only magnetic resonance angiography, only bilateral lesions can be diagnosed as moyamoya disease. Patients with moyamoya disease and underlying diseases such as neurofibromatosis type 1, autoimmune diseases, or Down syndrome can also be regarded as having moyamoya disease (correctly known as quasi-moyamoya disease) in the broad classification [5, 6]. However, lesions caused by atherosclerosis or cranial irradiation should not be treated as moyamoya disease. Conventional angiography is necessary for the diagnosis of unilateral moyamoya disease because it is sometimes difficult to distinguish it from non-moyamoya arteriopathy and middle cerebral artery disease.

3.3 Clinical and Radiological Features

The proportion of unilateral moyamoya disease cases was 19.7% in a Japanese study comprising 180 patients [7]. In other studies, it was reported to be approximately 15% (9.4%–18.0%) [8–16]. The age distribution in unilateral moyamoya disease shows two peaks, similar to that in bilateral moyamoya disease, but the proportion of childhood-onset disease is smaller in unilateral moyamoya disease than in bilateral moyamoya disease [7]. A report from China showed only one peak distribution, with a mean age at diagnosis of 30.8 years [2]. Ikezaki et al. reported a female-to-male ratio of 1.65, which is not different from that in moyamoya disease [7]. However, many reports showed a ratio of >2.0. In contrast, Ogata et al. reported that the female-to-male ratio in unilateral moyamoya disease was lower and between those in moyamoya disease and atherosclerotic intracranial arteriopathy [17]. Because the ratio is affected by ethnicity, surgical case-only analysis, year of enrollment, and use of magnetic resonance imaging (MRI) screening for asymptomatic patients, it varies across studies. Furthermore, a nationwide comprehensive study is needed to clarify the difference in the female-to-male ratio between unilateral and bilateral moyamoya disease.

Clinical manifestation also varies across studies. Some reports showed that symptomatic cases and left-side involvement were higher or hemorrhagic onset was common in unilateral moyamoya disease, whereas others showed that asymptomatic cases were more common (55.6%) [10]. This is susceptible to diagnostic and reporting biases. In a series of surgical cases, there were no asymptomatic cases. Screening examination by MRI such as brain checkup increases the incidence rate of asymptomatic unilateral moyamoya disease. Yu et al. compared patterns of hemorrhagic stroke between adult patients with bilateral moyamoya disease and those with unilateral moyamoya disease [18]. Patients with unilateral moyamoya disease and acute intracranial hemorrhage were at the earlier Suzuki stage and had a higher incidence rate of hypertension than patients with bilateral moyamoya disease. Intraventricular hemorrhage was more common in bilateral moyamoya disease, whereas subarachnoid hemorrhage was more common in unilateral moyamoya disease.

Familial cases accounted for 4.1%–17.6% of cases of unilateral moyamoya disease and ranged between 5% and 10% in most studies [2, 7, 10–12, 19–21]. Zhang et al. reported that familial cases accounted for 12.2% of bilateral moyamoya disease cases and 5.5% of unilateral moyamoya disease cases [2], suggesting that the proportion is higher in bilateral moyamoya disease. In accordance with this finding, the rate of bilateral involvement was higher in mutants than in wild types for the *RNF213* p.R4810K mutation [22].

Only a few studies have assessed CBF in unilateral moyamoya disease. Ogata reported the differences in angiographic and CBF characteristics between unilateral and bilateral moyamoya disease [17]. Ethmoidal moyamoya vessels were more prominent in patients with moyamoya disease than in those with unilateral moyamoya disease. CBF at resting state in patients with unilateral moyamoya disease was significantly higher than that in patients with bilateral moyamoya disease or those with atherosclerotic arteriopathy. The vascular reserve capacity was higher in patients with unilateral moyamoya disease, but it was not statistically significant. It was speculated that collateral flow from the unaffected hemisphere prevents the decrease of blood flow. However, caution is advised when interpreting the results of this study because the patients with unilateral moyamoya disease were mostly asymptomatic, whereas most of the patients with bilateral moyamoya disease and those with atherosclerosis had a stroke.

Angiographic characteristics are common in both unilateral and bilateral moyamoya disease. Both show progressive steno-occlusive changes at the terminal region of the ICA, accompanied by fine collaterals at the base of the brain. Nevertheless, some reports suggested that the initiation of stenosis in unilateral moyamoya disease may be different, i.e., stenosis starts at the distal part of the MCA or anterior cerebral artery (ACA) but not at the terminal region of the ICA. For instance, Liu et al. reported a patient with unilateral moyamoya disease associated with the *RNF213* mutation who underwent vertebral artery dissection followed by MCA and ACA stenosis before developing the angiographic moyamoya phenotype [23]. However, MCA stenosis in patients with bilateral moyamoya disease is likely to be underestimated. Therefore, the finding does not necessarily indicate that the progression pattern of arterial stenosis differs between unilateral and bilateral moyamoya disease. Additional clinical studies or preclinical models are necessary to examine the difference between unilateral and bilateral moyamoya disease.

3.4 Biomarkers

Several studies aimed to identify biomarkers for unilateral moyamoya disease. Homocystinuria is a well-known cause of quasi-moyamoya disease. Ge et al. showed that serum homocysteine level was elevated in patients with moyamoya disease and was significantly higher in patients with unilateral moyamoya disease than in those with bilateral moyamoya disease [15]. Jeon et al. reported that CRABP-I expression levels in bilateral moyamoya disease were significantly higher than those in unilateral moyamoya disease ($p = 0.044$) [24]. Both homocysteine and CRABP-I regulate retinoic acid, which is important for the generation of regulatory T cells, suggesting the role of autoimmunity in the development of unilateral moyamoya disease. In accordance with this finding, Chen et al. showed that autoimmune disease was more common in patients with unilateral moyamoya disease than in those with bilateral moyamoya disease, although no specific disease was identified [25].

The R4810K mutation in *RNF213* has been reported to be associated with unilateral and bilateral moyamoya disease. The prevalence of the R4810K mutation was reported to be lower in patients with unilateral moyamoya disease [22]. To date, no specific gene has been identified to cause unilateral moyamoya disease. *MRV-1* has been reported to be associated with moyamoya disease in patients with NF1. Such genetic factors may be identified in unilateral moyamoya disease in future studies.

In summary, compared with patients with bilateral moyamoya disease, hypertension and autoimmune disease were more common and homocysteine levels were higher in hemorrhagic stroke cases, whereas *RNF213* mutation was less common in patients with unilateral moyamoya disease. These findings suggest that the balance of genetic and nongenetic factors may differ between unilateral and bilateral moyamoya disease.

3.5 Differentiation of Moyamoya Disease from Non-moyamoya Arteriopathy, Including FCA

Intracranial arteriopathy is a common condition that resembles moyamoya disease but does not fulfill the diagnostic criteria for moyamoya disease. Such an arteriopathy is regarded as non-moyamoya arteriopathy. However, no clear distinction can be made between moyamoya disease and non-moyamoya arteriopathy. In the case of rapid progression of unilateral arteriopathy within a family of familial moyamoya diseases, the development of moyamoya vessels was not evident [26]. Some patients with moyamoya disease exhibit a typical feature of moyamoya arteriopathy on one hemisphere and an atypical feature on the other hemisphere. The frequency of the R4810K mutation was reported to be correlated with a number of diagnostic criteria for moyamoya disease (bilateral and basal moyamoya vessels and involvement of the terminal ICA), suggesting that non-moyamoya arteriopathy may be a spectrum of moyamoya disease or RNF213-related vasculopathies. However, no specific factor was identified other than *RNF213*, and the rationale for this hypothesis is insufficient. In the same context, quasi-moyamoya disease was also shown to be associated with *RNF213* [5], but further evidence is needed if we classify it under the same entity as moyamoya disease.

In cases of unilateral pediatric arteriopathy, differential diagnosis from transient cerebral arteriopathy (FCA) is necessary. FCA is also known as transient cerebral arteriopathy. However, transient indicates that the arterial narrowing is not progressive, and symptoms are not necessarily transient. Moreover, most children are left with permanent arterial abnormalities and residual neurological deficits. Therefore, FCA would be the preferred technical term. Braun et al. reported that among children with FCA in Europe, only 6% had progressive arteriopathy including moyamoya disease [27]. Conversely, Yeon et al. reported that moyamoya disease is more prevalent in East Asian countries and that FCA was not well recognized. They reported that 20% of cases of childhood arteriopathy, whose features are distinct from those of moyamoya disease at diagnosis, were progressive [28]. Stroke was preceded by chickenpox in 44% of patients with FCA and in none of the patients with progressive arteriopathies [27]. Araki et al. reported a case of bilateral FCA with occlusion of the left ICA followed by focal narrowing of the right ACA [29]. The patient did not have the R4810K mutation. In contrast, Echizenya et al. reported a patient with FCA with the R4810K mutation in whom arteriopathy occurred after viral infection and who recovered completely [30]. Thus, a combination of genetic and nongenetic factors does not necessarily induce progression of the arteriopathy or formation of moyamoya collaterals, suggesting that more than two factors may be necessary for disease progression in moyamoya disease. Comparative analysis, especially comparison of genetic architecture, has not been conducted between unilateral moyamoya disease and FCA. Future studies are warranted.

3.6 Contralateral Progression

Sixteen studies have analyzed contralateral progression of unilateral moyamoya disease (Table 3.1) [2, 7–12, 19–21, 31–35]. Ten studies included only surgical cases, two included only adult cases, and five included only pediatric cases. The percentage of contralateral progression ranged from 17.8% to 66.6% (median 28.5%) in pediatric cases and from 0 to 50.0% (median 14.6%) in adult cases. Zhang et al. performed one of the largest studies enrolling both pediatric and adult patients with unilateral moyamoya disease (17 children and 84 adults); they reported that the rate of contralateral progression was 22.2% and 14.6%, respectively [2]. Three studies consistently showed that pediatric patients aged <7 years develop contralateral progression faster than older populations [11, 12, 19] as well as develop the contralateral lesion within 3 years. These findings indicate that children have a higher risk of contralateral progression and a shorter progression period.

Several candidates were determined as predictors of contralateral progression. Age at diagnosis is one of the most reliable factors, as discussed above. Angiographic abnormalities (equivocal findings of stenosis) at the MCA or ACA have been also reported in several studies, although some denied it [12]. Kuroda et al. compared the risk of progression between the untreated hemisphere of moyamoya disease and the unaffected side of unilateral moyamoya disease. They showed that the interval from diagnosis to progression was shorter in patients with moyamoya disease [8], supporting the notion that angiographic narrowing is a predictor of disease progression. Recently, Church et al. analyzed a large cohort of 217 patients with unilateral moyamoya disease including Asian and Caucasian populations and reported that hyperlipidemia is a risk of contralateral progression [21]. Comorbidities related to quasi-moyamoya disease such as NF1 have been proposed as risk factors for contralateral progression, but the results are inconsistent [19, 21]. Further replication studies are necessary to draw conclusions.

Table 3.1 Summary of previous studies analyzing contralateral progression of unilateral moyamoya disease

Author	Year	Surgery	Total number of cases	Progression rate (child)	Progression rate (adult)	F-M ratio	Age at diagnosis	Family history	Disease type[a]	Follow-up period	Time to progression	Risk of contralateral progression
Matsushima	1994	All cases	6	2/6 (33.3%)	NA	1	7.2	NA	1/5/0/0/0	4.7 y	2.16 y	
Kawano	1994	NA	32	12/18 (66.6%)	5/14 (35.7%)	2.6	6.6 (child), 36.6 (adult)	9.30%	5/17/7/3/0	2.8 y	2.6 y	
Houkin	1996	NA	10	1/4 (25%)	0/6 (0%)	1	9.0 (child), 40.3 (adult)	0%	1/5/4/0/0	3.5 y	0.5 y	
Hirotsune	1997	All cases	17	6/12 (50%)	0/5 (0%)	1.4	13.5	NA	0/12/2/3/0	20 m	20 m	
Ikezaki	1997	114 (63.3%)	180	12/180 (6.7%) in total		1.65	2 peaks	6.70%	25/61/68/26/0	6.6 y	78 m	
Kuroda	2004	7 (63.6%)	11	NA	4/11 (36.3%)	NA	NA	NA	NA	NA	60 m	
Seol	2006	All cases	7	2 (28.5%)	NA	2.5	5.1	0%	3/4/0/0/0	64.7 m	25.5 m	
Kelly	2006	All cases	18	2/5 (40%)	5/13 (38.4%)	2.6	29.8	NA	6/7/1/3/0	19.3 m	12.7 m	Contralateral abnormality
Nagata	2006	All cases	20	5/20 (25%)	NA	NA	6.2	NA	NA	126.8 m	42.8 m	
Smith	2008	All cases	33	8/29 (28%)	2/4 (50%)	1.2	8.1 (child) 26.8 (adult)	6.10%	11/16/1/2/4	5.3 y	2.2 y	<7 y, cardiac anomaly, Asian ancestry, family history
Hayashi	2010	2 (22.2%)	9	0/1 (0%)	0/8 (0%)	2	39	6.70%	1/2/1/0/5	55.7 m	NA	

(continued)

Table 3.1 (continued)

Author	Year	Surgery	Total number of cases	Progression rate (child)	Progression rate (adult)	F-M ratio	Age at diagnosis	Family history	Disease type[a]	Follow-up period	Time to progression	Risk of contralateral progression
Park	2011	All cases	34	20/34 (58.5%)	NA	0.88	8.7	17.60%	4/23/0/6/1	35.3 m	17.4 m	<8 y, family history, contralateral abnormality
Yeon	2011	All cases	45	8/45 (17.8%)	NA	0.88	9.9	13.00%	5 CI or ICH, 40 TIA or other	53.4 m	27 m	<9 y
Lee	2014	All cases	41	NA	6/41 (14.6%)	3.1	41.1	4.90%	31 CI or TIA/5/5/0	50.1 m	34 m	Contralateral abnormality
Zhang	2016	98 (89.9%)	109	6/27 (22.2%)	12/82 (14.6%)	1.1	30.8	5.50%	24/43/29/13/0	43.8 m	NA	Contralateral abnormality
Church	2020	All cases	217	18/217 (8.3%) in total		2.4	33.8	4.10%	NA	5.8 y		Contralateral abnormality, hyperlipidemia

[a]Disease type was divided into cerebral infarction/transient ischemic attacks/intracranial hemorrhage/others/asymptomatic. F-M ratio represents the female-to-male ratio

Although it has not been reported whether the mutation in *RNF213* is associated with the contralateral progression of unilateral moyamoya disease, it has now been examined in the SUPRA Japan study. Considering that Asian ancestry and family history of moyamoya disease are risk factors for contralateral progression, the *RNF213* R4810K mutation may also be considered a risk factor.

In terms of patient care, a periodical examination by MRI is recommended to detect progression at an early stage before the onset of symptoms. Pediatric patients, especially those aged less than 9 years, should undergo examinations within a year's interval at least for 3 years. Because some studies showed that contralateral progression occurs after 5 years, and because long-term follow-up data are insufficient, it is recommended that patients continue to undergo periodical examinations.

3.7 PCA Involvement

Involvement of the posterior cerebral artery (PCA) is associated with poor prognosis in moyamoya disease. Thus, it is important to understand the risk of PCA involvement in unilateral moyamoya disease as well. It has been reported that PCA involvement tends to occur on the ipsilateral side. Matsushima reported that two of six pediatric patients with unilateral moyamoya disease had PCA involvement on the ipsilateral side [31]. Mugikura showed that PCA involvement occurs predominantly on the ipsilateral hemisphere [36]. Furthermore, the mechanism of disease progression of posterior circulation on the side of the anterior circulation needs to be evaluated in future studies.

3.8 Perspectives

Unilateral moyamoya disease shares a common genetic background (*RNF213* mutation) with bilateral moyamoya disease. However, patients with unilateral moyamoya disease were shown to have a lower frequency of the R4810K mutation, and nongenetic factors such as homocysteine level, hyperlipidemia, hypertension, and autoimmune disease were more predominant. The balance or the number of risk factors may differ between unilateral and bilateral moyamoya disease. Given that even moyamoya disease exhibits laterality, both unilateral and bilateral moyamoya disease should reflect different phases or phenotypes of the same disease; however, current evidence is insufficient to prove this presumption. Further comprehensive analyses comparing bilateral and unilateral moyamoya disease, FCA, quasi-moyamoya disease, and intracranial atherosclerotic disease are warranted. After replicating the effect of hyperlipidemia or homocysteine on unilateral moyamoya disease progression, preclinical models will be strongly required to prove the clinical findings and test the efficacy of therapeutic drugs such as statin or folic acid. Further studies on unilateral moyamoya disease will help better our understanding of the pathophysiology of moyamoya disease and provide a therapeutic strategy.

References

1. Mineharu Y, Takenaka K, Yamakawa H, Inoue K, Ikeda H, Kikuta K-I, et al. Inheritance pattern of familial moyamoya disease: autosomal dominant mode and genomic imprinting. J Neurol Neurosurg Psychiatry [Internet]. 2006 [cited 2010 Aug 31];77(August):1025–1029. Available from: http://jnnp.bmj.com/content/77/9/1025.full
2. Zhang Q, Wang R, Liu Y, Zhang Y, Wang S, Cao Y, et al. Clinical features and long-term outcomes of unilateral Moyamoya disease. World Neurosurg. 2016;96:474–82. https://doi.org/10.1016/j.wneu.2016.09.018.
3. Guidelines for diagnosis and treatment of moyamoya disease (Spontaneous Occlusion of the Circle of Willis). Neurol Med Chir [Internet]. 2012 Jan [cited 2013 Feb 18];52(5):245–266. Available from http://www.ncbi.nlm.nih.gov/pubmed/22870528
4. Tominaga T, Suzuki N, Miyamoto S, Koizumi A, Kuroda S, Takahashi JC, et al. Recommendations for the management of moyamoya disease: a statement from research committee on spontaneous occlusion of the circle of Willis (Moyamoya disease) [2nd edition]. Surg Cereb Stroke. 2018;46:1–24.
5. Morimoto T, Mineharu Y, Kobayashi H, Harada KH, Funaki T, Takagi Y, et al. Significant association of the RNF213 p.R4810K polymorphism with quasi-moyamoya disease. J Stroke Cerebrovasc Dis. 2016;25(11):2632–6. https://doi.org/10.1016/j.jstrokecerebrovasdis.2016.07.004.
6. Zhang Q, Liu Y, Yu L, Duan R, Ma Y, Ge P, et al. The association of the RNF213 p.R4810K polymorphism with quasi-moyamoya disease and a review of the pertinent literature. World Neurosurg. 2017;99:701–708.e1. https://doi.org/10.1016/j.wneu.2016.12.119.
7. Ikezaki K, Inamura T, Kawano T, Fukui M. Clinical features of probable moyamoya disease in Japan. Clin Neurol Neurosurg. 1997;99(Suppl. 2):S173–7.
8. Kuroda S, Ishikawa T, Houkin K, Nanba R, Hokari M, Iwasaki Y. Incidence and clinical features of disease progression in adult moyamoya disease. Stroke. 2005;36(10):2148–53.
9. Kelly ME, Bell-Stephens TE, Marks MP, Do HM, Steinberg GK. Progression of unilateral moyamoya disease: a clinical series. Cerebrovasc Dis. 2006;22(2–3):109–15.
10. Hayashi K, Suyama K, Nagata I. Clinical features of unilateral moyamoya disease. Neurol Med Chir. 2010;50(5):378–85.
11. Park EK, Lee YH, Shim KW, Choi JU, Kim DS. Natural history and progression factors of unilateral moyamoya disease in pediatric patients. Childs Nerv Syst. 2011;27(8):1281–7.
12. Yeon JY, Shin HJ, Kong D-S, Seol HJ, Kim J-S, Hong S-C, et al. The prediction of contralateral progression in children and adolescents with unilateral moyamoya disease. Stroke [Internet]. 2011 Oct [cited 2014 Jun 6];42(10):2973–2976. Available from: http://www.ncbi.nlm.nih.gov/pubmed/21836096
13. Hayashi K, Horie N, Suyama K, Nagata I. An epidemiological survey of moyamoya disease, unilateral moyamoya disease and quasi-moyamoya disease in Japan. Clin Neurol Neurosurg [Internet]. 2012 Oct 4 [cited 2012 Oct 24];9–12. Available from: http://www.ncbi.nlm.nih.gov/pubmed/23041378
14. Cho W, Chung YS, Kim JE. The natural clinical course of hemodynamically stable adult moyamoya disease. J Neurosurg. 2015;122:82–9.
15. Ge P, Zhang Q, Ye X, Liu X, Deng X, Wang J, et al. Modifiable risk factors associated with moyamoya disease: a case-control study. Stroke. 2020;51:2472–9.
16. Jee TK, Yeon JY, Kim SM, Bang OY, Kim J-S, Hong C-C. Prospective screening of extracranial systemic arteriopathy in young adults with. J Am Hear Assoc. 2020;9:e016670.
17. Ogata T, Yasaka M, Inoue T, Yasumori K, Ibayashi S, Iida M, et al. The clinical features of adult unilateral moyamoya disease: does it have the same clinical characteristics as typical moyamoya disease? Cerebrovasc Dis [Internet]. 2008 Jan [cited 2013 Jan 2];26(3):244–249. Available from: http://www.ncbi.nlm.nih.gov/pubmed/18648196
18. Yu Z, Zheng J, Guo R, Li H, You C, Ma L. Patterns of acute intracranial hemorrhage in adult patients with bilateral and unilateral moyamoya disease. Curr Neurovasc Res [Internet].

2019 Jun 21 [cited 2020 Oct 5];16(3):202–207. Available from: https://pubmed.ncbi.nlm.nih.gov/31223087/
19. Smith ER, Scott RM. Progression of disease in unilateral moyamoya syndrome. Neurosurg Focus [Internet]. 2008 Jan [cited 2010 Jul 30];24(2):E17. Available from: http://www.ncbi.nlm.nih.gov/pubmed/18275294
20. Lee SC, Jeon JS, Kim JE, Chung YS, Ahn JH, Cho W-S, et al. Contralateral progression and its risk factor in surgically treated unilateral adult moyamoya disease with a review of pertinent literature. Acta Neurochir [Internet]. 2014 Nov 8 [cited 2013 Nov 18];156:103–11. Available from: http://www.ncbi.nlm.nih.gov/pubmed/24201757
21. Church EW, Bell-Stephens TE, Bigder MG, Gummidipundi S, Han SS, Steinberg GK. Clinical course of unilateral moyamoya disease. Neurosurgery. 2020;0(0):1–7.
22. Moteki Y, Onda H, Kasuya H, Yoneyama T, Okada Y, Hirota K, et al. Systematic validation of RNF213 coding variants in Japanese patients with moyamoya disease. J Am Hear Assoc [Internet]. 2015;4(5):e001862–e001862. Available from: http://jaha.ahajournals.org/cgi/doi/10.1161/JAHA.115.001862
23. Liu Y, Wu X, Fan Z, Cheng J, Zhong L, Lin Y, et al. Development of atherosclerotic-moyamoya syndrome with genetic variant of RNF213 p.R4810K and p.T1727M: a case report. Clin Neurol Neurosurg [Internet]. 2018;168(October 2017):163–6. Available from: https://doi.org/10.1016/j.clineuro.2018.01.034
24. Jeon JS, Ahn JH, Moon Y-J, Cho W-S, Son Y-J, Kim S-K, et al. Expression of cellular retinoic acid-binding protein-I (CRABP-I) in the cerebrospinal fluid of adult onset moyamoya disease and its association with clinical presentation and postoperative haemodynamic change. J Neurol Neurosurg Psychiatry [Internet]. 2013 Nov 29 [cited 2013 Dec 17]; Available from: http://www.ncbi.nlm.nih.gov/pubmed/24292994
25. Chen J-B, Liu Y, Zhou L-X, Sun H, He M, You C. Increased prevalence of autoimmune disease in patients with unilateral compared with bilateral moyamoya disease. J Neurosurg [Internet]. 2015;124(May):1–6. Available from: http://www.ncbi.nlm.nih.gov/pubmed/26406790
26. Mineharu Y, Takagi Y, Takahashi JC, Hashikata H, Liu W, Hitomi T, et al. Rapid Progression of unilateral moyamoya disease in a patient with a family history and an RNF213 risk variant. Cerebrovasc Dis [Internet]. 2013 Jan [cited 2013 Oct 6];36(2):155–7. Available from: http://www.ncbi.nlm.nih.gov/pubmed/24029639
27. Braun KPJ, Bulder MMM, Chabrier S, Kirkham FJ, Uiterwaal CSP, Tardieu M, et al. The course and outcome of unilateral intracranial arteriopathy in 79 children with ischaemic stroke. Brain [Internet]. 2009 Mar [cited 2010 Jul 29];132(Pt 2):544–57. Available from: http://www.pubmedcentral.nih.gov/articlerender.fcgi?artid=2640213&tool=pmcentrez&rendertype=abstract
28. Yeon JY, Shin HJ, Seol HJ, Kim JS, Hong SC. Unilateral intracranial arteriopathy in pediatric stroke: course, outcome, and prediction of reversible arteriopathy. Stroke [Internet]. 2014 [cited 2020 Oct 5];45(4):1173–6. Available from: https://pubmed.ncbi.nlm.nih.gov/24549867/
29. Araki Y, Takagi Y, Mineharu Y, Kobayashi H, Miyamoto S, Wakabayashi T. Rapid contralateral progression of focal cerebral arteriopathy distinguished from RNF213-related moyamoya disease and fibromuscular dysplasia. Childs Nerv Syst [Internet]. 2017.; Available from: http://link.springer.com/10.1007/s00381-017-3451-9
30. Echizenya I, Tokairin K, Kawabori M, Kazumata K, Houkin K. Reversible cerebral angiopathy after viral infection in a pediatric patient with genetic variant of RNF213. J Stroke Cerebrovasc Dis. 2020;29(2):29–31.
31. Matsushima T, Inoue T, Natori Y, Fujii K, Fukui M, Hasuo K, et al. Children with unilateral occlusion or stenosis of the ICA associated with surrounding Moyamoya vessels – "unilateral" Moyamoya disease. Acta Neurochir [Internet]. 1994 Sep [cited 2020 Oct 4];131(3–4):196–202. Available from: https://pubmed.ncbi.nlm.nih.gov/7754820/
32. Kawano T, Fukui M, Hashimoto N, Yonekawa Y. Follow-up study of patients with "unilateral" moyamoya disease. Neurol Med Chir. 1994;34(11):744–7.

33. Houkin K, Abe H, Yoshimoto T, Takahashi A. Is “unilateral” moyamoya disease different from moyamoya disease? J Neurosurg [Internet]. 1996 Nov;85(5):772–776. Available from: http://www.ncbi.nlm.nih.gov/pubmed/8893713
34. Seol HJ, Wang K-C, Kim S-K, Lee CS, Lee DS, Kim I-O, et al. Unilateral (probable) moyamoya disease: long-term follow-up of seven cases. Childs Nerv Syst [Internet]. 2006 Mar [cited 2010 Jul 30];22(2):145–50. Available from: http://www.ncbi.nlm.nih.gov/pubmed/16220301
35. Nagata S, Matsushima T, Morioka T, Matsukado K, Mihara F, Sasaki T, et al. Unilaterally symptomatic moyamoya disease in children: long-term follow-up of 20 patients. Neurosurgery. 2006;59(4):830–6.
36. Mugikura S, Takahashi S, Higano S, Shirane R, Sakurai Y, Yamada S. Predominant involvement of ipsilateral anterior and posterior circulations in moyamoya disease. Stroke. 2002 Jun 1 [cited 2013 Nov 18];33(6):1497–500. Available from: https://doi.org/10.1161/01.STR.0000016828.62708.21.

Part II

Genetic Aspect of Moyamoya Disease

RNF213 as a Susceptibility Gene for Moyamoya Disease has Multifunctional Roles in Biological Processes

4

Hatasu Kobayashi, Kouji H. Harada, Toshiyuki Habu, Yasuhisa Nakamura, Jiyeong Kim, and Akio Koizumi

Abstract

RNF213 has been identified as a susceptibility gene for moyamoya disease (MMD), and a rare founder variant in RNF213 p. R4810K markedly increases the risk of MMD in East Asian populations. RNF213, a huge protein, harbors two tandem AAA+ ATPase domains and a ring finger domain. Although the physiological and pathological roles of RNF213 are largely obscure, RNF213 has been reported to be involved in various biological processes, and these processes are possibly linked to susceptibilities to several stressors. In this chapter, we review the functional properties of RNF213, focusing particularly on its vari-

H. Kobayashi
Department of Environmental and Molecular Medicine, Mie University Graduate School of Medicine, Tsu, Mie, Japan
e-mail: hatasuk@doc.medic.mie-u.ac.jp

K. H. Harada · Y. Nakamura
Department of Health and Environmental Sciences, Graduate School of Medicine, Kyoto University, Kyoto, Japan
e-mail: harada.koji.3w@kyoto-u.ac.jp; nakamura.yasuhisa.28r@st.kyoto-u.ac.jp

T. Habu · J. Kim
Department of Food Sciences and Nutrition, School of Food Sciences and Nutrition, Mukogawa Women's University, Nishinomiya, Hyogo, Japan
e-mail: habu@mukogawa-u.ac.jp; mw459156@mukogawa-u.ac.jp

A. Koizumi (✉)
Department of Health and Environmental Sciences, Graduate School of Medicine, Kyoto University, Kyoto, Japan

Institute of Public Health and Welfare Research, Kyoto, Japan
e-mail: koizumi@kyoto-hokenkai.or.jp

S. Kuroda (ed.), *Moyamoya Disease: Current Knowledge and Future Perspectives*, https://doi.org/10.1007/978-981-33-6404-2_4

ants such as p.R4810K, and the RNF213-associated susceptibilities reported in some stress models. The low penetrance of RNF213 p.R4810K, however, implies that environmental factors play an essential role in MMD development in addition to genetic predisposition. We also introduce our ongoing research and intermediate results on the environmental factors involved in RNF213-mediated MMD development.

Keywords

Moyamoya disease · RNF213 · p.R4810K · Ubiquitin ligase · ATPase · Environmental factors · Infection

4.1 Introduction: RNF213 and Moyamoya Disease

The incidence of Moyamoya Disease (MMD) is much higher in East Asia (0.94/10^5 person-years in Japan [1], 1.7/10^5 in Korea [2], 0.43/10^5 in China [3]) than in other parts of the world such as the USA (0.086/10^5) [4]. Furthermore, 10%–15% of Japanese patients with MMD have a family history of this disease [5]. Such regional differences and familial occurrences strongly suggest an important role for genetic predisposition to MMD etiology in the East Asian population. Since the 1990s, the genetic factors involved in MMD have been explored, and linkage and association studies have been conducted. The "skipping generation" phenomenon, which is unique to MMD inheritance, has not allowed linkage analyses to converge into a single locus for MMD [6]. Deep insight into the inheritance of MMD revealed the existence of a "carrier status," and this observation enabled us to identify a single robust MMD locus on 17q25.3 by extensive linkage analyses using three-generation Japanese families [6]. Additionally, positional cloning of this locus [7] and whole exome sequencing [8] identified p.R4810K (c.14429 G > A, rs112735431, hereafter called R4810K), as reported independently by a genome-wide association study [9].

Our previous study of sporadic MMD cases in Japan, Korea, and China showed that RNF213 R4810K is frequently found in Japanese (90%), Korean (79%), and Chinese (23%) patients and this variant dramatically increased the risk of MMD (odds ratio = 112) [8]. Following on from these studies, genetic screening for RNF213 R4810K and other RNF213 variants was conducted in MMD patients in Asia and other regions as well. Consequently, while many non-R4810K mutations have been identified in MMD patients worldwide, RNF213 R4810K was found to be absent in Caucasian, Hispanic and African populations including in control individuals and MMD cases alike, suggesting that RNF213 R4810K is an Asian-specific variant and may contribute to the high incidence of MMD in East Asia [10, 11]. Moreover, RNF213 R4810K recently emerged as a risk factor for several vascular diseases such as ischemic stroke [12], coronary artery disease [13], and pulmonary hypertension [14].

RNF213 R4810K, however, was also observed in 1%–2% of the general East Asian population [8, 15]. This indicates that there are numerous unaffected carriers of MMD in East Asia (estimated to be 15 million), and that there is a low penetrance of RNF213 R4810K in MMD (assuming that MMD occurs in 1/300 carriers), even though RNF213 R4810K substantially increases susceptibility to this disease [15]. Therefore, it is strongly suggested that in addition to R4810K, environmental factors play a critical role in MMD development (Fig. 4.1a).

RNF213, also called mysterin, encodes an extremely large protein (591 kDa) of 5207 amino acids (NP_001243000.2), and contains two tandem AAA+ ATPase domains and a ring finger (RING) domain (Fig.4.1b) [8, 18]. Biochemical assays have revealed the enzymatic activities of these domains, indicating that RNF213 is a unique protein containing a combination of ATPase and ubiquitin ligase activities [8]. The RNF213 protein forms a putative hexameric oligomer, the stabilization and destabilization of which is considered to be regulated by the first AAA+ domain or second AAA+ domain, respectively [18]. The ubiquitin ligase (E3) family mediates protein ubiquitination and resultant target protein degradation or regulating various signaling processes [19]. However, the substrate (or substrates) of RNF213 await identification. Notably, most of the MMD-associated rare RNF213 variants such as R4810K are located in the C-terminal portion, which includes the RING domain (Fig. 4.1b) [10, 11], indicating that the functional alterations caused by mutations in this region may be linked with MMD etiology.

After RNF213 was identified as a susceptibility gene for MMD, although its physiological and pathological roles remain largely unknown, many studies have shown that it is involved in various biological processes. Therefore, we review in this chapter

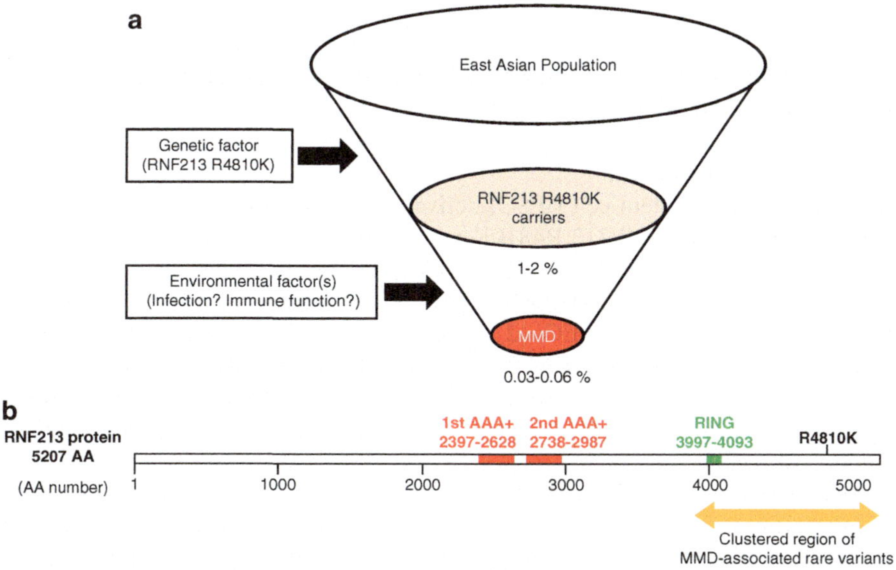

Fig. 4.1 RNF213 as a susceptibility gene for MMD. (**a**) Schematic model of the genetic and environmental factors involved in RNF213-mediated MMD in the East Asian population. MMD prevalence is described elsewhere [16, 17]. (**b**) Genomic structure and domains in RNF213. The domain structure is based on the study by Morito et al. [18]. *AA* amino acid, *AAA+* ATPase domain, *RING* ring finger domain

the functional properties of RNF213, focusing particularly on its variants (e.g., R4810K), and on the RNF213-associated susceptibilities that have been revealed by several stress models. We also introduce our ongoing research aimed at elucidating the environmental factors involved in RNF213-mediated MMD development.

4.2 Functional Properties of RNF213 and its Variants

4.2.1 Upregulation of RNF213 by Inflammatory Substances

Several studies using cultured cells have shown that RNF213 is induced by inflammatory substances [20–22]. Interferons (IFNs), antiviral cytokines, and viral mimic Poly(I:C) lead to marked upregulation of RNF213 in endothelial cells (ECs) [20–22]. However, lipopolysaccharide, a bacterial cell wall component, was found not to induce RNF213 expression in ECs, even though it elevated RNF213 levels in fibroblasts [20, 22]. These findings suggest that viral infections, but not bacterial ones, can result in RNF213 upregulation in ECs. Notably, IFNs have antiangiogenic activities [23] and RNF213 is associated with such activities. An RNF213 knockdown rescued the reduced angiogenesis induced by IFN-β in cultured ECs [21], indicating that RNF213 is a possible mediator of the antiangiogenic effects of IFNs. From these results, it is speculated that inflammation (especially that caused by viral infections) might be a candidate environmental factor associated with MMD.

4.2.2 Inhibitory Effects of RNF213 Variants on EC Functions and Cell Division

4.2.2.1 EC Dysfunction

Induced pluripotent stem cell (iPSC)-derived vascular ECs (iPSECs) from MMD patients carrying the RNF213 R4810K variant display reduced angiogenesis in an in vitro assay [24]. RNF213 R4810K overexpression, but not wild-type RNF213 overexpression or suppression of RNF213 by RNAi, inhibited angiogenesis and cell migration in human cultured ECs [21, 24]. Similar EC dysfunctions were observed in ECs overexpressing other RNF213 mutants (D4013N, R4019C, and V4146A) found in Caucasian MMD patients [25]. Furthermore, in mouse models, EC-specific overexpression of the Rnf213 mutant also inhibited hypoxia-induced cerebral angiogenesis [21].

Gene expression analysis of iPSECs shows that securin (otherwise called PTTG1; Pituitary Tumor Transforming Gene 1), a protein involved in angiogenesis in in vitro models and new vessel formation in in vivo models [26–28], is downregulated in MMD patients [24]. Securin levels have been found to decrease in ECs overexpressing RNF213 R4810K, but not in ECs overexpressing wild-type RNF213 [24]. Securin knockdown also led to angiogenesis inhibition in ECs, a situation similar to that invoked by RNF213 R4810K [24]. These results raise the possibility that securin plays a role in the EC dysfunction induced by RNF213 variants.

Smooth muscle cells (SMCs) are also involved in angiogenesis. iPSC-derived vascular SMCs derived from patients with MMD were tested for their angiogenic function [29]. Extensive studies on iPS SMCs derived from patients failed to reveal differences in their transcriptome profiles or cellular functions including proliferation, migration, and contractile ability. By contrast, significant differences in the transcriptome of iPS ECs derived from patients with MMD were observed.

Collectively, these studies suggest that patient-derived iPS ECs and SMCs could provide a novel tool for investigating the pathological processes in vivo. At present, these data also indicate that ECs may play a more pivotal role in MMD than SMCs.

4.2.2.2 Abnormal Mitosis

Apart from the inhibition of angiogenic activity in ECs, the observation of securin downregulation suggests that RNF213 R4810K is possibly linked with cell division and chromosome segregation abnormalities, prompting the hypothesis that RNF213 R4810K impairs mitosis, thereby resulting in mitotic failure during proliferation in MMD patients.

To elucidate the mechanism underlying mitotic failure, we investigated the possibility that RNF213 R4810K alters the reorganization process of cytoskeletal elements during cell division. Embryonic fibroblast cells from Rnf213 R4757K (corresponding to human R4810K) knock-in mice show abnormal mitotic spindle orientation and mitotic delay in anaphase (Fig. 4.2a). Overexpression of the R4810K variant led to fewer actin filaments in U2OS cells compared with those overexpressing wild type RNF213 protein (Fig. 4.2b).

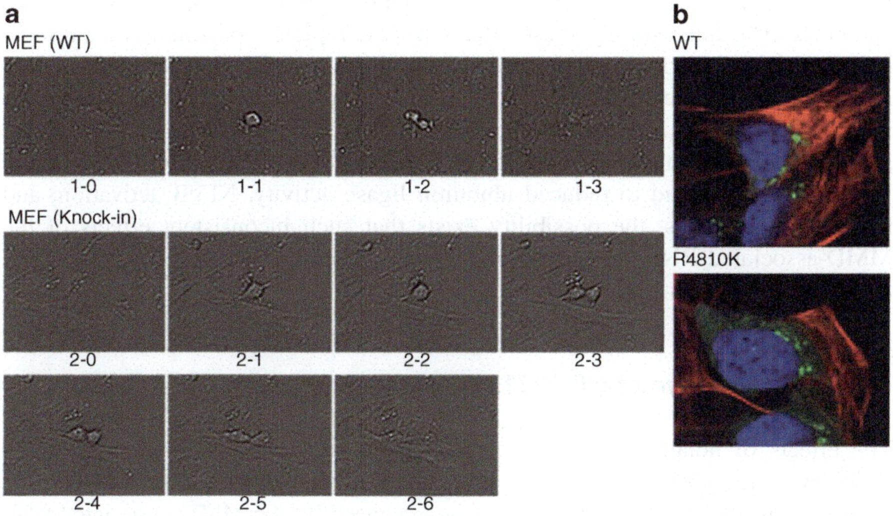

Fig. 4.2 Influence of the R4810K variant in the cell. (**a**) Live images of WT and knock-in mouse embryonic fibroblast (MEF) cells. Images were obtained every 15 min. (**b**) F-actin staining of cells overexpressing RNF213. U2OS cells expressing the wild type or variant RNF213. Actin (Red), RNF213 (Green), DNA (Blue)

4.2.3 Stabilizing Effect of RNF213 on Cytoplasmic Lipid Droplets

High-resolution microscopic imaging has revealed that RNF213 is located on the surface of cytoplasmic Lipid Droplets (LDs), the ubiquitous organelles that store neutral lipids and act as a source of metabolic energy and fat substances [30]. Overexpression and knockdown/knockout studies have shown that RNF213 stabilization of LDs occurs mainly by the elimination of adipose triglyceride lipase from LDs [30]. Loss-of-function mutations in the AAA+ domains and deletion of the RING domain both equally impaired this LD targeting, and led to different abnormal RNF213 distribution; diffusion throughout the cytosol and amorphous aggregate-like pattern formation, respectively [30]. Several MMD-related RNF213 variants in the RING domain (C3997Y, H4014N, C4017S, and C4032R) have also been reported to cause impaired LD targeting, while D4013N, another RING domain variant, and R4810K did not [30]. These results raise the possibility that fat metabolism may be potentially linked with MMD etiology.

4.2.4 NFκB Activation and Apoptosis by RNF213 Variants

Recently, in vitro ubiquitination analysis using the RNF213 RING domain showed that RNF213 generated K63-linked polyubiquitin chains through cooperation with Ubc13/Uev1A, a ubiquitin-conjugating enzyme [31]. Most of the MMD-associated variants in the RING domain of RNF213 (C3997Y, P4007Y, H4014N, C4017S, C4032R, and P4033L) reduce its ubiquitin ligase activity [31]. In cellular experiments using full-length RNF213, these variants enhanced NFκB activation and apoptosis [31]. Interestingly, these effects were completely prevented by a critical point mutation and deletion of the RNF213 AAA+ domain, indicating that these RING variants-induced NFκB activation and apoptosis were dependent on the AAA+ domain [31]. Nevertheless, in common with LD stabilization (Sect. 4.2.4.), some RING domain variants found in MMD patients (D4013N, R4019C, and W4024R) do not lead to reduced ubiquitin ligase activity, NFκB activation, and apoptosis [31]. Thus, the possibility exists that such inconsistent effects of the MMD-associated RNF213 variants may be related to the degree of genetic penetrance of the variants.

4.2.5 Roles Played by RNF213 Domains and Variants

The effects of ablating the domains and the MMD-associated rare variants in RNF213 on the above-described functions are summarized in Table 4.1. The EC dysfunctions and mitotic abnormalities were caused by the MMD-associated variants including R4810K, but not RNF213 knockdown [24, 32], suggesting that these deleterious effects are exerted through a gain-of-function mechanism. However, RNF213 knockdown, ablation of the AAA+ and RING domain activities, and the

Table 4.1 Effect of RNF213 knockdown, ablation of AAA+, and RING domain activities and rare MMD-associated variants on RNF213 functions

Genetic variant or modification		Function: EC function [21, 24, 25]	Mitosis [32]	LD targeting and stabilization [30]	NFκB activation and apoptosis [31]
RNF213 knockdown		*No effect*	*No effect*	**Impaired**	n.d.
AAA+ domain	Loss-of-function mutations and/ or ΔAAA	*No effect*	n.d.	**Impaired**	**Impaired***
RING domain	ΔRING	n.d.	n.d.	**Impaired#** **(incomplete)**	n.d.
	C3997Y	n.d.	n.d.	**Impaired#** **(incomplete)**	**Induced**
	P4007Y	n.d.	n.d.	n.d.	**Induced**
	D4013N	**Impaired**	n.d.	*No effect*	*No effect*
	H4014N	n.d.	n.d.	**Impaired#** **(incomplete)**	**Induced**
	C4017S	n.d.	n.d.	**Impaired#** **(incomplete)**	**Induced**
	R4019C	**Impaired**	n.d.	n.d.	*No effect*
	W4024R	n.d.	n.d.	n.d.	*No effect*
	C4032R	n.d.	n.d.	**Impaired#** **(incomplete)**	**Induced**
	P4033L	n.d.	n.d.	n.d.	**Induced**
V4146A		**Impaired**	n.d.	n.d.	n.d.
R4810K		**Impaired**	**Impaired**	*No effect*	n.d.

EC endothelial cells, *LD* lipid droplet; *n.d.* not determined. *Impaired NFκB activation and apoptosis induced by the variants indicated in the RING domain. #LD targeting and stabilization were lost in most cells (~80%), but they remained intact in a small portion of them (~20%)

presence of some MMD-associated variants led to impaired LD targeting and stabilization [30]. Furthermore, the degree of these suppressive effects varies; RNF213 knockdown and nulling of the AAA+ domain completely abolished LD targeting and stabilization, deletion, and some variants in the RING domain induce incomplete inhibition, but other definitive MMD-associated variants (D4013N and R4810K) have no effect [30]. In the case of NFκB activation and apoptosis, a similar variety of inducing effects of the RNF213 variants in the RING domain was reported [31]. Interestingly, AAA+ domain deletion or mutations greatly suppressed such NFκB activation and apoptosis induction, suggesting that these NFκB- and apoptosis-inducing activities of the RNF213 variants are dependent on the RNF213 AAA+ domain [31]. These variable roles of the RNF213 domains and variants suggest that RNF213 is a multifunctional protein involved in several biological processes, possibly through different mechanisms. To elucidate the role of RNF213 in MMD pathology, future studies will be required to uncover the mode of action by which MMD-associated RNF213 variants affect gene functions and lead to MMD development.

4.3 Susceptibilities Related to RNF213

4.3.1 Hypoxia and Hypoperfusion

Several studies using genetically modified mice have suggested that RNF213 is linked with susceptibilities to hypoxia and hypoperfusion. After exposure to hypoxia, Rnf213 R4757K (corresponding to human R4810K) EC-specific transgenic (EC-Tg) mice display inhibited compensatory cerebral angiogenesis, whereas Rnf213 knockout (KO) and Rnf213 wild-type EC-Tg mice did not [21]. The RNF213 R4757K variant also had an effect on hypoxia-induced extracranial vasculopathy. In a hypoxia-induced mouse model of pulmonary hypertension, overexpression of the Rnf213 R4757K variant in ECs aggravated their physiological and histopathological phenotypes [14]. These vascular abnormalities under hypoxia may be associated with the above-mentioned EC dysfunction caused by R4810K (Sect. 4.2.2). Furthermore, Banh et al. reported that RNF213 coordinates protein tyrosine phosphatase-1B (PTP1B) and hypoxia-inducible factor-1 (HIF1), and plays a role in the cellular response to hypoxia by controlling non-mitochondrial oxygen consumption in cancer cells [33]. PTP1B and HIF1 signaling could also be a pathway through which the RNF213 R4810K variant affected vascular function under hypoxia.

In contrast to hypoxia, both the RNF213 KO and the RNF213 R4757K variants are able to increase hypoperfusion susceptibility. In chronic cerebral hypoperfusion mouse models based on bilateral common carotid artery stenosis, Rnf213 KO mice, but not Rnf213 R4757K EC-Tg ones, show a markedly worsened decrease in cerebral blood flow (CBF) during the early phase, while CBF restoration was impaired in both KO and EC-Tg mice during the late phase [34]. During the early phase of cerebral hypoperfusion, arteriogenesis which is expansion and remodeling of preexisting arterioles play a critical role in the maintenance of CBF [35]. Therefore, suppressing RNF213 potentially leads to lowered arteriogenesis under cerebral hypoperfusion, a notion supported by the finding that the vascular remodeling induced by artery ligation is prevented in Rnf213 KO mice [36].

The above evidence supports the notion that RFN213 likely affects susceptibility to hypoxia and hypoperfusion, as is observed in steno-occlusive diseases including MMD via angiogenesis and arteriogenesis. Further animal and molecular studies are needed to elucidate the mechanisms by which RNF213 affects the vascular system under hypoxia and hypoperfusion stress.

4.3.2 Endoplasmic Reticulum Stress in Diabetes

RNF213 ablation has been reported to improve diabetes in Akita mice [37]. Akita mice are a well-known mouse model of Endoplasmic Reticulum (ER) stress-associated diabetes in which misfolding of mutant insulin results in ER stress and pancreatic β cell death [38, 39]. Male Rnf213 KO/Akita mice, which are generated by interbreeding Rnf213 KO with Akita mice, have lowered blood glucose levels and improved glucose tolerance in comparison with male Akita mice [37]. Notably, improved pancreatic β cell damage in Rnf213 KO/Akita mice was revealed by electron microscopy and immunohistochemistry for insulin and for CHOP, a marker of ER stress-associated apoptosis [37]. These results raise the possibility that RNF213 influences the susceptibility of pancreatic β cells to ER stress by regulating insulin misfolding and/or the ER stress response in Akita mice.

4.3.3 Lipotoxicity

Recently, a genome-wide short hairpin screen identified RNF213 as a lipid metabolism modulating gene [40]. RNF213 knockdown almost completely normalized the cellular lipidome alterations caused by palmitate, a saturated fatty acid, and reduced palmitate-induced cellular toxicity by preventing the accumulation of di-saturated glycerophospholipids [40]. This protection against lipotoxicity is possibly associated with RNF213 function stabilizing LDs (Sect. 4.2.3.). Moreover, RNF213 was able to block ER stress and NF-kB pathway activation downstream of lipotoxic stress [40], which might be linked with the above-mentioned involvement of RNF213 in ER stress in Akita mice (Sect. 4.3.2) and in variant-mediated NFκB activation and apoptosis (Sect. 4.2.4).

4.4 Relationship with Infection and Immune Function in MMD

As already mentioned, approximately 1/300 carriers of the RNF213 p.R4810K variant develop MMD. It is therefore thought that certain environmental factors are likely to trigger its onset. Although the environmental factors relevant to MMD have not been specified, the age of onset is often 5–10 years, and the relatives of those with MMD who carry R4810K are much more likely to develop MMD. Hence, the potential factors affecting shared traits within the family members are worth investigating.

Until the 1980s, the prevailing hypothesis was that MMD was an acquired disease caused by prior infection. Currently, the development of moyamoya blood vessels caused by infections or autoimmunity (among other possibilities) is regarded as moyamoya syndrome. However, since the discovery of the RNF213 mutation, immunity, infection, and genetic interactions cannot be overlooked in the pathological process, and therefore merit further attention.

In case reports and case-controlled studies, various bacterial and viral infections have been proposed to cause moyamoya syndrome. They include Leptospira, *Neisseria pneumococcus*, *Propionibacterium acnes*, *Streptococcus pneumoniae*, beta-hemolytic group A *Streptococcus*, *Mycobacterium tuberculosis*, *Haemophilus influenzae*, *Mycoplasma pneumoniae*, varicella-zoster virus (VZV), measles virus (MeV), human immunodeficiency virus, cytomegalovirus (CMV), and Epstein-Barr virus (reviewed in [41, 42]). However, few confirmatory and systematic studies of infectious diseases and MMD have been published.

Previous studies exploring the relationships involved in immune function disorders, such as autoimmune diseases and human leukocyte antigen (HLA) abnormalities, have shown that antiphospholipid antibody syndrome, systemic lupus erythematosus, Graves' disease, and HLA class I/II allogeneic abnormalities are accompanied by moyamoya syndrome (Reviewed in [41]). Expression of the RNF213 gene, which has been reported to be induced by interferon, causes endothelial damage, suggesting a relationship between it and bacterial and viral infections. Moyamoya syndrome has been sometimes associated with Kawasaki disease, which is considered a systemic vasculitis associated with infection. Recent metagenomic analysis of patients with Kawasaki disease prominently detected the *Streptococcus* genus in their intestines during the acute phase of the disease, and an increase in the *Ruminococcus* genus in the remote period after recovery [43]. Although this example highlights an association between intestinal bacteria and vasculitis, no studies have reported an association between intestinal bacteria and MMD. However, the pattern of onset and familial segregation may be related to shared microflora in affected families.

Thus, we are conducting several research projects on the above hypotheses. Various viral antibody titers (past infection history) in MMD with RNF213 p.R4810K are compared with RNF213p.R4810K carrying controls (sporadic cases, $n = 66$; family cases, $n = 45$; and age and sex 1: 1 matched controls). This design is an important combination for eliminating the effects of different backgrounds from the presence or absence of the RNF213 R4810K mutation. The intermediate results of these experiments are shown in Table 4.2. VZV and MeV were positive in all the samples, making their comparison difficult. Rubella virus positivity was slightly higher in the patient group, and CMV was slightly higher in the controls in both sporadic and family cases. However, no significant differences were found. It is unlikely that such a common viral infection would make a difference, and we are searching for other viral antibody titers that may be associated with angiopathy.

Further evaluation of the intestinal microflora of patients with MMD is also ongoing in our laboratory. Preoperative fecal samples from MMD patients have been obtained, and the composition and diversity of the bacteria are undergoing evaluation by sequencing the 16S rRNA V3/V4 region of these microbes by next-generation sequencing (NGS) with comparisons performed on an age- and sex-matched control group.

As mentioned above, after the discovery of the RNF213 MMD susceptibility gene, the momentum for exploring its relationship with infection and immunity continues to increase. The advent of NGS has great potential for elucidating the involvement of intestinal flora in relation to MMD in the future.

Table 4.2 Seroprevalence of selected viral antibodies in MMD patients and age- and sex-matched controls

			VZV		MeV		RuV		CMV	
		n	(+)	(−)	(+)	(−)	(+)	(−)	(+)	(−)
Sporadic	Case	66	66	0	66	0	64	2	57	9
	Control	66	66	0	66	0	60	6	62	4
Familial	Case	45	45	0	45	0	42	3	39	6
	Control	45	45	0	45	0	39	6	42	3

VZV varicella-zoster virus, *MeV* measles virus, *RuV* rubella virus, *CMV* cytomegalovirus. (+): positive; (−): negative

4.5 Conclusions and Perspectives

RNF213 is one of the major genetic risk factors for MMD, especially in East Asian countries. Many rare RNF213 variants such as R4810K have been found in MMD patients worldwide. Attempts to elucidate MMD etiology have identified the roles played by these MMD-associated variants in RNF213 gene functions and associated biological processes. However, the diverse effects of the variants on distinct phenotypes (Table 4.1) make it difficult to understand how the variants cause MMD. Recently, Ahel et al. proposed that RNF213 contains a dynein-like core with six ATPase units and a multidomain E3 module comprising an E3-back, E3-RING, E3-shell, and E3-core, based on their cryo-electron microscopic analysis using mouse Rnf213 [44]; thereby providing a molecular framework to help further investigations on the role of the MMD-associated RNF213 variants in disease etiology. Their study provides a novel functional aspect for RNF213 whereby RNF213 stays as a monomer for functionality and contains an E3 ligase activity in an undefined C-terminal region. This contradicts the current concept that the primary structure of the RNF213 protein's sequence predicts that it functions as a hexamer forming AAA+ walker protein with E3 ligase activity. At present, however, it remains unknown how to evaluate their study. To obtain a clear understanding on the basis of unification of various hypothesis, we should evaluate roles of RNF213 mutations in the pathological process through robust phenotypes induced by RF213 mutations, suggesting importance of the development of in vivo animal models or cells derived from animal models rather than in vitro cellular model using gene transfection. More efforts are needed in this direction.

Finally, to clarify the role of RNF213 in MMD etiology, it will be essential to identify the environmental factors and elucidate the mechanisms in which these factors interact with RNF213 in the development of MMD. Infections and inflammatory states have been suggested as the candidates for environmental factors that trigger MMD onset. Both future epidemiological and experimental (especially animal experiments using RNF213 genetically modified models) studies will be needed to obtain clarity.

Acknowledgment This study is supported by the grant, Shin-Gakujyutu funded by the Ministry of Education, Culture, Sports, Science and Technology of Japan (17H06397).

References

1. Baba T, Houkin K, Kuroda S. Novel epidemiological features of moyamoya disease. J Neurol Neurosurg Psychiatry. 2008;79(8):900–4. https://doi.org/10.1136/jnnp.2007.130666.
2. Ahn IM, Park DH, Hann HJ, Kim KH, Kim HJ, Ahn HS. Incidence, prevalence, and survival of moyamoya disease in Korea: a nationwide, population-based study. Stroke. 2014;45(4):1090–5. https://doi.org/10.1161/strokeaha.113.004273.
3. Miao W, Zhao PL, Zhang YS, Liu HY, Chang Y, Ma J, et al. Epidemiological and clinical features of Moyamoya disease in Nanjing, China. Clin Neurol Neurosurg. 2010;112(3):199–203. https://doi.org/10.1016/j.clineuro.2009.11.009.

4. Uchino K, Johnston SC, Becker KJ, Tirschwell DL. Moyamoya disease in Washington state and California. Neurology. 2005;65(6):956–8. https://doi.org/10.1212/01.wnl.0000176066.33797.82.
5. Tominaga T, Suzuki N, Miyamoto S, Koizumi A, Kuroda S, Takahashi J. Recommendations for the management of moyamoya disease: a statement from research committee on spontaneous occlusion of the circle of Willis (moyamoya disease) [2nd edition]. Surg Cereb Stroke. 2018;46(1):1–24.
6. Mineharu Y, Liu W, Inoue K, Matsuura N, Inoue S, Takenaka K, et al. Autosomal dominant moyamoya disease maps to chromosome 17q253. Neurology. 2008;70(24 Pt 2):2357–63.
7. Koizumi A. Genetic analysis of familial moyamoya. In: Hashimoro N, editor. Annual report of the research committee on spontaneous occlusion of the circle of Willis (Moyamoya disease) by science research Grants of Ministry of Health. Japan: Labor and Welfare; 2010.
8. Liu W, Morito D, Takashima S, Mineharu Y, Kobayashi H, Hitomi T, et al. Identification of RNF213 as a susceptibility gene for moyamoya disease and its possible role in vascular development. PLoS One. 2011;6(7):e22542. https://doi.org/10.1371/journal.pone.0022542PONE-D-10-04031.
9. Kamada F, Aoki Y, Narisawa A, Abe Y, Komatsuzaki S, Kikuchi A, et al. A genome-wide association study identifies RNF213 as the first Moyamoya disease gene. J Hum Genet. 2011;56(1):34–40.
10. Liao X, Deng J, Dai W, Zhang T, Yan J. Rare variants of RNF213 and moyamoya/non-moyamoya intracranial artery stenosis/occlusion disease risk: a meta-analysis and systematic review. Environ Health Prev Med. 2017;22(1):75. https://doi.org/10.1186/s12199-017-0680-1.
11. Koizumi A, Kobayashi H, Hitomi T, Harada KH, Habu T, Youssefian S. A new horizon of moyamoya disease and associated health risks explored through RNF213. Environ Health Prev Med. 2016;21(2):55–70. https://doi.org/10.1007/s12199-015-0498-7.
12. Okazaki S, Morimoto T, Kamatani Y, Kamimura T, Kobayashi H, Harada K, et al. Moyamoya disease susceptibility variant RNF213 p.R4810K increases the risk of ischemic stroke attributable to large-artery atherosclerosis. Circulation. 2019;139(2):295–8. https://doi.org/10.1161/CIRCULATIONAHA.118.038439.
13. Morimoto T, Mineharu Y, Ono K, Nakatochi M, Ichihara S, Kabata R, et al. Significant association of RNF213 p.R4810K, a moyamoya susceptibility variant, with coronary artery disease. PLoS One. 2017;12(4):e0175649. https://doi.org/10.1371/journal.pone.0175649.
14. Kobayashi H, Kabata R, Kinoshita H, Morimoto T, Ono K, Takeda M, et al. Rare variants in RNF213, a susceptibility gene for moyamoya disease, are found in patients with pulmonary hypertension and aggravate hypoxia-induced pulmonary hypertension in mice. Pulm Circ. 2018;8(3):2045894018778155. https://doi.org/10.1177/2045894018778155.
15. Liu W, Hitomi T, Kobayashi H, Harada KH, Koizumi A. Distribution of moyamoya disease susceptibility polymorphism p.R4810K in RNF213 in east and southeast Asian populations. Neurol Med Chir. 2012;52(5):299–303. DN/JST.JSTAGE/nmc/52.299 [pii]
16. Kuriyama S, Kusaka Y, Fujimura M, Wakai K, Tamakoshi A, Hashimoto S, et al. Prevalence and clinicoepidemiological features of moyamoya disease in Japan: findings from a nationwide epidemiological survey. Stroke. 2008;39(1):42–7. https://doi.org/10.1161/strokeaha.107.490714.
17. Wakai K, Tamakoshi A, Ikezaki K, Fukui M, Kawamura T, Aoki R, et al. Epidemiological features of moyamoya disease in Japan: findings from a nationwide survey. Clin Neurol Neurosurg. 1997;99(Suppl 2):S1–5. https://doi.org/10.1016/s0303-8467(97)00031-0.
18. Morito D, Nishikawa K, Hoseki J, Kitamura A, Kotani Y, Kiso K, et al. Moyamoya disease-associated protein mysterin/RNF213 is a novel AAA+ ATPase, which dynamically changes its oligomeric state. Sci Rep. 2014;4:4442. https://doi.org/10.1038/srep04442.
19. Metzger MB, Pruneda JN, Klevit RE, Weissman AM. RING-type E3 ligases: master manipulators of E2 ubiquitin-conjugating enzymes and ubiquitination. Biochimica et Biophysica Acta (BBA)-molecular. Cell Res. 2014;1843(1):47–60.
20. Ohkubo K, Sakai Y, Inoue H, Akamine S, Ishizaki Y, Matsushita Y, et al. Moyamoya disease susceptibility gene RNF213 links inflammatory and angiogenic signals in endothelial cells. Sci Rep. 2015;5:13191. https://doi.org/10.1038/srep13191.

21. Kobayashi H, Matsuda Y, Hitomi T, Okuda H, Shioi H, Matsuda T, et al. Biochemical and functional characterization of RNF213 (Mysterin) R4810K, a susceptibility mutation of Moyamoya disease, in angiogenesis in vitro and in vivo. J Am Heart Assoc. 2015;4(7) https://doi.org/10.1161/JAHA.115.002146.
22. Key J, Maletzko A, Kohli A, Gispert S, Torres-Odio S, Wittig I, et al. Loss of mitochondrial ClpP, Lonp1, and Tfam triggers transcriptional induction of Rnf213, a susceptibility factor for moyamoya disease. Neurogenetics. 2020; https://doi.org/10.1007/s10048-020-00609-2.
23. Lindner DJ. Interferons as antiangiogenic agents. Curr Oncol Rep. 2002;4(6):510–4. https://doi.org/10.1007/s11912-002-0065-4.
24. Hitomi T, Habu T, Kobayashi H, Okuda H, Harada KH, Osafune K, et al. Downregulation of Securin by the variant RNF213 R4810K (rs112735431, G>A) reduces angiogenic activity of induced pluripotent stem cell-derived vascular endothelial cells from moyamoya patients. Biochem Biophys Res Commun. 2013;438(1):13–9. https://doi.org/10.1016/j.bbrc.2013.07.00 4S0006-291X(13)01144-3.
25. Kobayashi H, Brozman M, Kyselova K, Viszlayova D, Morimoto T, Roubec M, et al. RNF213 rare variants in Slovakian and Czech Moyamoya disease patients. PLoS One. 2016;11(10):e0164759. https://doi.org/10.1371/journal.pone.0164759.
26. Zhou C, Tong Y, Wawrowsky K, Melmed S. PTTG acts as a STAT3 target gene for colorectal cancer cell growth and motility. Oncogene. 2014;33(7):851–61. https://doi.org/10.1038/onc.2013.16.
27. Malik MT, Kakar SS. Regulation of angiogenesis and invasion by human pituitary tumor transforming gene (PTTG) through increased expression and secretion of matrix metalloproteinase-2 (MMP-2). Mol Cancer. 2006;5:61. https://doi.org/10.1186/1476-4598-5-61.
28. Ishikawa H, Heaney AP, Yu R, Horwitz GA, Melmed S. Human pituitary tumor-transforming gene induces angiogenesis. J Clin Endocrinol Metab. 2001;86(2):867–74. https://doi.org/10.1210/jcem.86.2.7184.
29. Tokairin K, Hamauchi S, Ito M, Kazumata K, Sugiyama T, Nakayama N, et al. Vascular smooth muscle cell Derived from IPS cell of Moyamoya disease - comparative characterization with endothelial cell Transcriptome. J Stroke Cerebrovasc Dis. 2020;29(12) https://doi.org/10.1016/j.jstrokecerebrovasdis.2020.105305.
30. Sugihara M, Morito D, Ainuki S, Hirano Y, Ogino K, Kitamura A, et al. The AAA+ ATPase/ubiquitin ligase mysterin stabilizes cytoplasmic lipid droplets. J Cell Biol. 2019;218(3):949–60. https://doi.org/10.1083/jcb.201712120.
31. Takeda M, Tezuka T, Kim M, Choi J, Oichi Y, Kobayashi H, et al. Moyamoya disease patient mutations in the RING domain of RNF213 reduce its ubiquitin ligase activity and enhance NFkappaB activation and apoptosis in an AAA+ domain-dependent manner. Biochem Biophys Res Commun. 2020; https://doi.org/10.1016/j.bbrc.2020.02.024.
32. Hitomi T, Habu T, Kobayashi H, Okuda H, Harada KH, Osafune K, et al. The moyamoya disease susceptibility variant RNF213 R4810K (rs112735431) induces genomic instability by mitotic abnormality. Biochem Biophys Res Commun. 2013;439(4):419–26. https://doi.org/10.1016/j.bbrc.2013.08.067S0006-291X(13)01414-9.
33. Banh RS, Iorio C, Marcotte R, Xu Y, Cojocari D, Rahman AA, et al. PTP1B controls non-mitochondrial oxygen consumption by regulating RNF213 to promote tumour survival during hypoxia. Nat Cell Biol. 2016;18(7):803–13. https://doi.org/10.1038/ncb3376.
34. Morimoto T, Enmi JI, Hattori Y, Iguchi S, Saito S, Harada KH, et al. Dysregulation of RNF213 promotes cerebral hypoperfusion. Sci Rep. 2018;8(1):3607. https://doi.org/10.1038/s41598-018-22064-8.
35. Lin C-Y, Chang C, Cheung W-M, Lin M-H, Chen J-J, Hsu CY, et al. Dynamic changes in vascular permeability, cerebral blood volume, vascular density, and size after transient focal cerebral ischemia in rats: evaluation with contrast-enhanced magnetic resonance imaging. J Cereb Blood Flow Metab. 2008;28(8):1491–501.
36. Sonobe S, Fujimura M, Niizuma K, Nishijima Y, Ito A, Shimizu H, et al. Temporal profile of the vascular anatomy evaluated by 9.4-T magnetic resonance angiography and histopathologi-

cal analysis in mice lacking RNF213: a susceptibility gene for moyamoya disease. Brain Res. 2014;1552:64–71. https://doi.org/10.1016/j.brainres.2014.01.011.
37. Kobayashi H, Yamazaki S, Takashima S, Liu W, Okuda H, Yan J, et al. Ablation of Rnf213 retards progression of diabetes in the Akita mouse. Biochem Biophys Res Commun. 2013;432(3):519–25. https://doi.org/10.1016/j.bbrc.2013.02.015S0006-291X(13)00238-6.
38. Wang J, Takeuchi T, Tanaka S, Kubo SK, Kayo T, Lu D, et al. A mutation in the insulin 2 gene induces diabetes with severe pancreatic beta-cell dysfunction in the Mody mouse. J Clin Invest. 1999;103(1):27–37. https://doi.org/10.1172/JCI4431.
39. Oyadomari S, Koizumi A, Takeda K, Gotoh T, Akira S, Araki E, et al. Targeted disruption of the Chop gene delays endoplasmic reticulum stress–mediated diabetes. J Clin Investig. 2002;109(4):525–32. https://doi.org/10.1172/jci0214550.
40. Piccolis M, Bond LM, Kampmann M, Pulimeno P, Chitraju C, Jayson CBK, et al. Probing the global cellular responses to lipotoxicity caused by saturated fatty acids. Mol Cell. 2019;74(1):32–44 e8. https://doi.org/10.1016/j.molcel.2019.01.036.
41. Houkin K, Ito M, Sugiyama T, Shichinohe H, Nakayama N, Kazumata K, et al. Review of past research and current concepts on the etiology of moyamoya disease. Neurol Med Chir. 2012;52(5):267–77.
42. Mikami T, Suzuki H, Komatsu K, Mikuni N. Influence of inflammatory disease on the pathophysiology of Moyamoya disease and quasi-moyamoya disease. Neurol Med Chir. 2019; https://doi.org/10.2176/nmc.ra.2019-0059.
43. Kinumaki A, Sekizuka T, Hamada H, Kato K, Yamashita A, Kuroda M. Characterization of the gut microbiota of Kawasaki disease patients by metagenomic analysis. Front Microbiol. 2015;6:824. https://doi.org/10.3389/fmicb.2015.00824.
44. Ahel J, Lehner A, Vogel A, Schleiffer A, Meinhart A, Haselbach D, et al. Moyamoya disease factor RNF213 is a giant E3 ligase with a dynein-like core and a distinct ubiquitin-transfer mechanism. elife. 2020;9 https://doi.org/10.7554/eLife.56185.

RNF213 and Clinical Feature

5

Shunsuke Nomura, Hiroyuki Akagawa, Koji Yamaguchi,
Akitsugu Kawashima, and Takakazu Kawamata

Abstract

RNF213 was identified as the susceptibility gene for moyamoya disease. Further, several studies have clarified genotype–phenotype correlation of *RNF213* in patients with moyamoya disease. Although the frequency or the influence of the genotype differed in each ethnic, but especially Asian founder p.R4810K homozygous variant of *RNF213* was associated with severe clinical manifestation at the disease onset or younger age at disease onset in Japanese and Korean patients with moyamoya disease. Also, the other rare variant of *RNF213* may influence severe phenotype. Moreover, it has been recently clarified that the other diseases such as intracranial artery stenosis, moyamoya syndrome, extracranial artery stenosis, or cerebral aneurysm were potentially influenced by *RNF213*.

Keywords

Genotype · Genotype–phenotype correlation · Moyamoya disease · Phenotype *RNF213* · Variant

---

S. Nomura (✉) · A. Kawashima
Department of Neurosurgery, Tokyo Women's Medical University Yachiyo Medical Center, Chiba, Japan
e-mail: shunsukesn20@gmail.com; kawashima18surg@yahoo.co.jp

H. Akagawa
Institute for Integrated Medical Sciences (TIIMS), Tokyo Women's Medical University, Tokyo, Japan
e-mail: akagawa.hiroyuki@twmu.ac.jp

K. Yamaguchi · T. Kawamata
Department of Neurosurgery, Tokyo Women's Medical University, Tokyo, Japan
e-mail: yamaguchi.koji@twmu.ac.jp; tkawamata@twmu.ac.jp

S. Kuroda (ed.), *Moyamoya Disease: Current Knowledge and Future Perspectives*, https://doi.org/10.1007/978-981-33-6404-2_5

5.1 Introduction

In 2011, *RNF213* was identified as the susceptibility gene for Moyamoya disease (MMD) [1, 2]. In particular, in East Asia, the most frequent variant is *RNF213* p.R4810K variant, which was thought to be the Asian founder variant in MMD. Also, other variants have been detected both in East Asia and other countries. There is a difference in the distribution of those variants of *RNF213* and the clinical phenotype between the countries.

In the last ten years, several studies have clarified genotype–phenotype correlation of *RNF213* in patients with MMD and the other diseases associated with *RNF213*. Here, we summarized the clinical phenotype of *RNF213* variant in MMD, the difference of the phenotype between the countries, and other *RNF213*-associated diseases. Through this manuscript, we describe genetic information using NM_001256071.1 as the reference transcriptional sequence of *RNF213* in the GRCh37 (hg19) assembly; *RNF213* founder variant was described p.R4810K.

5.2 *RNF213* p.R4810K Genotype–Phenotype Correlation in Moyamoya Disease in East Asia

Several studies reported genotype–phenotype correlation in East Asia. Although *RNF213* p.R4810K was identified as an Asian founder variant, there are differences in the distribution or the clinical manifestation with the clinical manifestation between Japan and Korea, and China. Therefore, we describe this genotype–phenotype correlation in each country (Table 5.1).

5.2.1 Japan and Korea

In Japan and Korea, the distribution of the p.R4810K founder variant and clinical feature in each genotype was similar. By the past studies with relatively large participants, [2–5] the frequency of this variant was reported to be 73.4–90%, and the homozygous variant was reported to be 5.3–7.9%. Furthermore, the other rare variants were detected.

In Japan and Korea, the homozygosity of the p.R4810K founder variant was associated with a severe phenotype, especially with cerebral infarction and early age at the disease onset. There are several important studies showing the genotype–phenotype correlation at the disease onset. Kim EH et al. reported that the homozygous p.R4810K variant was associated with younger age at the disease onset, cerebral infarction at the disease onset, and cognitive impairment [4]. Miyatake et al. reported that the homozygous p.R4810K variant was associated with younger age at the disease onset, cerebral infarction at the disease onset, and involvement of posterior cerebral artery [3]. Our past study also confirmed that p.R4810K homozygous variant was associated with clinical phenotype at the disease onset [5, 11].

Table 5.1 Summary of genotype–phenotype correlation of *RNF213* p.R4810K

	Nation	Patient	Age Mean ± SD or median (range or IQR)	*RNF213* p.R4810K			Major significantly associated factor (associated p.R4810K genotype)
				Homozygote	Heterozygote	Wild type	
Miyatake S. 2012 [3]	Japan	204	Under15: 72.6% (range 0–58)	15 (7.4%)	153 (75.0%)	36 (17.6%)	Younger age at the onset, cerebral infarction at the onset, and PCA involvement (homozygote)
Kim EH. 2016 [4]	Korea	165	21.3 (range 2.4–70.5)	13 (7.9%)	112 (67.9%)	40 (24.2%)	Younger age at the disease onset, cerebral infarction at the onset and cognitive impairment (homozygote)
Nomura S. 2019 [5]	Japan	94	27 (range 1–64)	5 (5.3%)	64 (68.1%)	25 (26.6%)	Younger age at onset (homozygote)
Kim WH. 2019 [6]	Korea	35	35.5 ± 20.0	0 (0%)	28 (80%)	7 (20%)	Leptomeningeal flow patterns from posterior circulation to anterior circulation (wild type), PCA involvement (heterozygote)
Zhang Q. 2017 [7]	China	255	26.7 ± 14.7	2	78	175	Younger age at the onset, ischemic symptom, PCA involvement (heterozygote)
Wang Y. 2020 [8]	China	1385	35.2 (range 1–71)	6 (0.5%)	313 (22.4%)	1066 (76.1%)	Younger age at the onset (homozygote and heterozygote), PCA involvement (heterozygote)
Ge P. 2019 [9]	China	254	29 (IQR13–42)	0 (0%)	63 (24.8%)	191 (75.2%)	Postoperative better collateral formation (heterozygote)
Ge P. 2019 [10]	China	498	33 (IQR15–43)	4 (0.8%)	133 (26.7%)	361 (72.5%)	Younger age at the onset, TIA at the onset, PCA involvement (heterozygote and homozygote)

Interestingly, in most studies in Japan and Korea, there is no significant difference in age at the disease onset and cerebral infarction at the disease onset between p.R4810K heterozygous variant and the wild type, although the presence of the family history in the p.R4810K homozygote and heterozygote was superior to the wild type.

About angiographical features, there are a few reports. Kim EH et al. reported that there was no difference in Suzuki stage, bilateral vasculopathy, involvement with posterior cerebral artery between the genotypes [4]. On the other hand, Miyatake et al. reported that PCA involvement in p.R4180K homozygous variant and bilateral vasculopathy in p.R4810K homozygous and heterozygous variant was significantly higher than the other genotypes [3].

Kim WH et al. reported collateral flow patterns in MMD were different between the *RNF213* p.R4810K genotype [6]. Leptomeningeal flow patterns from posterior circulation to anterior circulation are significantly observed in p.R4810K wild type in Korean patients with MMD. This result also may mean the pathogenicity of this variant.

There are fewer reports regarding the phenotypes in the long-term cohort. We previously reported that genotype–phenotype correlation of p.R4810K in 94 Japanese patients with MMD with a median follow-up period of 8 years after direct or combined bypass surgery [5]. In this study, the incidence rate of recurrent stroke was low regardless of p.R4810K genotype, even patients with p.R4810K homozygous variant, which has been thought the most pathogenic in Japanese and Korean patients. In other words, we consider that optimal bypass surgery can be effective for all genotypes. We consider that we have not to decide treatment strategy by using this genotype at the present knowledge. Despite the result of genotyping, we will have to do the best treatment and optimal bypass surgery. In the near future, a larger study is needed to validate.

5.2.2 China

The distribution of the p.R4810K genotype is quite different from Japan and Korea in East Asia. The frequency of *RNF213* p.R4810K heterozygous and homozygous variants in MMD patients in China was much lower, instead of that the wild type was much higher compared to those in Japan and Korea [7, 10]. In the largest recent study of Chinese population [8], the frequency of p.R4810K homozygous variant, heterozygous variant, and the wild type were 0.5%, 22.4%, and 76.1%, respectively. Furthermore, they reported that the p.R4810K homozygous and heterozygous variants were associated with early age at onset, but not with severe manifestation like cerebral infarction at onset. The initial symptom in 66.7% of Chinese patients with the p.R4810K homozygous variant was a transient ischemic attack, and only one out of six cases presented with cerebral infarction at onset. This finding was not suggestive of the link between p.R4810K homozygote and severe clinical manifestation in China, which were quite different with Japanese and Korean patients.

Q Zhang reported case descriptions of four MMD Chinese patients with p.R4810K homozygous variant. They described indirect bypass was effective for all patients and early surgical intervention should be considered under evaluation of the homozygote in Japan and Korea [12]. P Ge reported that in long-term cohort p.R4810K genotype was not associated with recurrent stroke or neurological status, and this genotype may not be the long-term outcome in Chinese patients. Their opinion was similar to our previous study with Japanese patients [5], but further investigations will be needed because the distribution of this genotype or type of bypass surgery between the studies [13]. P Ge also reported that association between p.R4810K variant and postoperative collateral formation [9]. They described that postoperative collateral formation was better in patients with p.R4810K heterozygous variant than those with the wild type.

5.3 The Other Rare Variants of *RNF213*

Rare variants in *RNF213* other than p.R4810K have been detected in several studies in Asian and Caucasian patients as mentioned later. In the past studies, the positive association of these rare variants with MMD was proven with variable threshold test using a C score of Combined Annotation Dependent Depletion (CADD) [11].

Few studies reported the clinical phenotype of the other rare variant except *RNF213* p.R4180K. We described Japanese pediatric patients with the other rare variant [14]. He had severe manifestation with infarction onset and progression of posterior cerebral arteries, but his genetic screening showed p.R4810K wild type in spite of the presence of family history. Instead of the founder variant, the other rare variant, p.R4062Q heterozygous variant, was detected. We describe another one-year patient with the other rare variant as a compound heterozygous variant together with p.R4810K, who presented recurrent stroke after initial bypass surgery [11]. C scores of CADD of these rare variants were higher than that of p.R4810K. The function of *RNF213* was not completely understood. Even in Japanese patients with the higher frequency of p.R4810K, we cannot explain all genetic factors using only *RNF213* p.R4810K because of the influence of the other rare variant than p.R4810K. If we would predict or diagnose this p.R4810K founder variant, there would be a risk for us to overlook the risk caused by the other rare variants.

5.4 *RNF213* Variant in Caucasian

The distribution in Caucasian MMD patients was quite different. Basically, *RNF213* p.R4180K Asian founder variant was not discovered in Caucasian patients.

By Guey et al. [15], the p.R4810K variant was not identified in 68 Caucasian MMD probands, but 23 other rare variants were identified in 19 probands (27.9%), most of which variants located in the C-terminal region of RING-finger domain. Kobayashi also reported that *RNF213* rare variants were identified in 22.2% (4/18) of patients from Slovakia and the Czech Republic, although p.R4810K was not identified [16]. Furthermore, Cecchi et al. [17] reported that the p.R4810K was not found in non-Asian patients, but the other rare variants were identified 5 of the 22 European American probands (23%) and in both of two the Hispanic American probands.

Their studies confirmed *RNF213* was one of the causative genes for MMD not only in Asians but also in Caucasians. However, how the rare variants affected clinical phenotype such as disease severity was not analyzed well. In the near future, reports regarding genotype–phenotype correlation of *RNF213* rare variants in different ethnic patients are expected for further elucidation.

5.5 *RNF213* and Diseases Other than Moyamoya Disease

After the discovery of *RNF213* as the susceptibility gene of moyamoya disease, the significant association between *RNF213* and the other diseases has recently been reported (Fig. 5.1). The functional roles of how *RNF213* have influenced is unknown, so it is important to understand the influence of *RNF213* on other diseases. We summarized *RNF213*-related diseases.

1. Moyamoya syndrome

Moyamoya syndrome (MMS, Quasi MMD), MMD based on the different underlying disorders such as Neurofibrosomasis Type1 (NF1) or hyperthyroidism, was distinguished from MMD [18]. However, several studies reported that *RNF213* was

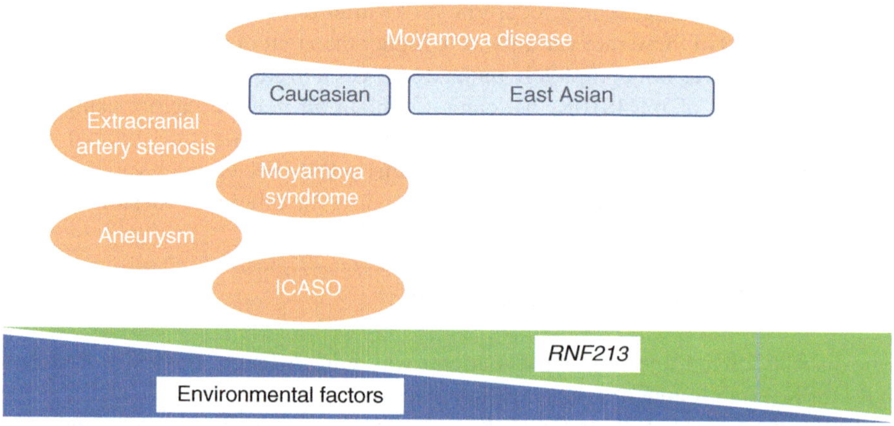

Fig. 5.1 The spectrum of moyamoya disease and the other diseases associated with *RNF213*. Pathology of each disease is composed of genetic factor and environmental factor. Involvement of *RNF213* with several diseases including moyamoya disease has been reported. The further to the left the disease located, the less the weight of genetic background of *RNF213* and the more the weight of the other environmental factor

significantly associated with these diseases [19–23]. The frequency of *RNF213* p.R4810K was reported to be widely from 0% to 66.7%, which differed in each study. This difference was caused by the extreme rarity of this type of disease and these studies included the various kinds of underlying entities.

The study of NF1-associated MMS showed that *RNF213* might be a susceptible gene for moyamoya development of patients with NF1 [21]. *RNF213* p.R4810K variant was detected in 3 (18.7%) out of 16 patients with NF1-associated MMS, on the other hand, none in 97 NF1 patients without MMS. Another genetic study with 15 patients with hyperthyroidism-associated MMS showed not only p.R4810K variant in six patients but also four other rare variants of *RNF213* in four patients [23].

Totally, the frequency of *RNF213* in MMS was less than MMD although there was a difference between the studies. These results suggest that *RNF213* may contribute to the pathogenesis of MMS in addition to the environmental factor of the underlying disease.

2. Intracranial artery stenosis and occlusion (ICASO)

Following the discovery of *RNF213* in MMD, Miyawaki et al. reported for the first time that *RNF213* was detected in 20/84 Japanese patients (23.8%) with non-MMD intracranial artery stenosis and occlusion (ICASO) [24, 25]. Then, several studies confirmed a similar association in East Asia [26–28]. Although ICASO was often founded from middle-aged to elderly, in particular, *RNF213* p.R4810K variant was common in early-onset stroke patients with intracranial artery stenosis (24%) [29].

Matsuda et al. investigated 59 relatives of patients with MMD and showed that six of 34 individuals with p.R4810K heterozygous variant intracranial artery steno-occlusive lesions [30]. On the other hand, none of the family members with the p.R4810K wild type showed intracranial stenotic lesions. As they mentioned, the significance of *RNF213* p.R4810K genotyping for screening was limited because of low rate that this variant penetrates and high rate of this among normal population, but genotyping for family members of patient with MMD may be useful.

Also, Cerebral Autosomal Dominant Arteriopathy with Subcortical Infarcts and Leukoencephalopathy (CADASIL) was known to primarily affect small cerebral arteries caused by *NOTCH3*. However, stenosis of major intracranial arteries is reportedly sometimes affected. Interestingly, the frequency of p.R4810K variant in CADASIL patients with ICAS (4/17; 23.5%) was significantly higher than those without ICAS (2/107; 1.9%) [31].

Moreover, the studies with high-resolution MRI showed that outer vessel diameter in ICASO patients with *RNF213* p.R4810K variant than those with the wild type [27, 32]. These results may suggest the important role of *RNF213* in patients with ICASO, although further studies are needed to validate these results.

3. Extracranial artery stenosis

Although there has been no large studies regarding the association regarding extracranial artery stenosis in MMD because of its rarity, the most recent study by TK Jee [33] revealed the frequency of extracranial arteriopathy and *RNF213* in patient with MMD for the first time. Among 63 Korean young adult patients with MMD, 11 patients (17%) had significant stenosis of extracranial arteries with coronary and aorta computed tomography angiography: Coronary in six patients, superior mesenteric in two, celiac in two, renal in one, and/or internal iliac artery in one. Importantly, four out of six (67%) patients with *RNF213* p.R4180K homozygous variant presented with extracranial arteriopathy, which was higher than 14% with the heterozygous variant and 8% in the wild type. They clarified that moyamoya disease and *RNF213* are linked with extracranial artery stenosis. As they mention, we may consider investigation of extracranial arteries for MMD patients with the homozygous variant.

Morimoto et al. revealed a significant association of *RNF213* p.R4810K with coronary artery disease, not MMD [34]. In their study, the allele frequency of p.R4810K was 2.04% in patients with coronary artery disease to 0.98% in control. The frequency of the p.R4810K carrier was 3.87% to 0.98% in control, including two p.R4810K homozygous variant.

Besides these studies, there are several case reports to support the association between *RNF213* and extracranial artery stenosis. In particular, the involvement of *RNF213* p.R4810K homozygous variant was the most frequently reported. We experienced middle-aged female patients with several extracranial artery stenoses harboring p.R4810K homozygous variant, instead of having no manifestation of MMD [35]. She also had coronary artery stenosis followed by coronary artery bypass surgery, and stenosis of the abdominal artery and superior mesenteric artery. Her two children and her uncle had typical MMD with p.R4810K heterozygous variant, but she had no evidence of MMD in spite of the presence of the homozygous variant. Further, Y Bang reported a similar case with p.R4810K homozygous variant presenting with systemic vasculopathy instead of MMD [36]. Chang et al. reported five patients with pulmonary artery stenosis associates with *RNF213* and MMD [37]. Three out of those five patients have MMD and the others did not have MMD, but genotyping of four patients of five revealed *RNF213* p.R4810K homozygous variant. Fukushima et al. also reported two patients with *RNF213* p.R4810K homozygous variant suffering from MMD and pulmonary artery stenosis [38]. Further, Hara et al. reported that two MMD patients with renal artery stenosis with *RNF213* p.R4810K heterozygous variant [39].

On the other hand, negative correlation of *RNF213* with some other arterial diseases was reported. In the report by Tashiro et al., *RNF213* p.R4810K was positive in 69% of the MMD patients (40/58), none of the intracranial vertebral artery dissection have p.R4810K (0/24) [40]. Also, only one out of 34 patients with extracranial carotid atherosclerosis was positive for *RNF213* p.R4810K by Miyawaki et al., the frequency of which was almost equal to control population [25]. Further, Araki et al. reported one pediatric patient with focal cerebral arteriopathy with *RNF213* p.R4810K Wild type, [41] but further larger study will be needed to validate the association.

4. Aneurysm

Not only stenotic arterial diseases but also cerebral aneurysms may be influenced by *RNF213*. S Zhou reported that *RNF213* was significantly associated with intracranial aneurysms in the French-Canadian Population [42]. Their genetic analysis using discovery cohort of affected family and validation cohort revealed that rare variant of *RNF213* was significantly associated with intracranial aneurysm in French-Canadian. Among 25 affected individuals from 249 discovery and validation cohorts, 14 rare variants in *RNF213* were detected. Most of the rare variants of *RNF213* in intracranial aneurysm were located in the entire exon including 2 AAA+ functional domains, although those in MMD were located posteriorly near RING finger domain. Also, Sauvigny T reported that four variants in *RNF213* (three patients) in 35 unrelated individuals and three affected members of a family performed by exome sequencing in Germany [43]. As they mentioned, genetic drift or ethnic-specific variant in *RNF213* may influence the difference of phenotype of this gene. In other words briefly, the role of *RNF213* may differ in each ethnic or district, however, the mechanism has still not been elucidated.

5. Others

Intracranial artery dissection or de novo MMD after stereotactic radiosurgery after arteriovenous malformation were reported in Japanese patients with *RNF213* p.R4810K variant [44]. Also, reversible cerebral angiopathy after viral infection leading to cerebral infarction was reported in those with *RNF213* p.R4810K [45]. However, they all were single case reports and this variant was founded in 2–3% of normal population in Japan. Therefore, further studies or accumulation of similar cases will be needed to validate their associations.

5.6 Conclusion

We described the correlation between *RNF213* and clinical features in MMD and the other diseases. MMD has complicated pathology because of multifactorial disease composed of genetic and environmental factors, but there was a certain tendency of genotype–phenotype correlation of *RNF213* in MMD in each ethnic. Furthermore, recent studies revealed *RNF213* was associated with other diseases except MMD, which means the spectrum of *RNF213* was broader than expected before. In the present era after the discovery of *RNF213*, unknown mechanism regarding MMD and *RNF213* was still remain. Further research such as epigenomic or environmental factors will be needed to clarify the mechanism of them.

References

1. Kamada F, Aoki Y, Narisawa A, Abe Y, Komatsuzaki S, Kikuchi A, et al. A genome-wide association study identifies RNF213 as the first moyamoya disease gene. J Hum Genet. 2011;56(1):34–40.
2. Liu W, Morito D, Takashima S, Mineharu Y, Kobayashi H, Hitomi T, et al. Identification of RNF213 as a susceptibility gene for moyamoya disease and its possible role in vascular development. PLoS One. 2011;6(7):e22542.

3. Miyatake S, Miyake N, Touho H, Nishimura-Tadaki A, Kondo Y, Okada I, et al. Homozygous c.14576G>A variant of RNF213 predicts early-onset and severe form of moyamoya disease. Neurology. 2012;78(11):803–10.
4. Kim EH, Yum MS, Ra YS, Park JB, Ahn JS, Kim GH, et al. Importance of RNF213 polymorphism on clinical features and long-term outcome in moyamoya disease. J Neurosurg. 2016;124(5):1221–7.
5. Nomura S, Yamaguchi K, Akagawa H, Kawashima A, Moteki Y, Ishikawa T, et al. Genotype-phenotype correlation in long-term cohort of Japanese patients with moyamoya disease. Cerebrovasc Dis. 2019;47(3–4):105–11.
6. Kim WH, Kim SD, Nam MH, Jung JM, Jin SW, Ha SK, et al. Posterior circulation involvement and collateral flow pattern in moyamoya disease with the RNF213 polymorphism. Childs Nerv Syst. 2019;35(2):309–14.
7. Zhang Q, Liu Y, Zhang D, Wang R, Zhang Y, Wang S, et al. RNF213 as the major susceptibility gene for Chinese patients with moyamoya disease and its clinical relevance. J Neurosurg. 2017;126(4):1106–13.
8. Wang Y, Zhang Z, Wei L, Zhang Q, Zou Z, Yang L, et al. Predictive role of heterozygous p.R4810K of RNF213 in the phenotype of Chinese moyamoya disease. Neurology. 2020;94(7):e678–e86.
9. Ge P, Ye X, Liu X, Deng X, Wang J, Wang R, et al. Association between p.R4810K variant and postoperative collateral formation in patients with moyamoya disease. Cerebrovasc Dis. 2019;48(1–2):77–84.
10. Ge P, Ye X, Liu X, Deng X, Wang R, Zhang Y, et al. Association between p.R4810K variant and long-term clinical outcome in patients with moyamoya disease. Front Neurol. 2019;10:662.
11. Moteki Y, Onda H, Kasuya H, Yoneyama T, Okada Y, Hirota K, et al. Systematic validation of RNF213 coding variants in Japanese patients with moyamoya disease. J Am Heart Assoc. 2015;4(5):e001862.
12. Zhang Q, Ge P, Ma Y, Zhang D, Wang R, Zhang Y, et al. Clinical features and surgical outcomes of patients with moyamoya disease and the homozygous RNF213 p.R4810K variant. J Child Neurol. 2019;34(13):793–800.
13. Nomura S, Akagawa H, Yamaguchi K, Kawashima A, Kawamata T. Surgical options and genetic screening of a patient with moyamoya disease harboring the RNF213 p.R4180 K homozygous variant. J Child Neurol. 2020; 883073820913373
14. Nomura S, Kawashima A, Akagawa H, Kawamata T. Letter to the editor. Influence of rare RNF213 variants other than p.R4810K on the clinical outcomes of moyamoya disease. J Neurosurg. 2018;129:1–2.
15. Guey S, Kraemer M, Herve D, Ludwig T, Kossorotoff M, Bergametti F, et al. Rare RNF213 variants in the C-terminal region encompassing the RING-finger domain are associated with moyamoya angiopathy in Caucasians. Eur J Hum Genet. 2017;25(8):995–1003.
16. Kobayashi H, Brozman M, Kyselova K, Viszlayova D, Morimoto T, Roubec M, et al. RNF213 rare variants in Slovakian and Czech moyamoya disease patients. PLoS One. 2016;11(10):e0164759.
17. Cecchi AC, Guo D, Ren Z, Flynn K, Santos-Cortez RL, Leal SM, et al. RNF213 rare variants in an ethnically diverse population with moyamoya disease. Stroke. 2014;45(11):3200–7.
18. Scott RM, Smith ER. Moyamoya disease and moyamoya syndrome. N Engl J Med. 2009;360(12):1226–37.
19. Miyawaki S, Imai H, Shimizu M, Yagi S, Ono H, Nakatomi H, et al. Genetic analysis of RNF213 c.14576G>A variant in nonatherosclerotic quasi-moyamoya disease. J Stroke Cerebrovasc Dis. 2015;24(5):1075–9.
20. Morimoto T, Mineharu Y, Kobayashi H, Harada KH, Funaki T, Takagi Y, et al. Significant association of the RNF213 p.R4810K polymorphism with quasi-moyamoya disease. J Stroke Cerebrovasc Dis. 2016;25(11):2632–6.
21. Phi JH, Choi JW, Seong MW, Kim T, Moon YJ, Lee J, et al. Association between moyamoya syndrome and the RNF213 c.14576G>A variant in patients with neurofibromatosis type 1. J Neurosurg Pediatr. 2016;17(6):717–22.

22. Zhang Q, Liu Y, Yu L, Duan R, Ma Y, Ge P, et al. The association of the RNF213 p.R4810K polymorphism with quasi-moyamoya disease and a review of the pertinent literature. World Neurosurg. 2017;99:701–8 e1.
23. Nomura S, Akagawa H, Yamaguchi K, Ishikawa T, Kawashima A, Kasuya H, et al. Rare and low-frequency variants in RNF213 confer susceptibility to Moyamoya syndrome associated with hyperthyroidism. World Neurosurg. 2019;127:e460–e6.
24. Miyawaki S, Imai H, Takayanagi S, Mukasa A, Nakatomi H, Saito N. Identification of a genetic variant common to moyamoya disease and intracranial major artery stenosis/occlusion. Stroke. 2012;43(12):3371–4.
25. Miyawaki S, Imai H, Shimizu M, Yagi S, Ono H, Mukasa A, et al. Genetic variant RNF213 c.14576G>a in various phenotypes of intracranial major artery stenosis/occlusion. Stroke. 2013;44(10):2894–7.
26. Bang OY, Chung JW, Cha J, Lee MJ, Yeon JY, Ki CS, et al. A polymorphism in RNF213 is a susceptibility gene for intracranial atherosclerosis. PLoS One. 2016;11(6):e0156607.
27. Choi EH, Lee H, Chung JW, Seo WK, Kim GM, Ki CS, et al. Ring finger protein 213 variant and plaque characteristics, vascular remodeling, and hemodynamics in patients with intracranial atherosclerotic stroke: a high-resolution magnetic resonance imaging and hemodynamic study. J Am Heart Assoc. 2019;8(20):e011996.
28. Okazaki S, Morimoto T, Kamatani Y, Kamimura T, Kobayashi H, Harada K, et al. Moyamoya disease susceptibility variant RNF213 p.R4810K increases the risk of ischemic stroke attributable to large-artery atherosclerosis. Circulation. 2019;139(2):295–8.
29. Kamimura T, Okazaki S, Morimoto T, Kobayashi H, Harada K, Tomita T, et al. Prevalence of RNF213 p.R4810K variant in early-onset stroke with intracranial arterial stenosis. Stroke. 2019;50(6):1561–3.
30. Matsuda Y, Mineharu Y, Kimura M, Takagi Y, Kobayashi H, Hitomi T, et al. RNF213 p.R4810K variant and intracranial arterial stenosis or occlusion in relatives of patients with Moyamoya disease. J Stroke Cerebrovasc Dis. 2017;26(8):1841–7.
31. Yeung WTE, Mizuta I, Watanabe-Hosomi A, Yokote A, Koizumi T, Mukai M, et al. RNF213-related susceptibility of Japanese CADASIL patients to intracranial arterial stenosis. J Hum Genet. 2018;63(5):687–90.
32. Hongo H, Miyawaki S, Imai H, Shinya Y, Ono H, Mori H, et al. Smaller outer diameter of atherosclerotic middle cerebral artery associated with RNF213 c.14576G>A variant (rs112735431). Surg Neurol Int. 2017;8:104.
33. Jee TK, Yeon JY, Kim SM, Bang OY, Kim JS, Hong SC. Prospective screening of extracranial systemic arteriopathy in young adults with moyamoya disease. J Am Heart Assoc. 2020;9:e016670.
34. Morimoto T, Mineharu Y, Ono K, Nakatochi M, Ichihara S, Kabata R, et al. Significant association of RNF213 p.R4810K, a moyamoya susceptibility variant, with coronary artery disease. PLoS One. 2017;12(4):e0175649.
35. Nomura S, Aihara Y, Akagawa H, Chiba K, Yamaguchi K, Kawashima A, et al. Can moyamoya disease susceptibility gene affect extracranial systemic artery stenosis? J Stroke Cerebrovasc Dis. 2019;29:104532.
36. Bang OY, Chung JW, Kim DH, Won HH, Yeon JY, Ki CS, et al. Moyamoya disease and spectrums of RNF213 vasculopathy. Transl Stroke Res. 2020;11(4):580–9.
37. Chang SA, Song JS, Park TK, Yang JH, Kwon WC, Kim SR, et al. Nonsyndromic peripheral pulmonary artery stenosis is associated with homozygosity of RNF213 p.Arg4810Lys regardless of co-occurrence of moyamoya disease. Chest. 2018;153(2):404–13.
38. Fukushima H, Takenouchi T, Kosaki K. Homozygosity for moyamoya disease risk allele leads to moyamoya disease with extracranial systemic and pulmonary vasculopathy. Am J Med Genet A. 2016;170(9):2453–6.
39. Hara S, Shimizu K, Nariai T, Kishino M, Kudo T, Umemoto T, et al. De novo renal artery stenosis developed in initially normal renal arteries during the long-term follow-up of patients with moyamoya disease. J Stroke Cerebrovasc Dis. 2020;29(8):104786.

40. Tashiro R, Fujimura M, Sakata H, Endo H, Tomata Y, Sato-Maeda M, et al. Genetic analysis of ring finger protein 213 (RNF213) c.14576G>A polymorphism in patients with vertebral artery dissection: a comparative study with moyamoya disease. Neurol Res. 2019;41(9):811–6.
41. Araki Y, Takagi Y, Mineharu Y, Kobayashi H, Miyamoto S, Wakabayashi T. Rapid contralateral progression of focal cerebral arteriopathy distinguished from RNF213-related moyamoya disease and fibromuscular dysplasia. Childs Nerv Syst. 2017;33(8):1405–9.
42. Zhou S, Ambalavanan A, Rochefort D, Xie P, Bourassa CV, Hince P, et al. RNF213 is associated with intracranial aneurysms in the French-Canadian population. Am J Hum Genet. 2016;99(5):1072–85.
43. Sauvigny T, Alawi M, Krause L, Renner S, Spohn M, Busch A, et al. Exome sequencing in 38 patients with intracranial aneurysms and subarachnoid hemorrhage. J Neurol. 2020;267(9):2533–45.
44. Torazawa S, Miyawaki S, Shinya Y, Kawashima M, Hasegawa H, Dofuku S, et al. De novo development of moyamoya disease after stereotactic radiosurgery for brain arteriovenous malformation in a patient with RNF213 p.Arg4810Lys (rs112735431). World Neurosurg. 2020;140:276–82.
45. Shinya Y, Miyawaki S, Nakatomi H, Shin M, Teraoka A, Saito N. Hemorrhagic onset intracranial artery dissection of middle cerebral artery followed by progressive arterial stenosis with genetic variant RNF213 p.Arg4810Lys (rs112735431). World Neurosurg. 2020;141:192–5.

RNF213 Variant as a Biomarker of Cerebrovascular Disease

6

Satoru Miyawaki and Nobuhito Saito

Abstract

Although originally associated with susceptibility to moyamoya disease (MMD), the *RNF213* c.14429G > A (p.Arg4810Lys, rs112735431) variant is reportedly significantly associated with Intracranial Artery Stenosis (ICAS), not diagnosed as MMD, and with noncardiac ischemic stroke in the Japanese population. The *RNF213* p.Arg4810Lys variant is generally found in about 2% of East Asian populations, including the Japanese and Korean, but is almost completely absent in other populations, including Europeans. Thus, the *RNF213* p.Arg4810Lys variant is thought to be a genetic characteristic of ischemic stroke in East Asian populations. In addition, associations have been identified in coronary stenosis/ renal artery stenosis and pulmonary hypertension. The *RNF213* p.Arg4810Lys variant continues to attract attention as a potential cause of systemic vascular disease. As functional analysis of *RNF213* continues to progress, molecular cascades related to the regulation of *RNF213* expression and cell activity are gradually being clarified, although the mechanisms underlying disease development remain unclear, thus further analysis is warranted.

Keywords

RNF213 · Moyamoya disease · Intracranial artery stenosis · Noncardiac ischemic stroke · Pulmonary hypertension

S. Miyawaki (✉) · N. Saito
Department of Neurosurgery, Faculty of Medicine, The University of Tokyo, Tokyo, Japan
e-mail: miyawaki-tky@umin.ac.jp; nsaito-nsu@m.u-tokyo.ac.jp

S. Kuroda (ed.), *Moyamoya Disease: Current Knowledge and Future Perspectives*, https://doi.org/10.1007/978-981-33-6404-2_6

6.1 *Ring Finger Protein 213 (RNF213)*

The *RNF213* gene was originally associated with susceptibility to moyamoya disease (MMD), which is a cerebrovascular disorder characterized by chronic progressive stenosis of the terminal portions of the bilateral internal carotid arteries and the formation and development of abnormal vascular networks (moyamoya vessels) at the base of the brain as collateral tracts [1–3]. MMD has long been suspected to have a genetic background due to the predominant occurrence among family members and the higher incidence among populations in Japan and other East Asian countries. In 2011, two different groups reported that the *RNF213* gene, located at 17q25.3, was associated with susceptibility to MMD with the use of different methods [4, 5]. The protein encoded by RNF213 contains a novel RING finger domain at the C-terminus of the gene and an AAA ATPase domain at the central part of the gene. Hence, the gene product is considered a new type of protein with E3 ubiquitin ligase and ATP degradation functions. Among the variants of *RNF213*, only one has been strongly associated with MMD in East Asian populations, including the Japanese. The variant c. 14429G > A, p.Arg4810Lys, rs112735431, the reference sequence of *RNF213* in this chapter, is currently the most common reference sequence (National Center for Biotechnology Information Reference Sequences NM_001256071 and NP_00124300). In this *RNF213* missense variant, which was reportedly detected in about 80% of Japanese patients with MMD, the arginine residue at amino acid position 4810 is changed to a lysine residue. Notably, about 2% of the Japanese population have this variant [4].

The *RNF213* p.Arg4810Lys variant in MMD has been detected in various populations in East Asia, including Japan, Korea, and China [5, 6]. On the other hand, the *RNF213* p.Arg4810Lys variant is rare and not associated with MMD in European populations [7–9]. A summary of past reports on the associations of the *RNF213* p.Arg4810Lys variant with MMD in Japanese [8, 10–16], Korean [8, 11, 17–21], and Chinese populations [8, 11, 22–27] is shown in Table 6.1. Interestingly, the frequency of the *RNF213* p.Arg4810Lys variant in patients with MMD is similar to that in Japanese and Korean populations, but slightly lower than in the Chinese population, suggesting differences in the genetic background of MMD among these populations.

6.2 *RNF213* and Intracranial Artery Stenosis

Intracranial Artery Stenosis (ICAS), as a leading cause of ischemic stroke, is mostly caused by arteriosclerotic changes in the intracranial blood vessels due to lifestyle-related diseases, such as hypertension, diabetes, and dyslipidemia, as well as various acquired factors associated with disease onset [12]. However, the prevalence of ICAS differs among different populations and is most predominant in East Asian, Hispanic, and African populations, suggesting the involvement of genetic factors in the onset of ICAS [28–32].

There are strict diagnostic criteria for MMD [33], which include [1] the presence of a progressive stenotic lesion at the terminus of the internal carotid artery [2], the

Table 6.1 Summary of previous association studies of the *RNF213* p.Arg4810Lys variant with various vascular diseases

	Japanese population				Korean population				Chinese population			
	Rate of the carrier of *RNF213* p.Arg4810Lys		Odds ratio (95% CI)	*P* value	Rate of the carrier of *RNF213* p.Arg4810Lys		Odds ratio (95% CI)	*P* value	Rate of the carrier of *RNF213* p.Arg4810Lys		Odds ratio (95% CI)	*P* value
	Case	Control			Case	Control			Case	Control		
Moyamoya disease	545 / 661 (82.4%)	40/1459 (2.7%)	166.6 (114.8–241.9)	<0.0001*	657/922 (71.2%)	54/2278 (2.3%)	102.1 (75.2–138.5)	<0.0001*	461/2081 (22.1%)	25/4562 (0.5%)	51.6 (34.3–77.5)	<0.0001*
References	4, 5, 11–16				5, 11, 17–21				5, 11, 22–27			
Intracranial artery stenosis	39/229 (17.0%)	4/235 (1.7%)	11.8 (4.16–33.7)	<0.0001*	176/970 (18.1%)	75/2938 (2.5%)	8.46 75.2–11.2)	<0.0001*	27/1570 (1.7%)	4/1500 (0.2%)	6.54 (2.28–18.74)	<0.0001*
References	13, 14, 16				17, 19, 20, 34–36				37–40			
Noncarid-iogenic ischemic stroke	20/383 (5.2%)	21/1011 (2.1%)	2.60 (1.39–4.85)	0.0019*								
References	52											
Coronary artery stenosis	37/956 (3.8%)	13/716 (1.8%)	2.18 (1.15–4.13)	0.014*								
References	53											
Pulmonary hyperten-sion	7/76 (9.2%)	–	–	–								
References	58											

*Statistically significant (Chi-square test)

development of moyamoya vessels in the basal ganglia as collateral circulation, and [3] the lack of underlying diseases that may cause arteriostenosis, such as chromosomal disorders, genetic diseases, inflammatory diseases, trauma, and tumors.

Imaging and exclusion of other diagnoses are the basis of the diagnostic criteria for MMD. However, it may be difficult to arrive at a clear diagnosis of MMD in actual clinical practice. Especially in the elderly, atherosclerotic changes occur to some extent. So, it is sometimes difficult to diagnose ICAS in old age as compared with MMD or atherosclerosis. Through analysis of *RNF213* p.Arg4810Lys in various cerebrovascular diseases in Japanese populations, about 23% of ICASs those do not meet the diagnostic criteria for moyamoya disease and are usually diagnosed as atherosclerosis were reported to have *RNF213* p.Arg4810Lys. Thus, *RNF213* p.Arg4810Lys variant was proven to be significantly associated with ICAS [13, 14, 16].

To date, similar analyses have been performed in Korea [17, 19, 20, 34–36] and China [37–40], which have demonstrated a significant association between ICAS and the *RNF213* p.Arg4810Lys variant [5]. A summary of the results of previous studies is presented in Table 6.1. Similar to MMD, there was a similar frequency of the *RNF213* p.Arg4810Lys variant between ICAS patients and controls in studies of Japanese and Korean populations, but a lower frequency in Chinese populations. Reportedly, the *RNF213* p.Arg4810Lys variant is present in about 2% of the Japanese and Korean populations, and about 1% of the Chinese population, but is rarely found in other populations, such as Europeans [41]. This difference in the frequency of the *RNF213* p.Arg4810Lys variant is considered an important genetic factor underlying the high incidences of MMD and ICAS in East Asian populations.

6.3 Variants of *RNF213* Other than p.Arg4810Lys Associated with ICAS

The *RNF213* gene is located on the long arm of chromosome 17 and encodes a large protein consisting of 5207 amino acids. The *RNF213* p.Arg4810Lys variant is absent in about 20% of MMD patients in Japan and most MMD patients in Europe. Several studies have been performed to identify *RNF213* variants, other than p.Arg4810Lys, associated with MMD [8–12, 15, 22, 24, 26, 42].

Our group analyzed the entire *RNF213* sequence of 168 ICAS patients and 1194 controls with the use of a next-generation sequencing to search for variants other than p.Arg4810Lys related to ICAS [43]. A total of 138 missense variants were identified in this cohort. In a case control association study that statistically examined differences in the frequency of variants between cases and controls, only the p.Arg4810Lys variant was significantly associated with ICAS. Analysis of the entire *RNF213* sequence also reconfirmed the association of the p.Arg4810Lys variant with ICAS [43].

Other *RNF213* variants, which are extremely rare in the general population, were also identified in ICAS patients. There have been many reports of rare *RNF213* variants in MMD, which were reviewed and compared with the rare variants identified in the ICAS patients in the present study (Fig. 6.1). The *RNF213* variants p.Cys118Arg

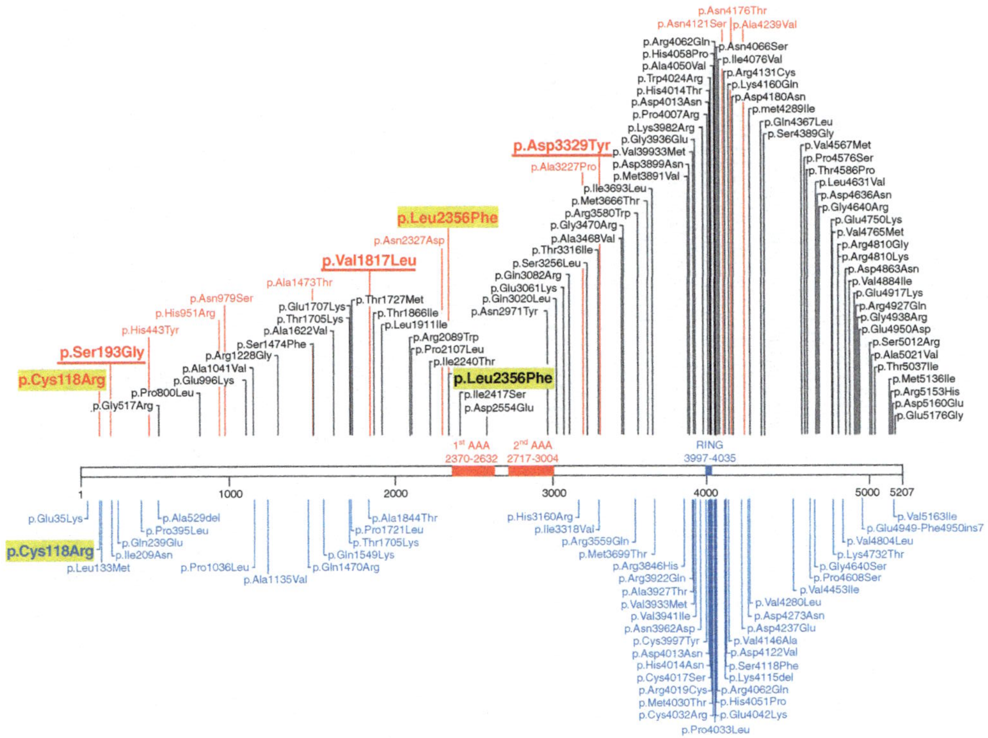

Fig. 6.1 *RNF213* nonsynonymous rare variants identified in ICAS patients without the p.Arg4810Lys variant and MMD patients in previous studies. Variants identified in the present study are marked in red, and previously reported *RNF213* variants in MMD patients in the Asian population and non-Asian population are marked in black and blue, respectively. The p.Cys118Arg and p.Leu2356Phe variants were identified in MMD patients. The p.Ser193Gly, p.Val1817Leu, and p.Asp3329Tyr variants were not detected in control subjects or the Single Nucleotide Polymorphism Database (Source: Comprehensive investigation of RNF213 nonsynonymous variants associated with intracranial artery stenosis. Author: Hiroki Hongo et al. Publication: Scientific Reports. Publisher: Springer Nature. Date: Jul 20, 2020)

and p.Leu2356Phe, which were identified in the present study, were previously reported in MMD, suggesting a correlation with ICAS. On the other hand, the variants p.Ser193Gly, p.Val1817Leu, and p.Asp3329Tyr were not found in the controls or reported in the Single Nucleotide Polymorphism Database (https://www.ncbi.nlm.nih.gov/snp/), suggesting that this is the first report of these variants in ICAS [43].

The pathogenicity of these rare variants was predicted by in silico analysis with the Polymorphism Phenotyping v2 tool (http://genetics.bwh.harvard.edu/pph2/) and the Combined Annotation Dependent Depletion tool (https://cadd.gs.washington.edu/). However, it is essential to determine if these rare variants are actually involved in the onset and progression of MMD and/or ICAS. To date, an animal model of MMD by genetic modification of *RNF213* has not yet been established, which should be addressed in future studies. Reportedly, rare variants with a RING finger domain located on the C-terminus of the *RNF213* gene are significantly more abundant in MMD in European populations. It has been suggested that dysfunction of the C-terminus of the *RNF213* gene is involved in the development of MMD [44]. In the present study, the rare variants identified in ICAS were not necessarily concentrated on the C-terminus, suggesting that the difference in the position of the *RNF213* mutation may influence the phenotype.

6.4 Features of ICAS with the *RNF213* p.Arg4810Lys Variant

ICAS with the *RNF213* p.Arg4810Lys variant is characterized by negative remodeling, in which the outer diameter of blood vessels is reduced at the stenosis site [45, 46]. The most common stenotic sites of ICAS with the *RNF213* p.Arg4810Lys variant occur in the internal and middle cerebral arteries of the anterior cerebral circulation, rather than the vertebral and basilar arteries in the posterior cerebral circulation [16, 35, 47]. Also, ICAS with the *RNF213* p.Arg4810Lys variant is reportedly more common in females, as with MMD [47].

The vascular smooth muscles of the internal carotid artery in the anterior circulation are developmentally derived from the neural crest, whereas those of the vertebral basilar artery in the posterior circulation are derived from the mesoderm [48, 49]. This difference in embryological background may be related to the site where the *RNF213* p.Arg4810Lys variant is likely to cause vascular stenosis.

In addition, a Korean group reported that MMD and ICAS with the *RNF213* p.Arg4810Lys variant are long-term risk factors for the recurrence of cerebral infarction [50]. Hence, further large-scale analyses are expected.

6.5 Associations of General Ischemic Stroke and the *RNF213* p.Arg4810Lys Variant

Recently, it has been reported that the *RNF213* p.Arg4810Lys variant is a genetic risk factor for general ischemic stroke and an important genetic factor related to cerebrovascular disease in the Japanese population [51]. In this report, association analysis of the *RNF213* p.Arg4810Lys variant with noncardiogenic stroke among 383 patients and 1011 controls reported the *RNF213* p.Arg4810Lys variant in 5.2% of noncardiogenic ischemic stroke patients and 2.1% of the controls, indicating a significant association with noncardiogenic ischemic stroke. This result was reconfirmed in two other large Japanese cohorts. Among the subtypes of noncardiogenic ischemic stroke, large artery atherosclerosis was most significantly associated with the *RNF213* p.Arg4810Lys variant.

6.6 Associations of Systemic Vascular Diseases with the *RNF213* p.Arg4810Lys Variant

Other than ICAS, the *RNF213* p.Arg4810Lys variant has been associated with systemic vascular stenosis, renal artery stenosis, coronary artery stenosis, pulmonary artery stenosis [52–56], and pulmonary hypertension [57–59] (Table 6.1). Notably, the prognosis of pulmonary hypertension with the *RNF213* p.Arg4810Lys variant is relatively poor, thus early lung transplantation should be considered in such cases [60]. Thus *RNF213* p.Arg4810Lys variant has attracted increased attention as a possible cause of systemic vascular disease.

6.7 Functional Analysis of the *RNF213* Gene

As mentioned earlier, the *RNF213* gene is located on the long arm of chromosome 17 and encodes a protein consisting of 5207 amino acids [10, 11]. The RNF213 protein contains a RING finger domain and an AAA ATPase domain, and, therefore, is considered a new type of protein with E3 ubiquitin ligase and ATP degradation functions [10, 11]. The *RNF213* p.Arg4810Lys variant reportedly can reduce angiogenic potential at the endothelial cell level in vitro [61], which results in the dysfunction of vascular endothelial cells in vivo [34]. Dysfunction of *RNF213* alone does not damage the blood vessels or cause the development of vascular lesions in vivo, as determined with the use of knockout and brain in knock-in mice [62, 63]. On the other hand, angiogenesis was reportedly suppressed in *RNF213* variant knock-in mice in response to hypoxic stress, suggesting that factors other than the *RNF213* variant are required for the development of vascular lesions [64]. Known molecular cascades, such as the INFβ and WNT signaling pathways, are related to the regulation of *RNF213* expression and cell activity [65, 66]. In addition, *RNF213* is involved in intracellular lipid metabolism [67]. Recently, the mouse RNF213 protein structure was clarified using a cryo-electron microscope [68]. It has been reported that the MMD-related variants on the C-terminus of the *RNF213* gene act as an E3 ubiquitin ligase and generally ameliorate the functions of *RNF213*. A decrease in the function of *RNF213* as an E3 ubiquitin ligase has been associated with the onset of MMD and ICAS [69]. However, the precise mechanisms by which *RNF213* and its variant cause intracranial arterial stenosis in humans has not been clarified, thus further studies are warranted.

6.8 Future Perspectives and Issues

The *RNF213* gene continues to attract attention due to associations with systemic vascular disease, as well as ICAS and MMD. *RNF213* p.Arg4810Lys variant is present in about 2% of the Japanese population. So it is not necessarily associated with the development of ICAS and MMD, as other additional factors are necessary. Therefore, the identification of such factors should be addressed in future functional analysis studies of the *RNF213* gene.

References

1. Kuroda S, Houkin K. Moyamoya disease: current concepts and future perspectives. Lancet Neurol. 2008;7:1056–66.
2. Scott RM, Smith ER. Moyamoya disease and moyamoya syndrome. N Engl J Med. 2009;360:1226–37.
3. Suzuki J, Takaku A. Cerebrovascular “moyamoya” disease. Disease showing abnormal net-like vessels in base of brain. Arch Neurol. 1969;20:288–99.
4. Liu W, Hitomi T, Kobayashi H, Harada KH, Koizumi A. Distribution of moyamoya disease susceptibility polymorphism p.R4810k in rnf213 in east and southeast asian populations. Neurol Med Chir. 2012;52:299–303.
5. Liao X, Deng J, Dai W, Zhang T, Yan J. Rare variants of rnf213 and moyamoya/non-moyamoya intracranial artery stenosis/occlusion disease risk: a meta-analysis and systematic review. Environ Health Prev Med. 2017;22:75.
6. Wang X, Wang Y, Nie F, Li Q, Zhang K, Liu M, et al. Association of genetic variants with moyamoya disease in 13 000 individuals: a meta-analysis. Stroke. 2020;51:1647–55.
7. Grami N, Chong M, Lali R, Mohammadi-Shemirani P, Henshall DE, Rannikmae K, et al. Global assessment of mendelian stroke genetic prevalence in 101 635 individuals from 7 ethnic groups. Stroke. 2020;51:1290–3.
8. Shoemaker LD, Clark MJ, Patwardhan A, Chandratillake G, Garcia S, Chen R, et al. Disease variant landscape of a large multiethnic population of moyamoya patients by exome sequencing. G3 (Bethesda, MD). 2015;6:41–9.
9. Cecchi AC, Guo D, Ren Z, Flynn K, Santos-Cortez RL, Leal SM, et al. Rnf213 rare variants in an ethnically diverse population with moyamoya disease. Stroke. 2014;45:3200–7.
10. Kamada F, Aoki Y, Narisawa A, Abe Y, Komatsuzaki S, Kikuchi A, et al. A genome-wide association study identifies rnf213 as the first moyamoya disease gene. J Hum Genet. 2011;56:34–40.
11. Liu W, Morito D, Takashima S, Mineharu Y, Kobayashi H, Hitomi T, et al. Identification of rnf213 as a susceptibility gene for moyamoya disease and its possible role in vascular development. PLoS One. 2011;6:e22542.
12. Miyatake S, Miyake N, Touho H, Nishimura-Tadaki A, Kondo Y, Okada I, et al. Homozygous c.14576g>a variant of rnf213 predicts early-onset and severe form of moyamoya disease. Neurology. 2012;78:803–10.
13. Miyawaki S, Imai H, Takayanagi S, Mukasa A, Nakatomi H, Saito N. Identification of a genetic variant common to moyamoya disease and intracranial major artery stenosis/occlusion. Stroke. 2012;43:3371–4.
14. Miyawaki S, Imai H, Shimizu M, Yagi S, Ono H, Mukasa A, et al. Genetic variant rnf213 c.14576g>a in various phenotypes of intracranial major artery stenosis/occlusion. Stroke. 2013;44:2894–7.
15. Moteki Y, Onda H, Kasuya H, Yoneyama T, Okada Y, Hirota K, et al. Systematic validation of rnf213 coding variants in japanese patients with moyamoya disease. J Am Heart Assoc. 2015;4:e001862.

16. Shinya Y, Miyawaki S, Imai H, Hongo H, Ono H, Takenobu A, et al. Genetic analysis of ring finger protein 213 (rnf213) c.14576g>a in intracranial atherosclerosis of the anterior and posterior circulations. J Stroke Cerebrovasc Dis. 2017;26:2638–44.
17. Bang OY, Ryoo S, Kim SJ, Yoon CH, Cha J, Yeon JY, et al. Adult moyamoya disease: a burden of intracranial stenosis in east asians? PLoS One. 2015;10:e0130663.
18. Kim EH, Yum MS, Ra YS, Park JB, Ahn JS, Kim GH, et al. Importance of rnf213 polymorphism on clinical features and long-term outcome in moyamoya disease. J Neurosurg. 2016;124:1221–7.
19. Bang OY, Chung JW, Cha J, Lee MJ, Yeon JY, Ki CS, et al. A polymorphism in rnf213 is a susceptibility gene for intracranial atherosclerosis. PLoS One. 2016;11:e0156607.
20. Park MG, Shin JH, Lee SW, Park HR, Park KP. Rnf213 rs112735431 polymorphism in intracranial artery steno-occlusive disease and moyamoya disease in koreans. J Neurol Sci. 2017;375:331–4.
21. Jang MA, Chung JW, Yeon JY, Kim JS, Hong SC, Bang OY, et al. Frequency and significance of rare rnf213 variants in patients with adult moyamoya disease. PLoS One. 2017;12:e0179689.
22. Wu Z, Jiang H, Zhang L, Xu X, Zhang X, Kang Z, et al. Molecular analysis of rnf213 gene for moyamoya disease in the chinese han population. PLoS One. 2012;7:e48179.
23. Wang X, Zhang Z, Liu W, Xiong Y, Sun W, Huang X, et al. Impacts and interactions of pdgfrb, mmp-3, timp-2, and rnf213 polymorphisms on the risk of moyamoya disease in han chinese human subjects. Gene. 2013;526:437–42.
24. Lee MJ, Chen YF, Fan PC, Wang KC, Wang K, Wang J, et al. Mutation genotypes of rnf213 gene from moyamoya patients in Taiwan. J Neurol Sci. 2015;353:161–5.
25. Huang Y, Cheng D, Zhang J, Zhao W. Association between the rs112735431 polymorphism of the rnf213 gene and moyamoya disease: a case-control study and meta-analysis. J Clin Neurosci. 2016;32:14–8.
26. Zhang Q, Liu Y, Zhang D, Wang R, Zhang Y, Wang S, et al. Rnf213 as the major susceptibility gene for chinese patients with moyamoya disease and its clinical relevance. J Neurosurg. 2017;126:1106–13.
27. Wang Y, Zhang Z, Wei L, Zhang Q, Zou Z, Yang L, et al. Predictive role of heterozygous p.R4810k of rnf213 in the phenotype of chinese moyamoya disease. Neurology. 2020;94:e678–86.
28. Banerjee C, Chimowitz MI. Stroke caused by atherosclerosis of the major intracranial arteries. Circ Res. 2017;120:502–13.
29. Holmstedt CA, Turan TN, Chimowitz MI. Atherosclerotic intracranial arterial stenosis: risk factors, diagnosis, and treatment. Lancet Neurol. 2013;12:1106–14.
30. White H, Boden-Albala B, Wang C, Elkind MS, Rundek T, Wright CB, et al. Ischemic stroke subtype incidence among whites, blacks, and hispanics: the northern Manhattan study. Circulation. 2005;111:1327–31.
31. Gorelick PB, Wong KS, Bae HJ, Pandey DK. Large artery intracranial occlusive disease: a large worldwide burden but a relatively neglected frontier. Stroke. 2008;39:2396–9.
32. Suri MFK, Zhou J, Qiao Y, Chu H, Qureshi AI, Mosley T, et al. Cognitive impairment and intracranial atherosclerotic stenosis in general population. Neurology. 2018;90:e1240–7.
33. Research Committee on the P, Treatment of Spontaneous Occlusion of the Circle of W, Health Labour Sciences Research Grant for Research on Measures for Infractable D. Guidelines for diagnosis and treatment of moyamoya disease (spontaneous occlusion of the circle of Willis). Neurol Med Chir. 2012;52:245–66.
34. Kim YJ, Lee JK, Ahn SH, Kim BJ, Kang DW, Kim JS, et al. Nonatheroscleotic isolated middle cerebral artery disease may be early manifestation of moyamoya disease. Stroke. 2016;47:2229–35.
35. Kim YJ, Kim BJ, Lee MH, Lee HB, Lee JS, Chang DI, et al. Are genetic variants associated with the location of cerebral arterial lesions in stroke patients? Cerebrovasc Dis. 2020;49:262–8.
36. Kim J, Park YS, Woo MH, An HJ, Kim JO, Park HS, et al. Distribution of intracranial major artery stenosis/occlusion according to rnf213 polymorphisms. Int J Mol Sci. 2020;21:1956.

37. Zhang T, Guo C, Liao X, Xia J, Wang X, Deng J, et al. Genetic analysis of rnf213 p.R4810k variant in non-moyamoya intracranial artery stenosis/occlusion disease in a chinese population. Environ Health Prev Med. 2017;22:41.
38. Xue S, Cheng W, Wang W, Song X, Wu J, Song H. The association between the ring finger protein 213 gene r4810k variant and intracranial major artery stenosis/occlusion in the han chinese population and high-resolution magnetic resonance imaging findings. Brain Circ. 2018;4:33–9.
39. Zhang Q, Yu L, Ge P, Ma Y, Zhang D, Zhang Y, et al. Association of ring finger protein 213 gene p.R4810k polymorphism with intracranial major artery stenosis/occlusion. J Stroke Cerebrovasc Dis. 2018;27:1556–64.
40. Sun X, Luo M, Li J, Lai R, Lin J, Wang Y, et al. Prevalence of rnf213 variants in symptomatic intracranial arterial stenosis/occlusion in China. Mol Gen Genomics. 2020;295:635–43.
41. Cao Y, Kobayashi H, Morimoto T, Kabata R, Harada KH, Koizumi A. Frequency of rnf213 p.R4810k, a susceptibility variant for moyamoya disease, and health characteristics of carriers in the japanese population. Environ Health Prev Med. 2016;21:387–90.
42. Kobayashi H, Brozman M, Kyselova K, Viszlayova D, Morimoto T, Roubec M, et al. Rnf213 rare variants in slovakian and czech moyamoya disease patients. PLoS One. 2016;11:e0164759.
43. Hongo H, Miyawaki S, Imai H, Shimizu M, Yagi S, Mitsui J, et al. Comprehensive investigation of rnf213 nonsynonymous variants associated with intracranial artery stenosis. Sci Rep. 2020;10:11942.
44. Guey S, Kraemer M, Herve D, Ludwig T, Kossorotoff M, Bergametti F, et al. Rare rnf213 variants in the c-terminal region encompassing the ring-finger domain are associated with moyamoya angiopathy in caucasians. Eur J Hum Genet. 2017;25:995–1003.
45. Hongo H, Miyawaki S, Imai H, Shinya Y, Ono H, Mori H, et al. Smaller outer diameter of atherosclerotic middle cerebral artery associated with rnf213 c.14576g>a variant (rs112735431). Surg Neurol Int. 2017;8:104.
46. Choi EH, Lee H, Chung JW, Seo WK, Kim GM, Ki CS, et al. Ring finger protein 213 variant and plaque characteristics, vascular remodeling, and hemodynamics in patients with intracranial atherosclerotic stroke: a high-resolution magnetic resonance imaging and hemodynamic study. J Am Heart Assoc. 2019;8:e011996.
47. Kamimura T, Okazaki S, Morimoto T, Kobayashi H, Harada K, Tomita T, et al. Prevalence of rnf213 p.R4810k variant in early-onset stroke with intracranial arterial stenosis. Stroke. 2019;50:1561–3.
48. Komiyama M. Cardio-cephalic neural crest syndrome: a novel hypothesis of vascular neurocristopathy. Interv Neuroradiol. 2017;23:572–6.
49. Komiyama M. Rnf213 genetic variant and the arterial circle of Willis. J Stroke Cerebrovasc Dis. 2018;27:2892–3.
50. Kim HJ, Choi EH, Chung JW, Kim JH, Kim YS, Seo WK, et al. Luminal and wall changes in intracranial arterial lesions for predicting stroke occurrence. Stroke. 2020;51:2495–504.
51. Okazaki S, Morimoto T, Kamatani Y, Kamimura T, Kobayashi H, Harada K, et al. Moyamoya disease susceptibility variant rnf213 p.R4810k increases the risk of ischemic stroke attributable to large-artery atherosclerosis. Biomed Res Int. 2019;139:295–8.
52. Morimoto T, Mineharu Y, Ono K, Nakatochi M, Ichihara S, Kabata R, et al. Significant association of rnf213 p.R4810k, a moyamoya susceptibility variant, with coronary artery disease. PLoS One. 2017;12:e0175649.
53. Bang OY, Chung JW, Kim DH, Won HH, Yeon JY, Ki CS, et al. Moyamoya disease and spectrums of rnf213 vasculopathy. Transl Stroke Res. 2019;11:580–9.
54. Hara S, Shimizu K, Nariai T, Kishino M, Kudo T, Umemoto T, et al. De novo renal artery stenosis developed in initially normal renal arteries during the long-term follow-up of patients with moyamoya disease. J Stroke Cerebrovasc Dis. 2020;29:104786.
55. Koyama S, Ito K, Terao C, Akiyama M, Horikoshi M, Momozawa Y, et al. Population-specific and trans-ancestry genome-wide analyses identify distinct and shared genetic risk loci for coronary artery disease. Nat Genet. 2020;52(11):1169–77.

56. Chang SA, Song JS, Park TK, Yang JH, Kwon WC, Kim SR, et al. Nonsyndromic peripheral pulmonary artery stenosis is associated with homozygosity of rnf213 p.Arg4810lys regardless of co-occurrence of moyamoya disease. Chest. 2018;153:404–13.
57. Suzuki H, Kataoka M, Hiraide T, Aimi Y, Yamada Y, Katsumata Y, et al. Genomic comparison with supercentenarians identifies rnf213 as a risk gene for pulmonary arterial hypertension. Circ Genom Precis Med. 2018;11:e002317.
58. Kobayashi H, Kabata R, Kinoshita H, Morimoto T, Ono K, Takeda M, et al. Rare variants in rnf213, a susceptibility gene for moyamoya disease, are found in patients with pulmonary hypertension and aggravate hypoxia-induced pulmonary hypertension in mice. Pulm Circ. 2018;8. 2045894018778155
59. Fukushima H, Takenouchi T, Kosaki K. Homozygosity for moyamoya disease risk allele leads to moyamoya disease with extracranial systemic and pulmonary vasculopathy. Am J Med Genet A. 2016;170:2453–6.
60. Hiraide T, Kataoka M, Suzuki H, Aimi Y, Chiba T, Isobe S, et al. Poor outcomes in carriers of the rnf213 variant (p.Arg4810lys) with pulmonary arterial hypertension. J Heart Lung Transplant. 2019;39(2):103–12.
61. Koizumi A, Kobayashi H, Hitomi T, Harada KH, Habu T, Youssefian S. A new horizon of moyamoya disease and associated health risks explored through rnf213. Environ Health Prev Med. 2016;21:55–70.
62. Sonobe S, Fujimura M, Niizuma K, Fujimura T, Furudate S, Nishijima Y, et al. Increased vascular mmp-9 in mice lacking rnf213: Moyamoya disease susceptibility gene. Neuroreport. 2014;25:1442–6.
63. Kanoke A, Fujimura M, Niizuma K, Ito A, Sakata H, Sato-Maeda M, et al. Temporal profile of the vascular anatomy evaluated by 9.4-tesla magnetic resonance angiography and histological analysis in mice with the r4859k mutation of rnf213, the susceptibility gene for moyamoya disease. Brain Res. 2015;1624:497–505.
64. Morimoto T, Enmi JI, Hattori Y, Iguchi S, Saito S, Harada KH. Dysregulation of rnf213 promotes cerebral hypoperfusion. Sci Rep. 2018;8:3607.
65. Scholz B, Korn C, Wojtarowicz J, Mogler C, Augustin I, Boutros M, et al. Endothelial rspo3 controls vascular stability and pruning through non-canonical wnt/ca(2+)/nfat signaling. Dev Cell. 2016;36:79–93.
66. Kobayashi H, Matsuda Y, Hitomi T, Okuda H, Shioi H, Matsuda T, et al. Biochemical and functional characterization of rnf213 (mysterin) r4810k, a susceptibility mutation of moyamoya disease, in angiogenesis in vitro and in vivo. J Am Heart Assoc. 2015;4:e002146.
67. Sugihara M, Morito D. The aaa+ atpase/ubiquitin ligase mysterin stabilizes cytoplasmic lipid droplets. J Cell Biol. 2019;218:949–60.
68. Ahel J, Lehner A, Vogel A, Schleiffer A, Meinhart A, Haselbach D, et al. Moyamoya disease factor rnf213 is a giant e3 ligase with a dynein-like core and a distinct ubiquitin-transfer mechanism. elife. 2020;9:e56185.
69. Bhardwaj A, Banh RS, Zhang W, Sidhu SS, Neel BG. Moyamoya disease-associated <em>rnf213</em> alleles encode dominant negative alleles that globally impair ubiquitylation. bioRxiv. 2020;2020:113795.

Part III

Pathophysiology of Moyamoya Disease

TIA and Headache in Pediatric Moyamoya Disease

7

Satoshi Kuroda

Abstract

This chapter precisely reviews the pathophysiology and clinical features of transient ischemic attack (TIA) and headache in pediatric moyamoya disease. Clinical features of TIA and headache are unique and almost specific for pediatric moyamoya disease. Therefore, the author strongly believes that the understanding of the mechanisms through which TIA and headache occur is quite important to know the moyamoya disease in depth and to perform appropriate surgical treatment for pediatric patients with moyamoya disease.

Keywords

Moyamoya disease · Children · TIA · Headache · Cerebral hemodynamics

7.1 Introduction

Moyamoya disease is known to frequently cause transient neurological symptoms such as transient ischemic attack (TIA) and headache attack in pediatric patients with moyamoya disease [1, 2]. The mechanisms through which these attacks occur are not fully understood, but we strongly believe that early diagnosis and early, appropriate surgical revascularization is the most important factor in preventing the neurological sequelae due to ischemia stroke in children with moyamoya disease.

S. Kuroda (✉)
Department of Neurosurgery, Graduate School of Medicine and Pharmaceutical Science, University of Toyama, Toyama, Japan
e-mail: skuroda@med.u-toyama.ac.jp

S. Kuroda (ed.), *Moyamoya Disease: Current Knowledge and Future Perspectives*, https://doi.org/10.1007/978-981-33-6404-2_7

In this chapter, we will discuss the mechanisms of TIAs and headache attacks in pediatric moyamoya disease by reviewing in detail previous studies on TIAs and headache attacks in pediatric patients with moyamoya disease.

7.2 Transient Ischemic Attack

7.2.1 Clinical Features and Mechanism

Moyamoya disease is known to cause transient ischemic attacks in many patients, both children and adults [1–3]. Since moyamoya disease essentially begins with a narrowing of the arteries around the terminal portion of the internal carotid artery, many of the neurological symptoms such as hemiparesis and aphasia are often attributed to the cerebral cortex in the frontal and/or temporal lobe. Especially in severe pediatric cases, however, unusual paraparesis, tetraparesis, or loss of consciousness may occur due to dense cerebral ischemia in the bilateral hemispheres [1]. In such cases, we should not misdiagnose it as epilepsy. On the other hand, it is well known that about 30% of patients with moyamoya disease also have stenotic lesions in the posterior cerebral artery (PCA) [4–9]. Disease progression in PCA has been reported to occur up to 15 years after surgical revascularization [10]. Because the PCA is a crucial source of collateral circulation in moyamoya disease, the involvement of PCA often causes neurological symptoms originating from not only the occipital lobe but also the adjacent parietal and posterior temporal lobes [7, 11]. The former includes visual symptoms such as homonymous hemianopsia, while the latter includes sensory aphasia and the numbness of the contralateral face and extremities.

The mechanism by which TIA occurs in moyamoya disease has not been specified. However, it is well known that cerebral hemodynamics is moderately impaired in pediatric moyamoya patients with TIA, but is markedly disturbed in them with ischemic stroke [12]. In addition, many of the infarcts are localized in the MCA-ACA or MCA-PCA watershed zone when TIA progresses to ischemic stroke (Fig. 7.1). These facts strongly suggest that hemodynamic ischemia is more likely involved in the occurrence of TIA than artery-to-artery embolism. This speculation is supported by the fact that the efficacy of antiplatelets is still controversial to prevent TIA and ischemic stroke [13, 14].

Clinical presentation of TIA in pediatric moyamoya disease is highly specific. It is widely known that TIA readily occurs after hyperventilation, such as crying or blowing a whistle or harmonica. However, there are almost no reports proving that TIA occurs after hyperventilation in adult cases of moyamoya disease, which suggests that the mechanism through which TIA occurs may differ between pediatric and adult cases. Previously, there are excellent reports on the mechanism of TIA in pediatric cases. Thus, it was already reported by several investigators in the 1970s, soon after the discovery of this disease, that hyperventilation-induced hypocapnia more distinctly reduced cerebral blood flow in patients with moyamoya disease than in healthy controls. It has also been reported that hypercapnia due to CO_2 loading causes little or no change in cerebral blood flow, or leads to an increase in cerebral

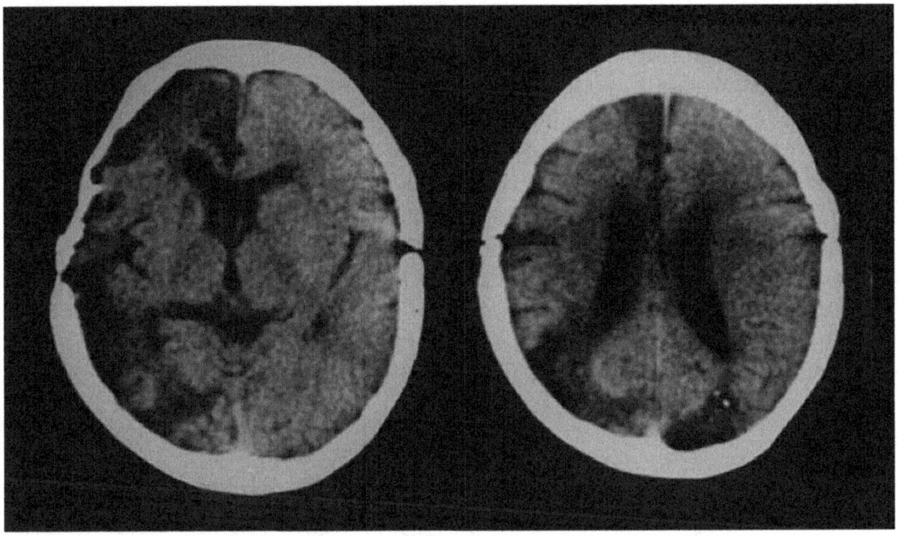

Fig. 7.1 Typical finding of plain CT scan in a 8-year-old boy who developed ischemic stroke. Note that cerebral infarction is mainly located in the borderzone between the MCA and ACA territories or between the MCA and PCA territories

blood flow in the temporo-occipital area but not in the frontal area [15–18]. Surgical revascularization improves the response of cerebral blood flow to hypercapnia [15]. At this time, Takeuchi et al. (1983) already hypothesized that *"a decrease in cerebral perfusion pressure may induce a maximally dilated state of the peripheral arterioles, leading to a loss of response to hypercapnia and an excessive reaction to hypocapnia*" and "*the pathophysiology may be most prominent in the frontal lobe in moyamoya disease*" (author's translation). These speculations are still true even in today's world where measurement techniques of cerebral blood flow and metabolism have advanced dramatically, and the author believes that the depth of the thinking of researchers at that time is extraordinary [18]. Then, Karasawa et al. (1986) precisely evaluated the findings on cerebral angiography during hypercapnia/hypocapnia. As the results, hypocapnia led to a decrease in arterial diameter in the arteries of the brain surface and in the moyamoya vessels of the basal ganglia. This change was more pronounced in the moyamoya vessels of the basal ganglia. Contrast opacification was also reduced in the MCA-ACA watershed zone [15]. Similar results have been reported by Takahashi et al. (1985) [19].

Specific response to hyperventilation in pediatric moyamoya disease has been also studied in the field of electrophysiology. Hyperventilation is known to induce synchronous slow waves on EEG in healthy children, which is observed in almost all parts of the brain and disappears with the cessation of hyperventilation. This phenomenon is called as "build up" phenomenon. In pediatric moyamoya disease, however, a few minutes after the build up disappears after hyperventilation, non-synchronous slow waves with higher amplitude occur, which is completely different from the build up phenomenon. This phenomenon, called re-build up phenomenon, is very specific to childhood moyamoya disease, and does not occur in adults with moyamoya disease (Fig. 7.2a). Because TIA has been often observed during re-build up phenomenon in pediatric moyamoya patients, several investigators have studied its pathophysiology using a variety of modalities to elucidate the mechanisms through which TIA develops in pediatric moyamoya disease [20]. Using ^{15}O positron emission tomography (PET), Kameyama et al. (1986) serially measured cerebral blood flow (CBF) and cerebral metabolic rate for oxygen ($CMRO_2$) before and after hyperventilation in three pediatric cases of moyamoya disease. As the results, both CBF and $CMRO_2$ significantly decreased in response to 3-min hyperventilation. A decrease in $CMRO_2$ was more pronounced than that in CBF. More interestingly, continuous measurement of PaO_2 and $PaCO_2$ revealed that hyperventilation led to an increase in PaO_2 as well as a decrease in $PaCO_2$ during

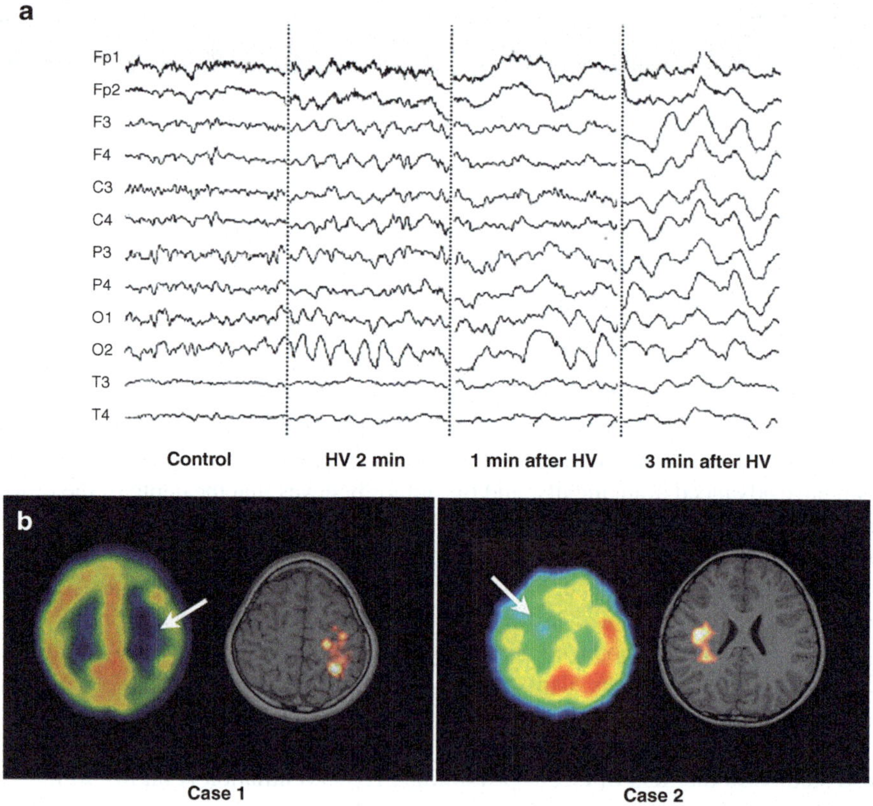

Fig. 7.2 (**a**) Typical EEG finding in a 4-year-old girl demonstrating the build up phenomenon during hyperventilation (HV) and the re-build up phenomenon after the cessation of HV. (**b**) Representative findings of acetazolamide-loaded cerebral blood flow map on SPECT and MEG in a 8-year-old girl (*left*) and a 12-year-old boy (*right*). Note a strong correlation between the area with impaired reactivity to acetazolamide (arrows) and the localization of original current dipoles of re-build up phenomenon

hyperventilation, and then the cessation of hyperventilation induced a rapid fall of PaO_2 as well as a gradual recovery of $PaCO_2$. They speculated that re-build up phenomenon may occur through not only ischemic hypoxia but also hypoxic hypoxia probably because of respiratory inhibition in response to PaO_2 elevation during hyperventilation [21]. Using ^{133}xenon inhalation method and single photon emission tomography (SPECT), Isobe and co-workers measured CBF before and after hyperventilation in 11 pediatric patients with moyamoya disease, and found a strong correlation between the areas where the re-build up phenomenon emerges on EEG and the areas where CBF markedly decreases after hyperventilation [22, 23]. Kuroda et al. (1995) reported that the re-build up phenomenon originated from the cerebral cortex where cerebrovascular reactivity to acetazolamide is severely impaired and disappeared after effective surgical revascularization [24]. In addition, they first applied near-infrared spectroscopy (NIRS) into this research field and continuously measured cerebral oxygenation state before and after hyperventilation in two pediatric patients. NIRS is known capable to monitor the changes in the concentrations of oxidized hemoglobin (oxy-Hb), deoxidized hemoglobin (deoxy-Hb), and total Hb (tHb) through the detectors put on the scalp noninvasively and to have a good time resolution (one datum per second). As the results, hyperventilation promptly decreased the concentrations of oxy-Hb and tHb in the frontal area on NIRS, causing the build up phenomenon. When the hyperventilation was stopped, the build up phenomenon disappeared, but the concentrations of oxy-Hb and tHb remained lower than the control value. Then, the concentration of oxy-Hb further decreased and the concentration of deoxy-Hb started to increase, leading to the occurrence of the re-build up phenomenon. Thereafter, the re-build up phenomenon disappeared as the parameters on NIRS gradually recovered to their control values. The results strongly suggest that the involved brain is exposed to more severe hypoxia after the cessation of hyperventilation than during hyperventilation in pediatric moyamoya disease [25]. The findings on NIRS correlates very well with those on ^{15}O PET reported by Kameyama et al. [21]. Subsequently, Qiao et al. (2003) first analyzed the spontaneous magnetic brain activity on a whole-head magnetoencephalography (MEG) system during and after hyperventilation in four pediatric patients with moyamoya disease. They found that the original current dipoles of the re-build up slow waves were mainly originating from the deep cortical sulci in the area where cerebrovascular reserve was disturbed on SPECT (Fig. 7.2b) [26]. However, no subsequent studies have been reported to elucidate the mechanism of the re-build up phenomenon in moyamoya disease, probably because the risk of TIA and ischemic stroke due to hyperventilation has reduced the availability of EEG itself.

7.2.2 Natural Course of TIA

Many pediatric patients have been reported to develop ischemic stroke after they repeated TIAs. In fact, Maki et al. (1976) reported that 8 of 24 pediatric patients had a poor outcome. Of these, one patient died of acute subdural hematoma, two had a severe motor and mental deficits, and the other five required special education. They concluded that their functional outcome was "good" in one-thirds, "borderline" in one-third, and "poor" in one-thirds, and that repeated TIAs followed by ischemic stroke was one of the determinants to predict poor outcome [27]. Kurokawa et al. also reported that the prevalence of patients with mild-to-severe disabilities increased up to about 50% with duration of illness [28]. Such a transition from TIA to ischemic stroke may result from severe cerebral ischemia since the onset of the disease as well as from a stepwise deterioration of cerebral hemodynamics in response to a disease progression.

On the other hand, however, several reports have shown that the frequency of TIAs gradually declines through adolescence in patients with repeated TIAs only and no conversion to ischemic stroke [28–30]. In fact, Kurokawa et al. (1985) reported that TIAs frequently occurred during the first 4 years after the onset and the frequency decreased thereafter [28]. This phenomenon may be related to the fact that the incidence of moyamoya disease is high in children between the ages of 5 and 15 years, but is much lower in young adults around the age of 20 years. Although the mechanism is not entirely understood, the author speculates that it is closely related to the fact that cerebral blood flow in children drastically changes with growth. In children, cerebral blood flow is reported to greatly vary with growth; Using the ^{133}xenon inhalation method, Takeuchi et al. (1983) measured the mean CBF value in healthy children and found that the mean value of CBF was 67.7 ml/min/100 g in healthy children (7–17 years of age), but was 53.6 ml/min/100 g of CBF in healthy adults (22–67 years old). They also found a more pronounced decrease in CBF with growth in children than in adults [18]. Subsequently, Ogawa et al. (1990) also measured CBF in healthy children and adults, and reported that CBF was higher than 100 ml/min/100 g in infants, but rapidly declined by age of 20 years followed by a gradual decline thereafter. According to their data, the changes in CBF showed a nonlinear curve as follows [31]:

$$\mathrm{Y} = 146.5 - 58.4 \log \mathrm{X}, \text{where X is the age} \left(P < 0.01, \mathrm{R} = -0.903\right).$$

Kuroda et al. (1993) also reported a negative correlation between CBF and age in healthy children. More interestingly, they found that once surgical revascularization improved CBF in children with moyamoya disease, CBF gradually declined with growth, just as it does in healthy children [12]. These dynamic profiles of CBF in children are most likely linked to those of brain metabolism. Thus, Kennedy and Sokoloff (1957) showed that brain oxygen utilization was about 1.3 times higher in children than in adults [32]. Chugani et al. (1987) measured cerebral metabolic rate for glucose (CMRGlc) using PET, and concluded that the value was very low at birth, increased by 3 to 4 years old, and continued at high levels until 9 years old, when the value started to decrease, reaching adult value by the latter part of the second decade [33].

Based on these observations, I speculate the mechanism through which TIA decreases in frequency with growth as follows: Children with severely impaired cerebral hemodynamics since the onset of the disease repeat TIAs and develop ischemic stroke within several years, leading to a poor functional outcome. On the other

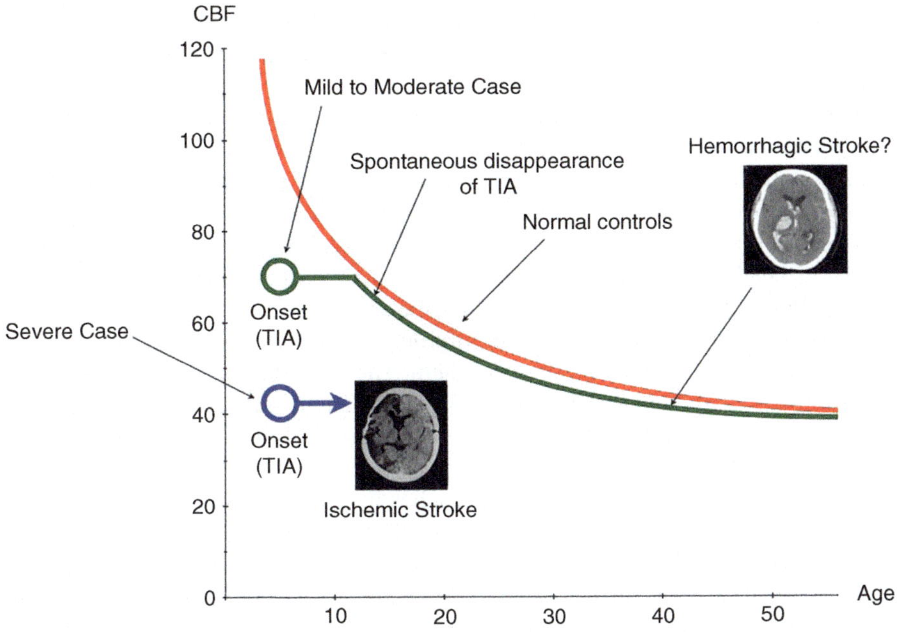

Fig. 7.3 A diagram demonstrating Kuroda's theory about the relationship between the age and cerebral blood flow (CBF) in healthy children (*red*) and moyamoya patients with severe (*blue*) and mild-to-moderate CBF decrease (*green*). See the text in detail

hand, children with mild-to-moderate impairment of cerebral hemodynamics at the onset will grow up with repeated TIAs. Because normal CBF levels gradually decline with growth, it is likely that patients' CBF levels will not differ much from healthy controls at some point in time and the frequency of TIAs may gradually decrease and even disappear (Fig. 7.3). So, it is not surprising that there are not a small number of cases of repeated mild TIAs in childhood that were not diagnosed as moyamoya disease in the hospital, but in time their TIAs disappeared and they became adults. Some of them may go their entire lives without experiencing any stroke. But, some others may develop the rupture of dilated, fragile moyamoya vessels due to a long-lasting hemodynamic stress, causing hemorrhagic stroke at around the age of 40 years (Fig. 7.3). In fact, a recent cohort study has found that adult moyamoya disease that may have occurred in childhood was associated with a higher incidence of hemorrhagic stroke than adult-onset moyamoya disease, with a higher incidence of lenticulostriate and choroidal channels as spontaneous collaterals [34].

7.3 Headache Attack

As with TIA, the clinical presentation of headache attacks in pediatric moyamoya disease is very different from that of adults. The occurrence of headache attacks in pediatric moyamoya disease appears to have been recognized soon after the disease was discovered, but scientific analysis did not start to be done until the 1990s. Since then, several case reports have pointed out that children with moyamoya disease develop migraine-like headaches [35–38].

For these two decades, there are several reports on headache attacks with relatively large cohorts [39–42]. According to these reports, the frequency of pediatric patients with headache attacks ranges from 22 to 38% of all pediatric patients. Their ages are distributed throughout childhood. There is no difference in age or gender between children with and without headache attacks [39–42]. Some children have recurrent headaches alone, while others have recurrent headaches and TIAs. In some patients, TIAs may occur with headache attacks [42].

Typically, their headache resembles migraine without aura and is associated with nausea and/or vomiting in one-thirds of them. Their headache usually occurs in the morning, especially when they woke up [39, 42]. Their headache attacks are often severe, because most of them cannot go to their school or kindergarten. The frequency of headache attacks was every day, every week, or every month in most of the cases. All of them repeat severe headaches in the unilateral or bilateral frontal and/or temporal area [39, 40]. Symptomatic drugs are not effective to relieve them [42]. Therefore, it should be stated that headache attacks in pediatric moyamoya disease are quite frequent and have a significant impact on daily life, including school [39]. Headache attacks usually resolve spontaneously in about 2–5 h [39, 40]. As a result, many pediatric patients complain of a headache in the morning and miss school but feel fine by noon, so their mothers who do not know that moyamoya disease is the cause may even suspect that their child is skipping school by pretending to have a headache.

These observations strongly suggest that the mechanisms of TIA and headache attack development are in very close proximity. Suzuki's angiographical stage is more advanced in pediatric patients with headache attacks than in those without [39]. Using cold xenon CT, Okada et al. (2012) measured CBF in the MCA territory, but found no significant difference in CBF between headache group and non-headache group. In pediatric patients, cerebrovascular reactivity (CVR) to acetazolamide was lower in headache group than in non-headache group, although statistical significance was borderline probably due to a small sample size [41]. Subsequently, however, Kawabori et al. (2012) reported that a decreased CBF and impaired CVR to acetazolamide were significant predictors for the occurrence of headache attacks. More importantly, there was a very strong correlation between the localization of headache and the area with impaired cerebral hemodynamics [39].

Several investigators have also evaluated the therapeutic effect of surgical revascularization on headache attacks in pediatric moyamoya disease. Thus, headache remained in 25 to 63% of patients after EDAS surgery [40, 42]. At least a 2-month period is required to resolve headaches after EDAS [43]. On the other hand, Okada et al. (2012) reported that headache markedly improved in 23 of 25 patients just after STA-MCA double anastomosis and advocated the superiority of direct bypass over EDAS in treating headache attacks. In their surgical procedures, two branches of the STA were anastomosed to two cortical branches of the MCA feeding to the frontal and temporal lobe, respectively [41]. Kawabori et al. (2013) demonstrated that headache completely disappeared in all patients within 2 weeks after STA-MCA single or double anastomosis and encephaloduro-myo-arterio-pericranial synangiosis (EDMAPS). They also anastomosed one of the STA branches to the frontal branch of the MCA. On postoperative cerebral angiography, surgical collaterals widely provided collateral blood flow to the operated hemispheres through direct and indirect bypass, including the area with a headache before surgery. Postoperative CBF study also revealed that both CBF and CVR significantly improved in the operated hemispheres, including the area where patients repeated headache before surgery [39].

These facts strongly suggest that persistent cerebral ischemia is closely involved in the development of migraine-like headache attacks in pediatric moyamoya disease [39, 41]. As mentioned above, most headache attacks occur primarily in the frontal region. However, EDAS primarily improves cerebral hemodynamics only in the parietal region, so a significant number of patients may still experience headache attacks even after EDAS. In addition, indirect bypass procedures such as EDAS require several months to complete angiogenesis between the donor tissues and brain surface (see Chap. 18), which may delay the resolution of headache after EDAS. On the other hand, STA-MCA anastomosis with or without indirect bypass has a great potential to improve cerebral hemodynamics in the frontal lobe just after surgery by anastomosing the STA branch to the frontal branch of the MCA. The fact may be able to explain the reason why headache attacks quickly disappear after STA-MCA anastomosis targeted to the frontal lobe [39, 41]. More scientifically, Olesen et al. (1993) reported three patients who had repeated migraine episodes because of severe stenosis or occlusion of the internal carotid artery. All of them had reduced cerebral blood flow in the involved hemispheres. They hypothesized that borderline ischemia may increase the risk of spreading cortical depression and lower the threshold for developing migraine, thereby inducing aura with or without headaches [44]. Their hypothesis is extremely interesting in considering the mechanism of headache attacks in pediatric moyamoya disease.

Acknowledgment This work was partly supported by a grant from the Research Committee on Moyamoya Disease, the Japanese Ministry of Health, Labour and Welfare.

References

1. Kuroda S, Houkin K. Moyamoya disease: current concepts and future perspectives. Lancet Neurol. 2008;7:1056–66.
2. Suzuki J, Takaku A. Cerebrovascular "moyamoya" disease. Disease showing abnormal net-like vessels in base of brain. Arch Neurol. 1969;20:288–99.
3. Fukui M. Current state of study on moyamoya disease in Japan. Surg Neurol. 1997;47:138–43.
4. Funaki T, Takahashi JC, Takagi Y, Yoshida K, Araki Y, Kikuchi T, Kataoka H, Iihara K, Miyamoto S. Impact of posterior cerebral artery involvement on long-term clinical and social outcome of pediatric moyamoya disease. J Neurosurg Pediatr. 2013;12:626–32.
5. Kuroda S, Ishikawa T, Houkin K, Iwasaki Y. Clinical significance of posterior cerebral artery stenosis/occlusion in moyamoya disease. No Shinkei Geka. 2002;30:1295–300.

6. Lee JY, Kim SK, Cheon JE, Choi JW, Phi JH, Kim IO, Cho BK, Wang KC. Posterior cerebral artery involvement in moyamoya disease: initial infarction and angle between PCA and basilar artery. Childs Nerv Syst. 2013;29:2263–9.
7. Miyamoto S, Kikuchi H, Karasawa J, Nagata I, Ihara I, Yamagata S. Study of the posterior circulation in moyamoya disease. Part 2: visual disturbances and surgical treatment. J Neurosurg. 1986;65:454–60.
8. Miyamoto S, Kikuchi H, Karasawa J, Nagata I, Ikota T, Takeuchi S. Study of the posterior circulation in moyamoya disease. Clinical and neuroradiological evaluation. J Neurosurg. 1984;61:1032–7.
9. Mugikura S, Takahashi S, Higano S, Shirane R, Kurihara N, Furuta S, Ezura M, Takahashi A. The relationship between cerebral infarction and angiographic characteristics in childhood moyamoya disease. AJNR Am J Neuroradiol. 1999;20:336–43.
10. Kuroda S, Nakayama N, Yamamoto S, Kashiwazaki D, Uchino H, Saito H, Hori E, Akioka N, Kuwayama N, Houkin K. Late (5-20 years) outcomes after STA-MCA anastomosis and encephalo-duro-myo-arterio-pericranial synangiosis in patients with moyamoya disease. J Neurosurg. 2020;1:1–8.
11. Saito H, Kashiwazaki D, Uchino H, Yamamoto S, Houkin K, Kuroda S. Specific clinical features and one-stage revascularization surgery for moyamoya disease with severe cerebral ischemia in the territory of posterior cerebral artery. Acta Neurochir. 2020;2020:1–10.
12. Kuroda S, Kamiyama H, Abe H, Yamauchi T, Kohama Y, Houkin K, Mitsumori K. Cerebral blood flow in children with spontaneous occlusion of the circle of Willis (moyamoya disease): comparison with healthy children and evaluation of annual changes. Neurol Med Chir (Tokyo). 1993;33:434–8.
13. Kraemer M, Berlit P, Diesner F, Khan N. What is the expert's option on antiplatelet therapy in moyamoya disease? Results of a worldwide survey. Eur J Neurol. 2012;19:163–7.
14. Yamada S, Oki K, Itoh Y, Kuroda S, Houkin K, Tominaga T, Miyamoto S, Hashimoto N, Suzuki N, Research Committee on Spontaneous Occlusion of Circle of W. Effects of surgery and antiplatelet therapy in ten-year follow-up from the registry study of research committee on Moyamoya disease in Japan. J Stroke Cerebrovasc Dis. 2016;25:340–9.
15. Karasawa J, Kikuchi H, Nagata I, Naruo Y, Ihara I, Nakagawara J, Miyamoto S, Hashimoto K, Kuriyama Y. Cerebral hemodynamics in moyamoya disease. Significance of cerebral blood flow in relation to changes in arterial CO2 tension. Neurol Med Chir (Tokyo). 1986;26:695–700.
16. Nagaya T, Nukui H, Miyagi O, Tamada J. Cerebral hemodynamics in cases with "moyamoya" disease. Neurol Med Chir (Tokyo). 1982;22:707–15.
17. Nishimoto A, Onbe H, Ueta K. Clinical and cerebral blood flow study in moyamoya disease with TIA. Acta Neurol Scand. 1979;60(Suppl 72):434–5.
18. Takeuchi S. Cerebral hemodynamics in patients with moyamoya disease (part II). Evaluation of regional cerebral blood flow by 133Xe inhalation methods. Neurol Med Chir (Tokyo). 1983;23:720–8.
19. Takahashi A, Fujiwara S, Suzuki J. Cerebral angiography following hyperventilation in moyamoya disease--in reference to the "re-build up" phenomenon on EEG. No Shinkei Geka. 1985;13:255–64.
20. Kodama N, Aoki Y, Hiraga H, Wada T, Suzuki J. Electroencephalographic findings in children with moyamoya disease. Arch Neurol. 1979;36:16–9.
21. Kameyama M, Shirane R, Tsurumi Y, Takahashi A, Fujiwara S, Suzuki J, Ito M, Ido T. Evaluation of cerebral blood flow and metabolism in childhood moyamoya disease: an investigation into "re-build-up" on EEG by positron CT. Childs Nerv Syst. 1986;2:130–3.
22. Isobe M, Kuroda S, Kamiyama H, Abe H, Mitumori K. Cerebral blood flow reactivity to hyperventilation in children with spontaneous occlusion of the circle of Willis (moyamoya disease). No Shinkei Geka. 1992;20:399–407.
23. Kazumata K, Kuroda S, Houkin K, Abe H, Mitumori K. Regional cerebral hemodynamics during re-build-up phenomenon in childhood moyamoya disease. An analysis using 99mTc-HMPAO SPECT. Childs Nerv Syst. 1996;12:161–5.

24. Kuroda S, Kamiyama H, Isobe M, Houkin K, Abe H, Mitsumori K. Cerebral hemodynamics and “re-build-up” phenomenon on electroencephalogram in children with moyamoya disease. Childs Nerv Syst. 1995;11:214–9.
25. Kuroda S, Houkin K, Hoshi Y, Tamura M, Kazumata K, Abe H. Cerebral hypoxia after hyperventilation causes “re-build-up” phenomenon and TIA in childhood moyamoya disease. A near-infrared spectroscopy study. Childs Nerv Syst. 1996;12:448–52. discussion 453
26. Qiao F, Kuroda S, Kamada K, Houkin K, Iwasaki Y. Source localization of the re-build up phenomenon in pediatric moyamoya disease-a dipole distribution analysis using MEG and SPECT. Childs Nerv Syst. 2003;19:760–4.
27. Maki Y, Nakada Y, Nose T, Yoshii Y. Clinical and radioisotopic follow-up study of 'Moyamoya. Childs Brain. 1976;2:257–71.
28. Kurokawa T, Tomita S, Ueda K, Narazaki O, Hanai T, Hasuo K, Matsushima T, Kitamura K. Prognosis of occlusive disease of the circle of Willis (moyamoya disease) in children. Pediatr Neurol. 1985;1:274–7.
29. Fukuyama Y, Umezu R. Clinical and cerebral angiographic evolutions of idiopathic progressive occlusive disease of the circle of Willis (“moyamoya” disease) in children. Brain and Development. 1985;7:21–37.
30. Imaizumi T, Hayashi K, Saito K, Osawa M, Fukuyama Y. Long-term outcomes of pediatric moyamoya disease monitored to adulthood. Pediatr Neurol. 1998;18:321–5.
31. Ogawa A, Yoshimoto T, Suzuki J, Sakurai Y. Cerebral blood flow in moyamoya disease. Part 1: correlation with age and regional distribution. Acta Neurochir. 1990;105:30–4.
32. Kennedy C, Sokoloff L. An adaptation of the nitrous oxide method to the study of the cerebral circulation in children; normal values for cerebral blood flow and cerebral metabolic rate in childhood. J Clin Invest. 1957;36:1130–7.
33. Chugani HT, Phelps ME, Mazziotta JC. Positron emission tomography study of human brain functional development. Ann Neurol. 1987;22:487–97.
34. Yamamoto S, Kashiwazaki D, Uchino H, Saito H, Akioka N, Kuwayama N, Kuroda S. Clinical and radiological features of childhood onset adult Moyamoya disease: implication for hemorrhagic stroke. Neurol Med Chir (Tokyo). 2020;60:360–7.
35. Aydin K, Okuyaz C, Gucuyener K, Serdaroglu A, Akpek S. Moyamoya disease presented with migrainelike headache in a 4-year-old girl. J Child Neurol. 2003;18:361–3.
36. Liu X-F, Jung DK. Moyamoya disease and migrain-like headaches. Schweiz Arch Neurol Psychiatr. 1999;150:272–4.
37. Park-Matsumoto YC, Tazawa T, Shimizu J. Migraine with aura-like headache associated with moyamoya disease. Acta Neurol Scand. 1999;100:119–21.
38. Sewell RA, Johnson DJ, Fellows DW. Cluster headache associated with moyamoya. J Headache Pain. 2009;10:65–7.
39. Kawabori M, Kuroda S, Nakayama N, Hirata K, Shiga T, Houkin K, Tamaki N. Effective surgical revascularization improves cerebral hemodynamics and resolves headache in pediatric Moyamoya disease. World Neurosurg. 2013;80:612–9.
40. Matsushima Y, Aoyagi M, Nariai T, Nojiri T, Ohno K. Headache in pediatric moyamoya patients: pre- and postoperative changes. Nerv Syst Child (Jpn). 2000;25:442–7.
41. Okada Y, Kawamata T, Kawashima A, Yamaguchi K, Ono Y, Hori T. The efficacy of superficial temporal artery-middle cerebral artery anastomosis in patients with moyamoya disease complaining of severe headache. J Neurosurg. 2012;116:672–9.
42. Seol HJ, Wang KC, Kim SK, Hwang YS, Kim KJ, Cho BK. Headache in pediatric moyamoya disease: review of 204 consecutive cases. J Neurosurg. 2005;103:439–42.
43. Matsushima Y. Facts and myths on indirect anastomosis as a treatment of moyamoya disease. Surg Cereb Stroke (Jpn). 2000;28:104–10.
44. Olesen J, Friberg L, Olsen TS, Andersen AR, Lassen NA, Hansen PE, Karle A. Ischaemia-induced (symptomatic) migraine attacks may be more frequent than migraine-induced ischaemic insults. Brain. 1993;116(Pt 1):187–202.

Ischemic Stroke

8

Haruto Uchino and Kiyohiro Houkin

Abstract

Ischemic stroke in moyamoya disease (MMD) is caused by cerebral hypoperfusion due to insufficient development of collateral circulation after the progression of steno-occlusive lesions. Although cerebral infarction is not a majority onset in ischemic MMD, its occurrence can cause severe neurological deficits or cognitive dysfunctions. Infarct patterns are greatly affected by collateral pathway. Therefore, patients with MMD may show different infarct patterns from those with conventional ischemic stroke due to atherosclerotic disease. In addition to cerebral blood flow, multiple parameters such as cerebrovascular reactivity, cerebral blood volume, and oxygen extraction fraction are generally measured using positron emission tomography or single photon emission computed tomography to evaluate hemodynamic or metabolic status and stratify the risk of future stroke. Magnetic resonance imaging and cerebral angiography are adjunctive modalities for that purpose. Thus, the assessment of hemodynamic compromise is essential for the optimal treatment and verification of performing revascularization surgery for patients with ischemic MMD.

Keywords

Cerebral infarction · Cerebral perfusion pressure · Cerebral blood flow · Cerebrovascular reactivity · Cerebral blood volume · Oxygen extraction fraction · Ischemic stroke

H. Uchino (✉) · K. Houkin
Department of Neurosurgery, Hokkaido University, Sapporo, Japan
e-mail: uchino-hok@umin.ac.jp; houkin@med.hokudai.ac.jp

S. Kuroda (ed.), *Moyamoya Disease: Current Knowledge and Future Perspectives*, https://doi.org/10.1007/978-981-33-6404-2_8

8.1 Introduction

The main mechanism for cerebral infarction in moyamoya disease (MMD) is cerebral hemodynamic ischemia due to insufficient development of collateral circulation caused by progression of the steno-occlusive lesions. Cerebral microembolism may also play an alternative role and transient embolic signals have been observed by transcranial Doppler sonography in a few cases [1]. However, cerebral hemodynamic compromise is considered as the main cause of ischemic symptoms, and the incidence of embolic signals in patients with MMD is lower than that in patients with atherosclerotic lesions [1]. Cerebral infarctions are often multiple and occur in watershed areas in MMD (Fig. 8.1). Ischemic events, such as transient ischemic attacks or cerebral infarction, are more frequent in pediatric patients than in adult patients, as adult patients may present with hemorrhagic as well as ischemic stroke. Furthermore, patients under 3 years of age often show an aggressive clinical course, presenting with sudden onset of infarction. Forty percent of them experience a recurrence of ischemic stroke in a short time span while awaiting revascularization surgery [2]. A registry study from Japan showed that cerebral infarction accounted

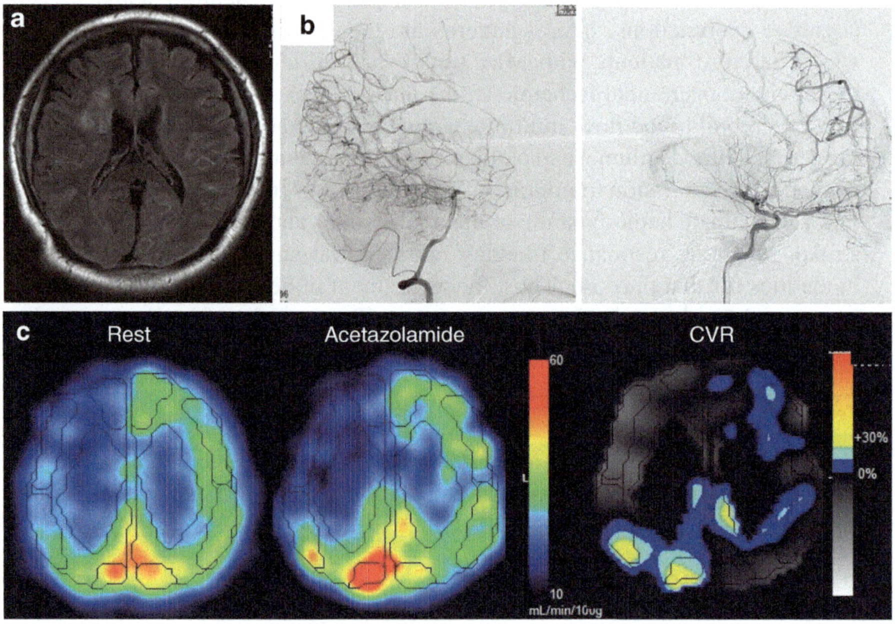

Fig. 8.1 Radiological findings of an adult patient. (**a**) Fluid-attenuated inversion-recovery imaging demonstrates subcortical infarction in anterior deep watershed area of the right frontal lobe and clear ivy signs in the sulci of bilateral hemispheres. (**b**) Lateral views of right internal carotid angiography and right vertebral angiography indicate insufficient collateral circulation in the anterior watershed area. (**c**) Single photon emission computed tomography scans reveal decline in the cerebral blood flow and cerebrovascular reactivity (CVR) in bilateral frontal lobes, where the hemodynamic status in the right hemisphere is worse than that in the left

for 22% of all patients with a recent onset of MMD, and that the proportion of adult patients with MMD experiencing initial ischemic events has been increasing recently [3]. In contrast to East Asian countries, including Japan, that have a greater proportion (~ 30%) of adult patients presenting with hemorrhage, the significant majority of adult patients in Western countries present with ischemic symptoms [3, 4]. Female patients and those with a prior history of stroke are reported to be at a greater risk of experiencing subsequent ischemic events [4].

8.2 Symptomatology

The initial clinical signs of infarction in patients with MMD rely on the location and size of the injury, and may include neurological deficits, recurrent transient ischemic attacks, headache, seizures, and alteration of consciousness [5]. When posterior cerebral artery (PCA) lesions progress and occipital infarction occurs, visual disturbances are frequently seen [6, 7]. Motor weakness affecting the lower extremities is also clinically relevant for ischemia resulting from PCA lesions since the posterior pericallosal arteries supply the medial part of the precentral area more so than the anterior cerebral artery does. One of the reasons infarction occurs more frequently in patients younger than 3 years of age may be because they cannot voice transient ischemic attack symptoms and these become apparent to their caregivers only after they develop infarction [8]. Multiple infarctions and chronic ischemic injury can lead to cognitive dysfunction and poor social outcomes in both pediatric and adult patients [9–12]. Intelligence is the main cognitive function adversely affected in pediatric patients, whereas adult patients commonly experience impaired executive function [11]. A previous study on pediatric patients showed that cortical infarction showed a more significant association with a poor intellectual outcome compared to white matter infarction [9]. While executive functioning is generally attributed to the frontal lobes [13], ischemic stroke in the parietal and occipital regions is also associated with impairment of executive function [10].

8.3 Radiological Features: Locations and Collateral Flows

Infarct patterns are greatly affected by the collateral pathway and vulnerability of the brain to ischemia and therefore patients with MMD may show different infarct patterns to patients with conventional ischemic stroke caused by atherosclerotic disease. The involvement of the PCAs is a key factor contributing to ischemic stroke in MMD and it is observed in approximately 30% of pediatric and adult patients at initial diagnosis [14, 15]. Thus, patients with PCA lesions experience cerebral infarction more frequently than those without [15]. The mechanism of cerebral ischemia in this case may mainly be due to a decrease in the collateral flow from the PCA. In MMD, the arteries of the posterior circulation are crucial in compensating for the weakened anterior circulation when stenosis of the internal carotid artery (ICA) and middle cerebral artery progresses. In addition, the collateral flow from the PCA via the posterior communicating artery is very important in reducing the incidence of border zone infarction, and the proximal ICA steno-occlusive lesion is reported to be significantly associated with the incidence of ischemic stroke [16, 17].

A North American study of pediatric patients categorized infarct patterns into cortical, subcortical, and watershed infarctions [5]. More than half of the patients showed infarction in the watershed border zone, in particular the deep watershed zone. This is because the watershed zone is especially vulnerable to reduction in cerebral perfusion in MMD. The location of ischemic stroke may further vary depending on the disease stage. Previous studies have shown that cerebral infarctions tend to be distributed throughout the anterior watershed area in less advanced cases, while lesions were often located in the posterior watershed area or the PCA territory in more advanced cases [18, 19]. In addition, the subcortical area of the watershed zone was likely involved in less advanced cases, whereas the outer cortical and wider area were involved in more advanced cases [19]. Another study done in Korea categorized the patterns of infarction in pediatric and adult patients into gyral, atypical territorial, honeycomb, classic territorial, multiple-dot, border zone, and deep lacunar [20]. This study demonstrated that the gyral pattern was the most common, while the deep lacunar was seen less frequently. Among the pediatric patients gyral and border zone infarcts were more frequent, whereas the classical territorial pattern was more frequently encountered in adult patients. The location of the infarct was confined to the cortex more frequently in pediatric patients, whereas simultaneous cortical and subcortical infarctions were more common in adult patients.

Lacunar infarction occurs less frequently and is reportedly detected in 11.8%–16.2% of adult patients and 2.5% of pediatric patients with MMD [20, 21]. The lower incidence of lacunar infarction, when compared to other patterns of infarction, may be attributed to chronic perfusion compromise and the development of basal moyamoya vessels. Another study showed a lower incidence of recurrent stroke and better functional outcome in patients with lacunar infarction compared to those with non-lacunar infarctions [21].

8.4 Cerebral Hemodynamic Compromise

Hemodynamic compromise plays a major role in the risk of ischemic stroke in patients with MMD. Surgical revascularization is an effective treatment to improve cerebral perfusion in such cases. Assessment of hemodynamic status is essential in deciding an optimal treatment plan for each patient and justifying an invasive surgical option when necessary.

8.4.1 Compensatory Mechanisms against Cerebral Perfusion Pressure Decrease

As arterial stenosis progresses, cerebral perfusion pressure (CPP) may decrease in the distal circulation. The extent of this decrease is affected by the degree of stenosis as well as the development of collateral flow. However, arterial stenosis does not always consistently predict the decrease in CPP. There are two autoregulatory mechanisms to maintain the supply of oxygen and glucose to the brain when CPP decreases.

The first mechanism is vascular autoregulation, which regulates vascular resistance via dilation of arterioles to maintain cerebral blood flow (CBF) within the normal range. This condition is detected by an increase in cerebral blood volume (CBV), and is described as Powers stage I [22, 23]. Vascular mean transit time (MTT) is defined as the ratio of CBV to CBF. Prolonged MTT is used to detect arteriolar dilation. The second mechanism is metabolic compensation, via an increased oxygen extraction fraction (OEF). OEF can increase to maintain normal oxygen metabolism (cerebral metabolic rate of oxygen [$CMRO_2$]), when there is a reduction in CBF or oxygen supply. This condition is called misery perfusion [24], or Powers stage II [23].

Derdeyn et al. proposed a modified model of compensatory responses to CPP reduction (Fig. 8.2) [25]. In the autoregulatory range, CBF decreases and OEF increases slightly to maintain $CMRO_2$. CBV may not change or may increase. When autoregulatory capacity is exceeded, it leads to a sharp decrease in CBF and increase in OEF and MTT. CBV may increase slightly, remain elevated, or continue to increase. Further decrease in CPP exceeds the capacity of compensation and results

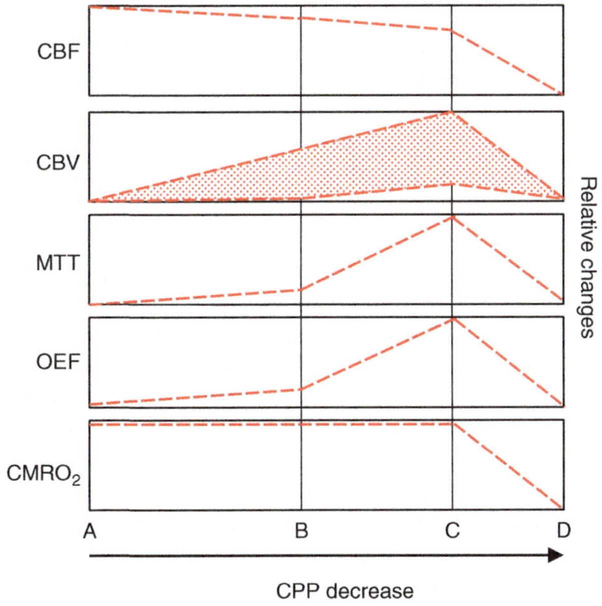

Fig. 8.2 Schema of hemodynamic and metabolic changes in response to reductions in cerebral perfusion pressure [25]. The area between points A and B represents the autoregulatory range. The area between points B and C represents the points that exceed the limits of autoregulation. The area between C and D represents the exhaustion of compensatory mechanisms to maintain normal oxygen metabolism. Point D represents neuronal death. *CBF* Cerebral blood flow, *CBV* Cerebral blood volume, *MTT* Mean transit time, *OEF* Oxygen extraction fraction

in cerebral infarction. In this model, the first modification is that a slight decrease in CBF leads to an increase in OEF through the autoregulatory range of CPP reduction. Second, CBV measurements may be variable through the autoregulatory range. This is because CBV is a complex physiological parameter; it is composed of arterial, capillary, and venous compartments. There may be individual biological variability in the cerebral vasodilatory response to reduced CPP. Thus, this modified model describes OEF and CBV as independent parameters and does not clearly define stages I and II as defined by Powers et al., reflecting the reality of hemodynamic status in patients with cerebral ischemia.

8.4.2 Evaluation of Cerebral Perfusion Pressure Decrease

Certain patterns of collateral blood flow are correlated with hemodynamic compromise in MMD. However, anatomical angiography does not always accurately reflect the amount of blood flow. Furthermore, the measurement of CBF alone is not sufficient to evaluate cerebral hemodynamics. This can be attributed to two reasons. First, CBF may be maintained at a normal range via autoregulation, even though CPP decreases. Second, CBF may be reduced when the metabolic demand is low, but CPP is normal. Considering these factors, there are three key parameters to assess hemodynamic compromise: cerebrovascular reactivity (CVR), CBV, and OEF. Although positron emission tomography (PET) is still the gold standard to evaluate hemodynamic parameters, the usefulness of perfusion computed tomography (CT) and perfusion magnetic resonance imaging (MRI), such as dynamic susceptibility contrast MRI and arterial spin-labeling MRI have been reported [26–28].

CVR measurement is obtained after the application of a cerebral vasodilatory stimulus such as acetazolamide by using a variety of modalities such as single photon emission computed tomography (SPECT), PET, and perfusion CT/MRI. Kuroda et al. categorized hemodynamic status into four types using measurements of CBF and CVR: Type 1, normal CBF and CVR; Type 2, normal CBF and reduced CVR; Type 3, reduced CBF and CVR (Fig. 8.1); and Type 4, reduced CBF and normal CVR [29]. Type 2 is considered to be similar to Powers stage I and Type 3 is similar to Powers stage II. Type 4 represents matched hypometabolism. However, it is also known that approximately 40% of affected hemispheres with abnormally reduced CBF and CVR (Type 3) do not exhibit increased OEF or misery perfusion [30, 31].

CBV can also be measured by PET and SPECT. When MTT is measured using perfusion CT/MRI, CBV is obtained in combination with the measurement of CBF using the equation: CBV = CBF × MTT. An increase in CBV and MTT indicates a lowering of CPP prior to CBF reduction. Measurement of MTT is considered to be more sensitive than that of CBV alone, but it is not very specific in detecting autoregulatory vasodilation. Normal CBV is often observed in patients with increased OEF (Fig. 8.2). This finding hints at the presence of a variable vasodilatory capacity or a chronic compensatory mechanism.

The hemodynamic status with increased OEF is defined as misery perfusion, and it indicates metabolic compensation in response to CPP reduction. Although OEF has been measured exclusively by ^{15}O-gas PET so far, OEF measurements using quantitative susceptibility mapping of MRI have recently been carried out, and a good correlation with PET-OEF has been reported [32].

The ability to maintain CPP during acute or chronic ischemia depends on the capacity of the cerebral collateral circulation. A recent study showed a correlation between the morphological features of angiography and the hemodynamic status using PET [33]. In this study, scanty or vacant blood flow was observed in the watershed area using fused three-dimensional digital subtraction angiography, which is consistent with the perfusion abnormality defined by decreased CBF, increased CBV, and prolonged MTT.

8.5 Ivy Sign

The ivy sign was first reported as a characteristic radiological marker of the pial network observed in MMD on post-contrast images and on fluid-attenuated inversion-recovery (FLAIR) images [34, 35]. The ivy sign is useful as an indirect indicator of hemodynamic status of the leptomeningeal collateral pathways in MMD (Fig. 8.1). Studies have shown the presence of the ivy sign on FLAIR images in 46–66% of involved hemispheres in patients with MMD [36–39]. Although the mechanism of the ivy sign has not been fully understood, it is generally considered to be a slow flow of blood within the pial arteries via leptomeningeal collaterals and dilated pial vasculature compensating for decreased CPP [40]. The ivy sign is associated with ischemic symptoms and hemodynamic compromise, such as a decrease in CBF and CVR when assessed by SPECT. PET studies have also shown a significant correlation between the ivy sign and increased CBV or OEF [40, 41]. Thus, the ivy sign can be a predictor of ischemic recurrence in patients with MMD. A recent study shows that it has a dose–response effect; hemispheres with ivy signs in broader regions have a greater likelihood of experiencing subsequent ischemic events [42]. Thus, the ivy sign could be an adjunctive radiological marker to screen for high-risk ischemic patients who need revascularization surgery.

8.6 Surgical Indications

The goal of using surgical revascularization to treat ischemic MMD is to prevent cerebral infarction and future cognitive dysfunction due to chronic ischemia by improving cerebral perfusion status. It is generally recommended for patients with clinical symptoms due to hemodynamic compromise indicated by parameters such as CBF, CVR, CBV, OEF, and MTT. Although the surgical indications and the definition of hemodynamic compromise vary among surgeons, it is important to diagnose hemodynamic compromise early and precisely, so that appropriate intervention can be taken before the occurrence of irreversible brain damages. This is especially important in pediatric patients who typically present a more progressive clinical course than adults.

8.7 Antiplatelet Therapy for Ischemic MMD

There is no clinical evidence for the efficacy of antiplatelet therapy in preventing ischemic stroke in MMD. One registry study from Japan showed that antiplatelet therapy does not decrease the recurrence rate of ischemic stroke [3]. In a worldwide survey of experts in the field of MMD treatment, 14% of Asian (Japanese and Korean) experts and 64% of non-Asian experts agreed with the usage of long-term antiplatelet drugs. On the other hand, 57% of Asian experts and 27% of non-Asian experts maintained that antiplatelet drugs are not needed to treat MMD [43]. Asian experts who do not prescribe antiplatelet therapy answered that they are afraid of the possibility of a cerebral hemorrhage, and they do not believe that it is useful against hemodynamic insufficiency. In contrast, the supporters of antiplatelet therapy answered that antiplatelet drugs improve microcirculation, prevent microembolism, and benefit the postoperative result by maintaining blood flow through the bypass.

References

1. Horn P, Lanczik O, Vajkoczy P, Daffertshofer M, Bueltmann E, Werner A, et al. Hemodynamic reserve and high-intensity transient signals in moyamoya disease. Cerebrovasc Dis. 2005;19(3):141–6. https://doi.org/10.1159/000083246.
2. Kim SK, Seol HJ, Cho BK, Hwang YS, Lee DS, Wang KC. Moyamoya disease among young patients: its aggressive clinical course and the role of active surgical treatment. Neurosurgery. 2004;54(4):840–4.; discussion 4–6. https://doi.org/10.1227/01.neu.0000114140.41509.14.
3. Yamada S, Oki K, Itoh Y, Kuroda S, Houkin K, Tominaga T, et al. Effects of surgery and antiplatelet therapy in ten-year follow-up from the registry study of research committee on Moyamoya disease in Japan. J Stroke Cerebrovasc Dis. 2016;25(2):340–9. https://doi.org/10.1016/j.jstrokecerebrovasdis.2015.10.003.
4. Gross BA, Du R. The natural history of moyamoya in a north American adult cohort. J Clin Neurosci. 2013;20(1):44–8. https://doi.org/10.1016/j.jocn.2012.08.002.
5. Rafay MF, Armstrong D, Dirks P, MacGregor DL, de Veber G. Patterns of cerebral ischemia in children with moyamoya. Pediatr Neurol. 2015;52(1):65–72. https://doi.org/10.1016/j.pediatrneurol.2014.10.007.
6. Kazumata K, Kamiyama H, Saito H, Maruichi K, Ito M, Uchino H, et al. Direct anastomosis using occipital artery for additional revascularization in Moyamoya disease after combined superficial temporal artery-middle cerebral artery and indirect bypass. Operative Neurosurgery. 2017;13(2):213–23. https://doi.org/10.1227/NEU.0000000000001346.
7. Saito H, Kashiwazaki D, Uchino H, Yamamoto S, Houkin K, Kuroda S. Specific clinical features and one-stage revascularization surgery for moyamoya disease with severe cerebral ischemia in the territory of posterior cerebral artery. Acta Neurochir. 2020; https://doi.org/10.1007/s00701-020-04580-7.
8. Mugikura S, Higano S, Shirane R, Fujimura M, Shimanuki Y, Takahashi S. Posterior circulation and high prevalence of ischemic stroke among young pediatric patients with Moyamoya disease: evidence of angiography-based differences by age at diagnosis. AJNR Am J Neuroradiol. 2011;32(1):192–8. https://doi.org/10.3174/ajnr.A2216.
9. Kuroda S, Houkin K, Ishikawa T, Nakayama N, Ikeda J, Ishii N, et al. Determinants of intellectual outcome after surgical revascularization in pediatric moyamoya disease: a multivariate analysis. Childs Nerv Syst. 2004;20(5):302–8. https://doi.org/10.1007/s00381-004-0924-4.

10. Mogensen MA, Karzmark P, Zeifert PD, Rosenberg J, Marks M, Steinberg GK, et al. Neuroradiologic correlates of cognitive impairment in adult Moyamoya disease. AJNR Am J Neuroradiol. 2012;33(4):721–5. https://doi.org/10.3174/ajnr.A2852.
11. Weinberg DG, Rahme RJ, Aoun SG, Batjer HH, Bendok BR. Moyamoya disease: functional and neurocognitive outcomes in the pediatric and adult populations. Neurosurg Focus. 2011;30(6):E21. https://doi.org/10.3171/2011.3.FOCUS1150.
12. Zhao M, Deng X, Gao F, Zhang D, Wang S, Zhang Y, et al. Ischemic stroke in young adults with Moyamoya disease: prognostic factors for stroke recurrence and functional outcome after revascularization. World Neurosurg. 2017;103:161–7. https://doi.org/10.1016/j.wneu.2017.03.146.
13. Kazumata K, Tokairin K, Sugiyama T, Ito M, Uchino H, Osanai T, et al. Association of cognitive function with cerebral blood flow in children with moyamoya disease. J Neurosurg Pediatr. 2019;25:1–7. https://doi.org/10.3171/2019.7.PEDS19312.
14. Funaki T, Takahashi JC, Takagi Y, Yoshida K, Araki Y, Kikuchi T, et al. Impact of posterior cerebral artery involvement on long-term clinical and social outcome of pediatric moyamoya disease. J Neurosurg Pediatr. 2013;12(6):626–32. https://doi.org/10.3171/2013.9.PEDS13111.
15. Hishikawa T, Tokunaga K, Sugiu K, Date I. Assessment of the difference in posterior circulation involvement between pediatric and adult patients with moyamoya disease. J Neurosurg. 2013;119(4):961–5. https://doi.org/10.3171/2013.6.JNS122099.
16. Ohkura A, Negoto T, Aoki T, Noguchi K, Okamoto Y, Komatani H, et al. Stenotic changes of the posterior cerebral artery are a major contributing factor for cerebral infarction in moyamoya disease. Surg Neurol Int. 2018;9:105. https://doi.org/10.4103/sni.sni_18_18.
17. Hendrikse J, Hartkamp MJ, Hillen B, Mali WP, van der Grond J. Collateral ability of the circle of Willis in patients with unilateral internal carotid artery occlusion: border zone infarcts and clinical symptoms. Stroke. 2001;32(12):2768–73. https://doi.org/10.1161/hs1201.099892.
18. Mugikura S, Takahashi S, Higano S, Shirane R, Kurihara N, Furuta S, et al. The relationship between cerebral infarction and angiographic characteristics in childhood moyamoya disease. AJNR Am J Neuroradiol. 1999;20(2):336–43.
19. Kim JM, Lee SH, Roh JK. Changing ischaemic lesion patterns in adult moyamoya disease. J Neurol Neurosurg Psychiatry. 2009;80(1):36–40. https://doi.org/10.1136/jnnp.2008.145078.
20. Cho HJ, Jung YH, Kim YD, Nam HS, Kim DS, Heo JH. The different infarct patterns between adulthood-onset and childhood-onset moyamoya disease. J Neurol Neurosurg Psychiatry. 2011;82(1):38–40. https://doi.org/10.1136/jnnp.2009.181487.
21. Zhao M, Deng X, Wang S, Zhang D, Zhang Y, Zhao J. Lacunar infarction in adult patients with moyamoya disease. Clin Neurol Neurosurg. 2018;164:81–6. https://doi.org/10.1016/j.clineuro.2017.10.040.
22. Powers WJ, Press GA, Grubb RL Jr, Gado M, Raichle ME. The effect of hemodynamically significant carotid artery disease on the hemodynamic status of the cerebral circulation. Ann Intern Med. 1987;106(1):27–34. https://doi.org/10.7326/0003-4819-106-1-27.
23. Powers WJ. Cerebral hemodynamics in ischemic cerebrovascular disease. Ann Neurol. 1991;29(3):231–40. https://doi.org/10.1002/ana.410290302.
24. Baron JC, Bousser MG, Rey A, Guillard A, Comar D, Castaigne P. Reversal of focal "misery-perfusion syndrome" by extra-intracranial arterial bypass in hemodynamic cerebral ischemia. A case study with 15O positron emission tomography. Stroke. 1981;12(4):454–9. https://doi.org/10.1161/01.str.12.4.454.
25. Derdeyn CP, Videen TO, Yundt KD, Fritsch SM, Carpenter DA, Grubb RL, et al. Variability of cerebral blood volume and oxygen extraction: stages of cerebral haemodynamic impairment revisited. Brain. 2002;125(Pt 3):595–607. https://doi.org/10.1093/brain/awf047.
26. Hara S, Tanaka Y, Ueda Y, Hayashi S, Inaji M, Ishiwata K, et al. Noninvasive evaluation of CBF and perfusion delay of Moyamoya disease using arterial spin-labeling MRI with multiple Postlabeling delays: comparison with (15)O-gas PET and DSC-MRI. AJNR Am J Neuroradiol. 2017;38(4):696–702. https://doi.org/10.3174/ajnr.A5068.

27. Kawano T, Ohmori Y, Kaku Y, Muta D, Uekawa K, Nakagawa T, et al. Prolonged mean transit time detected by dynamic susceptibility contrast magnetic resonance imaging predicts cerebrovascular reserve impairment in patients with Moyamoya disease. Cerebrovasc Dis. 2016;42(1–2):131–8. https://doi.org/10.1159/000445696.
28. Rim NJ, Kim HS, Shin YS, Kim SY. Which CT perfusion parameter best reflects cerebrovascular reserve?: correlation of acetazolamide-challenged CT perfusion with single-photon emission CT in Moyamoya patients. AJNR Am J Neuroradiol. 2008;29(9):1658–63. https://doi.org/10.3174/ajnr.A1229.
29. Kuroda S, Kamiyama H, Abe H, Houkin K, Isobe M, Mitsumori K. Acetazolamide test in detecting reduced cerebral perfusion reserve and predicting long-term prognosis in patients with internal carotid artery occlusion. Neurosurgery. 1993;32(6):912–8.; discussion 8-9. https://doi.org/10.1227/00006123-199306000-00005.
30. Nemoto EM, Yonas H, Kuwabara H, Pindzola RR, Sashin D, Meltzer CC, et al. Identification of hemodynamic compromise by cerebrovascular reserve and oxygen extraction fraction in occlusive vascular disease. J Cereb Blood Flow Metab. 2004;24(10):1081–9. https://doi.org/10.1097/01.WCB.0000125887.48838.37.
31. Kuroda S, Shiga T, Houkin K, Ishikawa T, Katoh C, Tamaki N, et al. Cerebral oxygen metabolism and neuronal integrity in patients with impaired vasoreactivity attributable to occlusive carotid artery disease. Stroke. 2006;37(2):393–8. https://doi.org/10.1161/01.STR.0000198878.66000.4e.
32. Kudo K, Liu T, Murakami T, Goodwin J, Uwano I, Yamashita F, et al. Oxygen extraction fraction measurement using quantitative susceptibility mapping: comparison with positron emission tomography. J Cereb Blood Flow Metab. 2016;36(8):1424–33. https://doi.org/10.1177/0271678X15606713.
33. Karakama J, Nariai T, Hara S, Hayashi S, Sumita K, Inaji M, et al. Unique angiographic appearances of Moyamoya disease detected with 3-dimensional rotational digital subtraction angiography imaging showing the hemodynamic status. J Stroke Cerebrovasc Dis. 2018;27(8):2147–57. https://doi.org/10.1016/j.jstrokecerebrovasdis.2018.03.006.
34. Maeda M, Tsuchida C. "Ivy sign" on fluid-attenuated inversion-recovery images in childhood moyamoya disease. AJNR Am J Neuroradiol. 1999;20(10):1836–8.
35. Ohta T, Tanaka H, Kuroiwa T. Diffuse leptomeningeal enhancement, "ivy sign," in magnetic resonance images of moyamoya disease in childhood: case report. Neurosurgery. 1995;37(5):1009–12. https://doi.org/10.1227/00006123-199511000-00024.
36. Yoon HK, Shin HJ, Chang YW. "Ivy sign" in childhood moyamoya disease: depiction on FLAIR and contrast-enhanced T1-weighted MR images. Radiology. 2002;223(2):384–9. https://doi.org/10.1148/radiol.2232011094.
37. Kawashima M, Noguchi T, Takase Y, Ootsuka T, Kido N, Matsushima T. Unilateral hemispheric proliferation of ivy sign on fluid-attenuated inversion recovery images in moyamoya disease correlates highly with ipsilateral hemispheric decrease of cerebrovascular reserve. AJNR Am J Neuroradiol. 2009;30(9):1709–16. https://doi.org/10.3174/ajnr.A1679.
38. Ideguchi R, Morikawa M, Enokizono M, Ogawa Y, Nagata I, Uetani M. Ivy signs on FLAIR images before and after STA-MCA anastomosis in patients with Moyamoya disease. Acta Radiol. 2011;52(3):291–6. https://doi.org/10.1258/ar.2011.100367.
39. Fujiwara H, Momoshima S, Kuribayashi S. Leptomeningeal high signal intensity (ivy sign) on fluid-attenuated inversion-recovery (FLAIR) MR images in moyamoya disease. Eur J Radiol. 2005;55(2):224–30. https://doi.org/10.1016/j.ejrad.2004.11.009.
40. Vuignier S, Ito M, Kurisu K, Kazumata K, Nakayama N, Shichinohe H, et al. Ivy sign, misery perfusion, and asymptomatic moyamoya disease: FLAIR imaging and (15)O-gas positron emission tomography. Acta Neurochir. 2013;155(11):2097–104. https://doi.org/10.1007/s00701-013-1860-4.

41. Kaku Y, Iihara K, Nakajima N, Kataoka H, Fukushima K, Iida H, et al. The leptomeningeal ivy sign on fluid-attenuated inversion recovery images in moyamoya disease: positron emission tomography study. Cerebrovasc Dis. 2013;36(1):19–25. https://doi.org/10.1159/000351143.
42. Nam KW, Cho WS, Kwon HM, Kim JE, Lee YS, Park SW, et al. Ivy sign predicts ischemic stroke recurrence in adult Moyamoya patients without revascularization surgery. Cerebrovasc Dis. 2019;47(5-6):223–30. https://doi.org/10.1159/000500610.
43. Kraemer M, Berlit P, Diesner F, Khan N. What is the expert's option on antiplatelet therapy in moyamoya disease? Results of a worldwide survey. Eur J Neurol. 2012;19(1):163–7. https://doi.org/10.1111/j.1468-1331.2011.03481.x.

Hemorrhagic Stroke and the Japan Adult Moyamoya Trial

9

Takeshi Funaki, Jun C. Takahashi, Susumu Miyamoto, and the JAM Trial Group

Abstract

The Japan Adult Moyamoya (JAM) Trial was a unique randomized controlled trial demonstrating the effectiveness of direct bypass surgery for hemorrhagic moyamoya disease. Prespecified subgroup analysis undertaken as part of the trial demonstrated that posterior-dominant initial hemorrhage is a significant predictor of rebleeding and an effect modifier for surgery. Periventricular anastomosis—fragile collaterals formed by the lenticulostriate arteries, thalamic perforators, and choroidal arteries—might present a clue to the mechanism of high rebleeding risk linked to posterior hemorrhage. Angiographic analyses of the JAM Trial revealed that choroidal collaterals and the involvement of the posterior cerebral artery are associated with posterior hemorrhage, and subsequent cohort analysis of the nonsurgical group has revealed that choroidal anastomosis is a strong predictor of rebleeding. A better understanding of periventricular anastomosis might contribute to further progress in the surgical treatment of hemorrhagic moyamoya disease.

Keywords

Moyamoya disease · Intracranial hemorrhage · Cerebral revascularization · Periventricular anastomosis · The Japan Adult Moyamoya Trial

---

the JAM Trial Group

T. Funaki (✉) · S. Miyamoto
Department of Neurosurgery, Kyoto University Graduate School of Medicine, Kyoto, Japan
e-mail: tfunaki@kuhp.kyoto-u.ac.jp; miy@kuhp.kyoto-u.ac.jp

J. C. Takahashi
Department of Neurosurgery, Faculty of Medicine, Kindai University, Osaka, Japan
e-mail: juntak@med.kindai.ac.jp

S. Kuroda (ed.), *Moyamoya Disease: Current Knowledge and Future Perspectives*, https://doi.org/10.1007/978-981-33-6404-2_9

9.1 Introduction

The Japan Adult Moyamoya (JAM) Trial is the only Randomized Controlled Trial (RCT) for moyamoya disease. The trial revealed the effectiveness of direct bypass in preventing rebleeding in adult hemorrhagic moyamoya disease. In this chapter, the authors discuss the mechanism and treatment of hemorrhagic moyamoya disease with a focus on the results of the JAM Trial (see also Chap. 13).

9.2 The JAM Trial

The rebleeding rate of hemorrhagic moyamoya disease can be as high as 7% per year, and the outcome after rebleeding is poor [1]. The rupturing of the fragile collateral vessels typical of the disease, the so-called moyamoya vessels, has been considered the mechanism of hemorrhage in moyamoya disease. The diminishing of such collateral vessels after bypass surgery is well known [2]. This recognition has given rise to the hypothesis that bypass surgery can prevent rebleeding by reducing the hemodynamic burden on the fragile collateral vessels typical of the disease. This hypothesis, however, had remained untested before the JAM Trial.

The JAM Trial was a multicentered RCT, the purpose of which was to test the above hypothesis [3, 4]. The inclusion criteria of the trial are shown in Table 9.1. At the beginning of the study, the optimal sample size was calculated on the assumption that the incidence of adverse neurological events was 8%/y in the nonsurgical group and 4%/y in the surgical group. The follow-up period was 5 years, and the sample size of 160 (80 patients per group) was expected to provide 80% of the statistical validity required to detect a difference between the two groups with a significance level of 0.05. However, this number was reduced to 80 in January 2006 when a far smaller number of patients were discovered to be eligible for the study, as indicated later [3]. Despite the change in sample size, the trial required 12 years to complete.

In the randomization process, the participants were classified as exhibiting either anterior or posterior hemorrhage: the former was defined as hemorrhage occurring in the putamen, caudate, or anterior half of the body of the lateral ventricle; the latter was defined as hemorrhage occurring in the thalamus, the posterior half of the body of the lateral ventricle, or the atrium. Accordingly, each participant was randomly assigned to either the surgical or the nonsurgical group. The JAM Trial Group adopted stratified randomization, which balanced the proportion of anterior and posterior hemorrhage patients assigned to each category, as it had been hypothesized that the surgical effects and rebleeding risk might vary between those with anterior hemorrhage and those with posterior hemorrhage.

The patients assigned to the surgical group underwent direct bypass, superficial temporal artery (STA) to middle cerebral artery (MCA) anastomosis, performed by registered neurosurgeons in different sessions for each side. Neither indirect bypass alone nor high-flow bypass using venous or radial artery graft was permitted. The

Table 9.1 Patient eligibility of the Japan Adult Moyamoya Trial, reprinted from the Japan Adult Moyamoya Trial Group (Neurol Med Chir 44:218–219, 2004)

1. Clinical requirements (1) Age: Between 18 and 60 years at the time of the initial bleeding episode (2) Independent in daily life (modified Rankin disability scale 0–2) (3) Intracranial hemorrhage, intraventricular hemorrhage, or subarachnoid hemorrhage within the preceding 12 months (4) At least one month has passed after the last stroke episode, either ischemic or hemorrhagic (5) At least one month has passed after the completion of acute phase treatment for the hemorrhage and for the related secondary pathophysiology (e.g., hydrocephalus)
2. Radiological requirements (1) Computed tomography/magnetic resonance imaging (a) Absence of extensive infarction spreading widely over the territory of a main arterial trunk (b) Absence of contrast enhancement in the infarcted area (2) Angiography Angiographic findings should satisfy the diagnostic criteria of the spontaneous occlusion of the circle of Willis (moyamoya disease) published by the Ministry of Health, Labor and Welfare of Japan: (a) Occlusive lesions are present in the terminal portion of the intracranial internal carotid artery, or in the proximal portion of the anterior or middle cerebral arteries. (b) Abnormal vascular network demonstrated in the region of basal ganglia and thalamus (moyamoya vessels) in the arterial phase (c) These findings are present bilaterally
3. Exclusion criteria (1) Not independent in daily life (modified Rankin disability 3–5) (2) Atherosclerotic carotid disease, or cardiac arrhythmia which may cause thromboembolic complications (3) Malignant tumors or organ failure of the heart, liver, kidney, or lung (4) Unstable angina or myocardial infarction within the past 6 months (5) Hematological abnormality showing bleeding diathesis (6) Uncontrolled diabetes with a serum fasting blood glucose level of more than 300 mg/dl, or requiring insulin (7) Hypertension with a diastolic blood pressure of more than 110 mmHg (8) Treated by extracranial–intracranial bypass surgery before enrollment (9) Pregnancy

*The Japan Adult Moyamoya Trial Group thereafter amended the inclusion criteria on age as that between 18 and 65 years

primary endpoint was defined as all adverse events, and the secondary endpoint was a rebleeding attack. All participants were followed for 5 years by a team comprising a particular neurologist and neurosurgeon.

9.3 Primary Results of the JAM Trial

A total of 80 participants, comprising 42 surgical and 38 nonsurgical patients, were eventually enrolled in the trial. All patients completed the 5-year follow-up, and no crossover or failure to follow-up occurred. Kaplan–Meier method revealed that the incidence of both endpoints was significantly lower in the surgical group than in the nonsurgical group (primary endpoint, $P = 0.048$; secondary endpoint, $P = 0.042$; Fig. 9.1). The rebleeding rate calculated according to the person-year method was 7.6% per year in the nonsurgical group versus 2.7% per year in the surgical group. The hazard ratio (HR) of the secondary endpoint estimated with the Cox proportional hazard model was 0.355, indicating that the rebleeding rate had decreased by two-thirds. On the other hand, the upper limit of 95% confidence interval of the HR slightly exceeded 1, and the primary report of the JAM Trial published in *Stroke* characterized the results as "statistically marginal." The discrepancy in statistical significance between the Kaplan–Meier method and Cox proportional hazard model is apparently attributable to the problem of sample size mentioned above. Conducting an RCT with a larger sample size, however, seems unfeasible considering the difficulty of participant recruitment for the JAM Trial. It should be noted that the primary report of the JAM Trial was accepted by *Stroke* in 2014 with the following

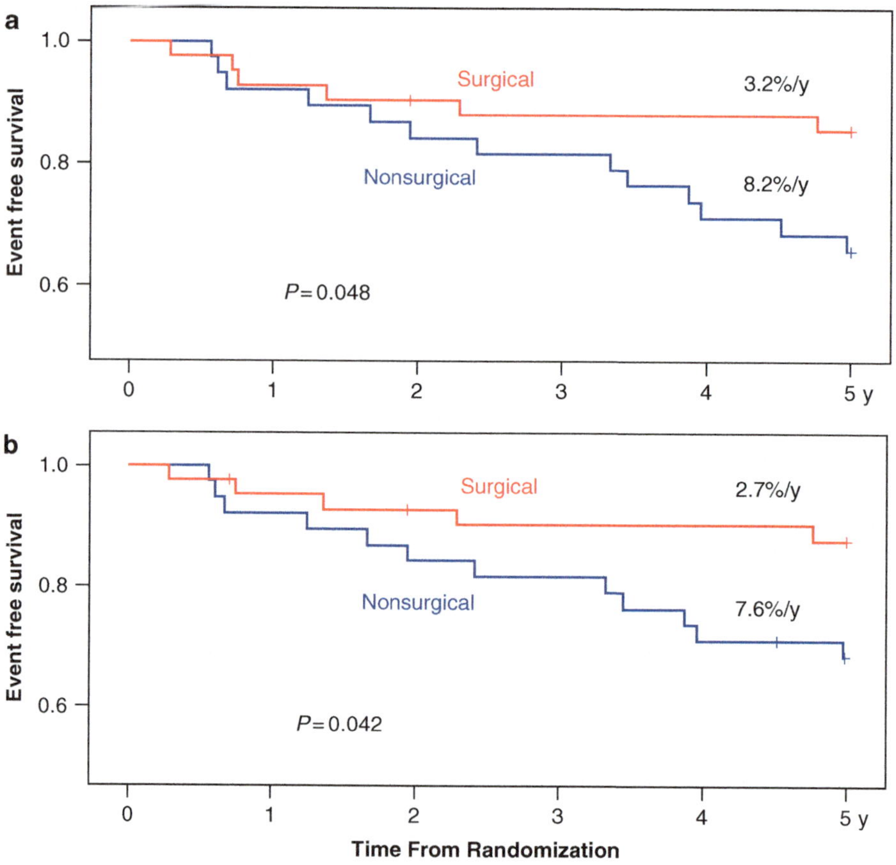

Fig. 9.1 Kaplan–Meier curves for the primary (**a**) and secondary (**b**) endpoints, modified with permission from Miyamoto et al. (*Nippon Rinsho* 2014;72; supple 7: 639–42 [Japanese])

conclusion: *Kaplan–Meier analysis revealed the significant difference between the surgical and nonsurgical group, suggesting the preventive effect of direct bypass against rebleeding* [3].

9.4 Prespecified Subgroup Analysis of the JAM Trial

The JAM Trial Group then investigated the prespecified question of whether the surgical effects and natural course varied with the hemorrhage site at onset, which had been the rationale for the stratified randomization. First, a subgroup analysis by hemorrhage site was performed for all 80 patients. As shown in Fig. 9.2, the HR for the surgical group relative to the nonsurgical group was very low (0.07) in the posterior hemorrhage group, suggesting a high degree of surgical effectiveness, whereas the HR exceeded 1 (1.62) in the anterior hemorrhage group. The test for interaction revealed that the surgical effects varied significantly with the hemorrhage site ($P = 0.013$).

The JAM Trial Group then limited the analysis to the nonsurgical group, which comprised 38 patients, including 21 exhibiting anterior hemorrhage and 17 exhibiting posterior hemorrhage. As shown in Fig. 9.3, the incidence rates for the primary end points were significantly higher for the posterior group than for the anterior group ($P = 0.003$). This indicates that the natural outcome also varied with the hemorrhage site.

These results suggest that patients with posterior hemorrhage have a poorer natural prognosis and accrue greater benefit from surgery. Direct bypass should be considered especially for the posterior hemorrhage group. These results were published

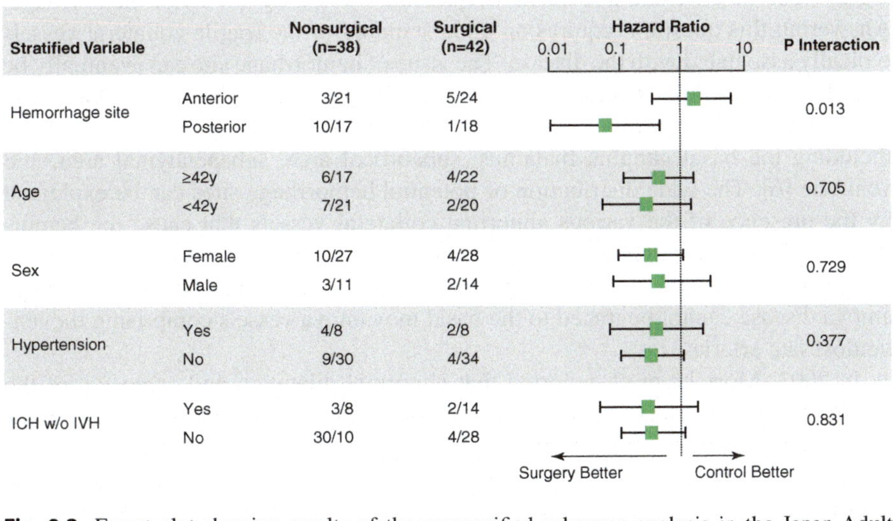

Fig. 9.2 Forest plot showing results of the prespecified subgroup analysis in the Japan Adult Moyamoya Trial, reprinted with permission from Funaki et al. (*Clin Neurosci* 2016;34:1218–1221 [Japanese])

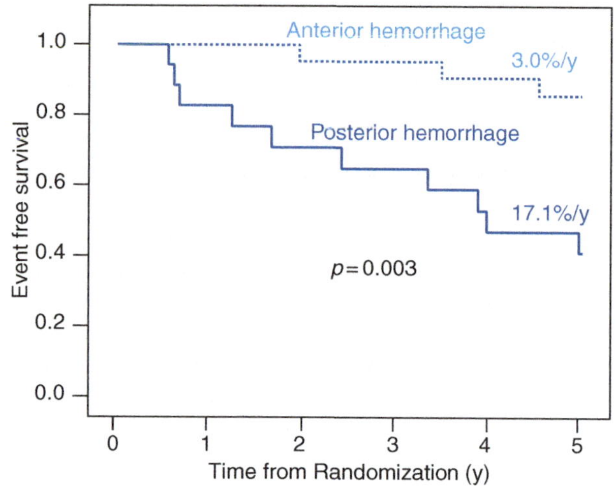

Fig. 9.3 Kaplan–Meier curves for the nonsurgical group in the Japan Adult Moyamoya Trial, reprinted with permission from Funaki e al (*Clin Neurosci* 34:1218–1221, 2016 [Japanese])

in *Stroke* in 2016 [5]. It should be noted that these results are not the product of post hoc analyses; they were obtained from "prespecified" analysis to test the predescribed hypothesis under stratified randomization.

9.5 Mechanism of Bleeding in Moyamoya Disease: Periventricular Anastomosis

The results of the subgroup analysis in the JAM Trial raise new questions about the higher risk of rebleeding evident in patients exhibiting posterior hemorrhage. Answering this question requires an understanding of the fragile collateral vessels typically associated with the disease. The issue of hemorrhage site can eventually be traced to the fragile collateral vessels responsible for bleeding (see also Chap. 13).

Hemorrhage in moyamoya disease occurs in various sites of the cerebrum, including the basal ganglia, thalamus, subcortical area, subependymal area, and ventricle [6]. The wide distribution of potential hemorrhage sites can be explained by the presence of the various abnormal collateral vessels that cause the hemorrhage. Although researchers had considered so-called "basal moyamoya vessels" as the vessels responsible for bleeding, some of the hemorrhages occurring in moyamoya disease cannot be traced to the basal moyamoya vessels comprising the lenticulostriate arteries.

In 2003, Morioka et al. reported that abnormal dilatation and extension of the anterior choroidal artery or the perforator from the posterior communicating artery were more commonly observed in hemorrhagic moyamoya disease than in the ischemic form of the disease [7]. This finding suggests that not only lenticulostriate arteries but also thalamic perforators and choroidal arteries are associated with hemorrhage in moyamoya disease. A recent study using high-resolution black-blood

MRA has demonstrated that all three arteries—lenticulostriate, thalamic perforating, and choroidal—share the common feature of serving as collaterals to the cortex [8]. These arteries anastomose to the medial end of the medullary or insular arteries, which supply blood from the cortex to the cerebral depths in normal anatomy. As a result of this change, the direction of blood flow in the medullary artery is reversed to supply blood from the depths to the cortex. This type of collateral system, typical of moyamoya disease, has been referred to as "periventricular anastomosis" (Fig. 9.4) [8, 9].

The formation of periventricular anastomosis is explained by the theory of ventriculofugal and ventriculopetal arteries [10]. According to this famous theory advocated by Van den Bergh in 1969, the deep white matter is supplied by two arterial systems: the ventriculopetal artery (i.e., medullary artery) from the surface to the ventricle; and the ventriculofugal artery form the ventricle to the surface (Fig. 9.5). The ventriculofugal artery, also known as the subependymal artery [11], is formed by the peripheral ends of the perforating or choroidal arteries [12].

The ventriculofugal and ventriculopetal arteries form no anastomosis in normal anatomy, as the border zone between these arteries is believed to be the cause of periventricular ischemia. In moyamoya disease, a long-standing cortical ischemia might induce an abnormal connection between these arteries and result in periventricular anastomosis. In the early 1970s, Kodama et al. suggested the possibility of such a connection forming between perforating and medullary arteries [13].

The results of recent studies shed light on the significance of periventricular anastomosis as a hemorrhage-prone collateral in moyamoya disease [8, 14–16]. Anastomotic sites in the periventricular collaterals are considered especially fragile because of the histopathological connection between vessels. Even microaneurysms frequently emerge at the sites of anastomoses because of the characteristic inflection points that typically form in the collaterals at these sites.

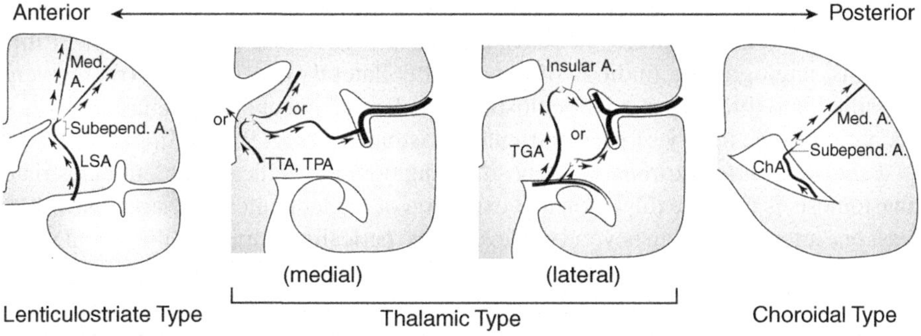

Fig. 9.4 Schematic illustration showing a coronal plane of the left hemisphere and three types of periventricular anastomosis, reprinted with permission from Funaki et al. (*Neurol Med Chir (Tokyo)* 2015;55(3):204–9)

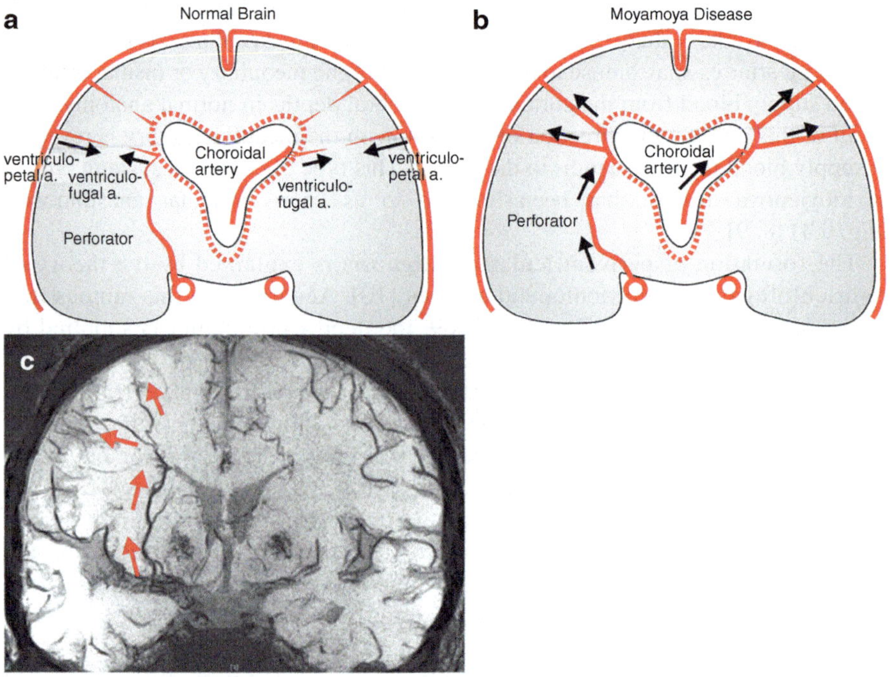

Fig. 9.5 (**a**, **b**) Schematic illustration showing ventriculopetal/ventriculofugal arterial system on a coronal plane for the normal brain (**a**) and moyamoya disease (**b**) (**c**) Flow-sensitive black-blood MR angiography showing lenticulostriate-type periventricular anastomosis, reprinted with permission from Funaki et al. (Jpn J Neurosurg 2017;26:4–11 [Japanese])

9.6 Why Does the Posterior Hemorrhage Group Have a Poor Natural Prognosis?

The JAM Trial Group performed additional analyses to answer the question of why patients exhibiting posterior hemorrhage are at higher risk of rebleeding. In this analysis, angiographic findings of abnormal collaterals causing hemorrhage were classified into three types—lenticulostriate, thalamic, and choroidal anastomoses—according to the theory of periventricular anastomosis (Fig. 9.6) [15].

Lenticulostriate anastomosis. A positive angiographic indicator of lenticulostriate anastomosis is extreme dilatation and extension of the lenticulostriate arteries with at least one artery extending beyond the level of the pericallosal artery in the lateral view. In such situations, the lenticulostriate arteries are reasonably considered to extend beyond the upper level of the lateral ventricle to connect to the medullary arteries.

Thalamic anastomosis. A positive angiographic indicator of thalamic anastomosis is extreme dilatation and extension of the thalamic perforators with at least one perforator extending beyond the position of the medial posterior choroidal artery in the lateral view. In such a situation, the thalamic perforators are reasonably considered to extend beyond the thalamus to connect to the medullary arteries.

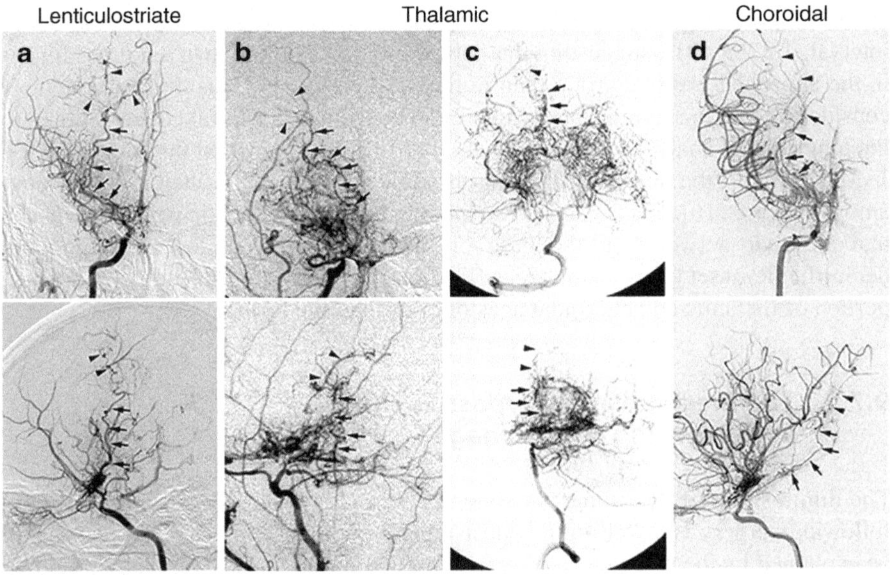

Fig. 9.6 Angiographic definition of collaterals in Japan Adult Moyamoya Trial. (**a**) Lenticulostriate anastomosis. (**b, c**) Thalamic anastomosis. (**d**) Choroidal anastomosis. Anterior–posterior and lateral views are shown in the upper and lower row, respectively. (**a**, **b**), and (**d**) are right carotid angiography; (**c**) is right vertebral angiography. The perforating or choroidal arteries are shown as arrows, the medullary arteries as arrowheads, reprinted with permission from Funaki et al. (Jpn J Neurosurg 2017;26:4–11 [Japanese])

Choroidal anastomosis. This is defined as an anastomosis between the choroidal artery and the medial end of the medullary artery. Both the anterior and the lateral posterior choroidal arteries can serve as the origin of such an anastomosis. Positive angiographic (lateral view) indicators of choroidal anastomosis are as follows: (1) extreme dilatation and extension of the choroidal artery with a sharp deviation of the lateral ventricle at its peripheral portion to connect to the medullary artery; (2) extreme extension of the anterior choroidal or lateral posterior choroidal artery beyond the atrium of the lateral ventricle to the body of the lateral ventricle; or (3) extension of the medial posterior choroidal artery penetrating the corpus callosum to the pericallosal artery.

Analysis of the 75 hemorrhagic hemispheres in the JAM Trial revealed that choroidal anastomosis and involvement of the posterior cerebral artery (PCA) were the significant characteristics of posterior hemorrhage [15]. Choroidal anastomosis typically forms around the atrium and is located in the most posterior of the collaterals [9]. This suggests that the high rebleeding risk of posterior hemorrhage is attributable to the extreme fragility of a choroidal anastomosis distributed posteriorly.

This hypothesis was tested with two additional analyses of the JAM Trial [14, 16]. First, an ancillary study using the 5-year follow-up data on the nonsurgical cohort of the JAM Trial revealed that the presence of choroidal anastomosis is an independent predictor of rebleeding [14]. The adjusted HR for rebleeding in the choroidal-positive group relative to the negative group was 11.10 (95% confidence interval, 1.37–89.91), suggesting that rebleeding risk is more than ten times higher in the choroidal-positive group than in the negative group. This finding is notable considering that the significance of choroidal anastomosis was first demonstrated in the longitudinal analysis. Second, a case control study compared the data set of the JAM Trial with the angiographic data of adult patients with ischemic-onset moyamoya disease [16]. This analysis revealed that the characteristic pattern of abnormal vascular networks at the base of the brain differ in the ischemic- and hemorrhagic-onset types, with the latter patients showing a significantly higher proportion of thalamic and choroidal anastomoses than the former.

9.7 The Mechanism of Bypass Surgery in Preventing Hemorrhage

The diminishing of the numerous abnormal vessels typical of moyamoya disease following surgery is a well-known postsurgical phenomenon. This can reasonably be explained by the mechanism of periventricular anastomosis. Our data reveal that retrograde flow in the medullary artery can be restored to normal (from surface to depth) after surgery, resulting in elimination of the pathological anastomosis and normalization of the perforating or choroidal arteries [17]. Accordingly, this change might be observed as shrinkage of the abnormal vessels because normograde flow in the medullary artery is almost invisible.

Such a change, which can be viewed as a *normalization* of periventricular vasculature, is considered a key mechanism of bypass surgery in preventing rebleeding, as suggested from the JAM Trial. In other words, a bypass whose perfusion overlaps the cortical distribution of the periventricular anastomosis can normalize the outflow of the medullary artery, resulting in successful shrinkage of the periventricular anastomosis.

According to our additional data of interest, among the three subtypes of periventricular anastomosis, choroidal anastomosis was the type most likely to normalize following bypass surgery [17]. This result corresponds well with the results of prespecified subgroup analysis in the JAM Trial, which suggests the posterior hemorrhage group accrues greater benefit from bypass surgery [5] because choroidal anastomosis is considered a typical bleeding source in posterior hemorrhage. The variance in the likelihood of normalization might be attributable to the differing cortical distribution patterns seen in the subtypes of periventricular anastomosis. Our most recent study revealed that choroidal anastomosis outflows were to the lateral cortex predominantly posterior to the central sulcus, whereas outflows of the lenticulostriate anastomosis were more likely to be characterized as medial and anterior [18].

The knowledge of periventricular anastomosis might promote a new direct-bypass strategy focusing on hemorrhage prevention, which targets the responsible periventricular anastomosis (Fig. 9.7) [19].

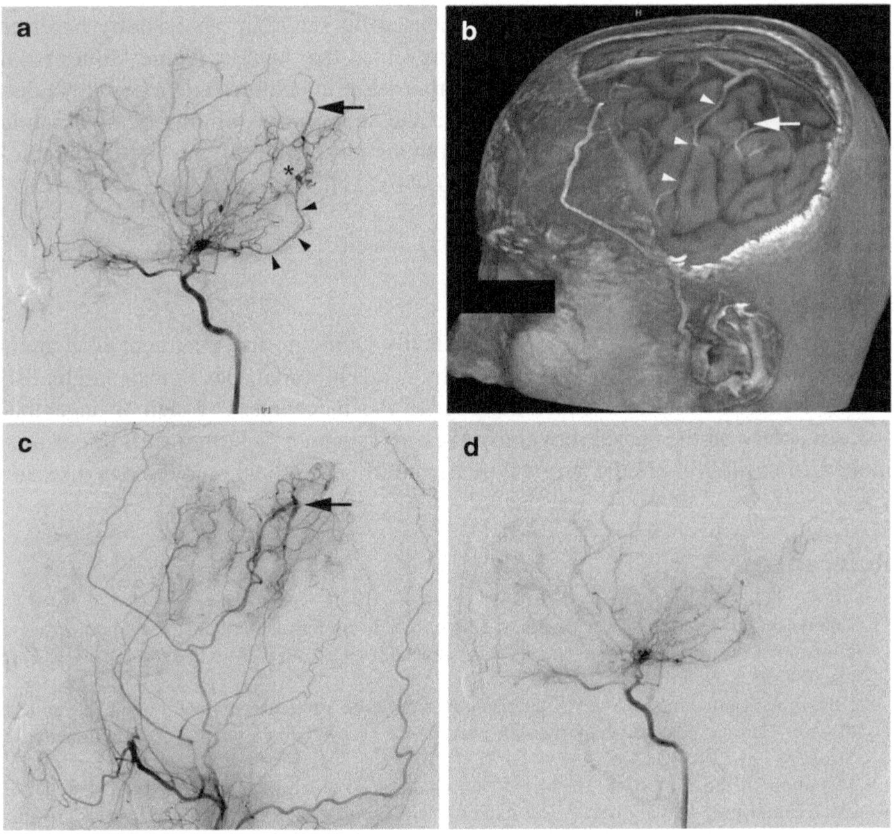

Fig. 9.7 (**a**) Lateral view angiography of the left internal carotid artery before surgery revealing choroidal anastomosis (black arrowheads), extending to the target vessel (arrow). Note the aneurysm observed at the site of the anastomosis (asterisk). (**b**) Corresponding brain surface image generated with MR angiography data. White arrowheads indicate the central sulcus. The target vessel is exposed on the postcentral gyrus (arrow). (**c**) Lateral view angiography of the left external carotid artery obtained 9 months after surgery revealing patency of the bypass and accurate anastomosis to the target vessel (arrow). (**d**) Lateral view angiography of the left internal carotid artery obtained 9 months after surgery revealing marked shrinkage of the choroidal anastomosis and aneurysm, reprinted with permission from Funaki et al. (Neurol Med Chir (Tokyo). 2019;59(12):517–22)

9.8 Additional Sub-analyses of the JAM Trial

Analysis of the nonhemorrhagic hemispheres included in the JAM Trial suggests that choroidal anastomosis is also a predictor of de novo hemorrhage [20]. The annual risk of de novo hemorrhage in the nonhemorrhagic hemispheres was relatively high (5.8% per year). Given that the nonhemorrhagic hemisphere in hemorrhagic moyamoya disease resembles a nonhemorrhagic hemisphere in asymptomatic or less-symptomatic patients, choroidal anastomosis might also be a predictor of de novo hemorrhage in asymptomatic individuals in these populations.

The last analysis of the JAM Trial focused on subgroup analysis by baseline hemodynamic failure [21]. This analysis revealed that hemodynamic failure is an independent risk factor for subsequent hemorrhage in hemorrhagic moyamoya disease. Moreover, the analysis revealed that the subgroup exhibiting hemodynamic failure tended to accrue greater benefit from surgery; however, the test for interaction was not statistically significant ($P = 0.056$) [21].

9.9 Summary

The results of the JAM Trial are dramatically changing the treatment of hemorrhagic moyamoya disease. The recent findings on choroidal anastomosis might also overturn the conventional understanding of the mechanism of hemorrhage that focuses solely on the "basal moyamoya vessels." Such a paradigm shift might promote further progress in the surgical treatment of hemorrhagic moyamoya disease.

References

1. Kobayashi E, Saeki N, Oishi H, Hirai S, Yamaura A. Long-term natural history of hemorrhagic moyamoya disease in 42 patients. J Neurosurg. 2000;93(6):976–80. https://doi.org/10.3171/jns.2000.93.6.0976.
2. Houkin K, Kamiyama H, Abe H, Takahashi A, Kuroda S. Surgical therapy for adult moyamoya disease. Can surgical revascularization prevent the recurrence of intracerebral hemorrhage? Stroke. 1996;27(8):1342–6.
3. Miyamoto S, Yoshimoto T, Hashimoto N, Okada Y, Tsuji I, Tominaga T, et al. Effects of extracranial-intracranial bypass for patients with hemorrhagic moyamoya disease: results of the Japan adult moyamoya trial. Stroke. 2014;45(5):1415–21. https://doi.org/10.1161/strokeaha.113.004386.
4. Miyamoto S. Study design for a prospective randomized trial of extracranial-intracranial bypass surgery for adults with moyamoya disease and hemorrhagic onset-the Japan Adult Moyamoya Trial Group. Neurol Med Chir (Tokyo). 2004;44(4):218–9.
5. Takahashi JC, Funaki T, Houkin K, Inoue T, Ogasawara K, Nakagawara J, et al. Significance of the hemorrhagic site for recurrent bleeding: prespecified analysis in the Japan adult moyamoya trial. Stroke. 2016;47(1):37–43. https://doi.org/10.1161/strokeaha.115.010819.
6. Kawaguchi S, Sakaki T, Kakizaki T, Kamada K, Shimomura T, Iwanaga H. Clinical features of the haemorrhage type moyamoya disease based on 31 cases. Acta Neurochir. 1996;138(10):1200–10.
7. Morioka M, Hamada J, Kawano T, Todaka T, Yano S, Kai Y, et al. Angiographic dilatation and branch extension of the anterior choroidal and posterior communicating arteries are predictors of hemorrhage in adult moyamoya patients. Stroke. 2003;34(1):90–5.
8. Funaki T, Takahashi JC, Yoshida K, Takagi Y, Fushimi Y, Kikuchi T, et al. Periventricular anastomosis in moyamoya disease: detecting fragile collateral vessels with MR angiography. J Neurosurg. 2016;124(6):1766–72. https://doi.org/10.3171/2015.6.jns15845.
9. Funaki T, Fushimi Y, Takahashi JC, Takagi Y, Araki Y, Yoshida K, et al. Visualization of periventricular collaterals in moyamoya disease with flow-sensitive black-blood magnetic resonance angiography: preliminary experience. Neurol Med Chir (Tokyo). 2015;55(3):204–9. https://doi.org/10.2176/nmc.oa.2014-0360.
10. Van den Bergh R. The ventriculofugal arteries. AJNR Am J Neuroradiol. 1992;13(1):413–5.

11. Marinkovic S, Gibo H, Filipovic B, Dulejic V, Piscevic I. Microanatomy of the subependymal arteries of the lateral ventricle. Surg Neurol. 2005;63(5):451–8.; discussion 8. https://doi.org/10.1016/j.surneu.2004.06.013.
12. De Reuck J. The human periventricular arterial blood supply and the anatomy of cerebral infarctions. Eur Neurol. 1971;5(6):321–34.
13. Kodama N, Suzuki J. Cerebrovascular moyamoya disease IIIrd report-the study on the aging of the perforating branches and the possibility of collateral pathway. Neurol Med Chir Part I. 1974;14(1):55–67. https://doi.org/10.2176/nmc.14pt1.SUPPLEMENT_55.
14. Funaki T, Takahashi JC, Houkin K, Kuroda S, Takeuchi S, Fujimura M, et al. High rebleeding risk associated with choroidal collateral vessels in hemorrhagic moyamoya disease: analysis of a nonsurgical cohort in the Japan adult Moyamoya trial. J Neurosurg. 2019;130(2):525–30. https://doi.org/10.3171/2017.9.jns17576.
15. Funaki T, Takahashi JC, Houkin K, Kuroda S, Takeuchi S, Fujimura M, et al. Angiographic features of hemorrhagic moyamoya disease with high recurrence risk: a supplementary analysis of the Japan adult Moyamoya trial. J Neurosurg. 2018;128(3):777–84. https://doi.org/10.3171/2016.11.jns161650.
16. Fujimura M, Funaki T, Houkin K, Takahashi JC, Kuroda S, Tomata Y, et al. Intrinsic development of choroidal and thalamic collaterals in hemorrhagic-onset moyamoya disease: case-control study of the Japan adult Moyamoya trial. J Neurosurg. 2018;130(5):1453–9. https://doi.org/10.3171/2017.11.Jns171990.
17. Miyakoshi A, Funaki T, Takahashi JC, Takagi Y, Kikuchi T, Yoshida K, et al. Restoration of periventricular vasculature after direct bypass for moyamoya disease: intra-individual comparison. Acta Neurochir. 2019;161(5):947–54. https://doi.org/10.1007/s00701-019-03866-9.
18. Miyakoshi A, Funaki T, Fushimi Y, Nakae T, Okawa M, Kikuchi T, et al. Cortical distribution of fragile periventricular anastomotic collateral vessels in moyamoya disease: an exploratory cross-sectional study on Japanese moyamoya patients. Am J Neuroradiol. 2020:5. https://doi.org/10.3174/ajnr.A6861. [Epub ahead of print]
19. Funaki T, Kataoka H, Yoshida K, Kikuchi T, Mineharu Y, Okawa M, et al. The targeted bypass strategy for preventing hemorrhage in moyamoya disease: technical note. Neurol Med Chir (Tokyo). 2019;59(12):517–22. https://doi.org/10.2176/nmc.tn.2019-0162.
20. Funaki T, Takahashi JC, Houkin K, Kuroda S, Fujimura M, Tomata Y, et al. Effect of choroidal collateral vessels on de novo hemorrhage in moyamoya disease: analysis of nonhemorrhagic hemispheres in the Japan adult moyamoya trial. J Neurosurg. 2019;132(2):408–14. https://doi.org/10.3171/2018.10.Jns181139.
21. Takahashi JC, Funaki T, Houkin K, Kuroda S, Fujimura M, Tomata Y, et al. Impact of cortical hemodynamic failure on both subsequent hemorrhagic stroke and effect of bypass surgery in hemorrhagic moyamoya disease: a supplementary analysis of the Japan adult Moyamoya trial. J Neurosurg. https://doi.org/10.3171/2020.1.Jns192392. [Epub ahead of print]

Cognitive Function in Pediatric Moyamoya Disease

10

Satoshi Kuroda

Abstract

Since the very early stage of moyamoya disease discovery, it has been known that cerebral infarction can cause cognitive dysfunction in children with moyamoya disease. In recent years, there are fewer children who develop cerebral infarction after a long period of repeated TIAs through the improved ability to diagnose moyamoya disease at an early stage. However, infants often have sudden onset of ischemic stroke, and the sequelae of cognitive dysfunction as well as motor dysfunction are still an issue that cannot be completely resolved. In this chapter, the author will review the pathophysiology of cognitive dysfunction in pediatric patients with moyamoya disease, their radiological findings, and effective surgical revascularization. The author strongly believes that early diagnosis and surgical revascularization should be performed before they still repeat TIAs or headache attacks and have not progressed to a completed stroke in order to improve the intellectual prognosis of pediatric patients with moyamoya disease. In addition, we should plan to perform surgical revascularization through "large" craniotomy covering the frontal lobes for this purpose.

Keywords

Moyamoya disease · Children · Cognitive dysfunction · Cerebral hemodynamics · Ischemic stroke · Surgical revascularization

S. Kuroda (✉)
Department of Neurosurgery, Graduate School of Medicine and Pharmaceutical Science, University of Toyama, Toyama, Japan
e-mail: skuroda@med.u-toyama.ac.jp

S. Kuroda (ed.), *Moyamoya Disease: Current Knowledge and Future Perspectives*, https://doi.org/10.1007/978-981-33-6404-2_10

10.1 Introduction

Since the very early stage of moyamoya disease discovery, it has been known that cerebral infarction can cause cognitive dysfunction in children with moyamoya disease. Cognitive dysfunction, along with motor dysfunction, is a factor that has a significant impact on the quality of later life of pediatric patients with moyamoya disease. Therefore, a detailed understanding of the causes, pathophysiology, and effective treatment of cognitive dysfunction in pediatric moyamoya disease is crucial for improving the long-term prognosis of pediatric patients with moyamoya disease.

10.2 Clinical Features

In the 1980s, cognitive dysfunction in pediatric moyamoya disease patients began to be studied in detail. Several investigators have reported that a significant subgroup of children with moyamoya disease develops cognitive dysfunction. In recent years, many pediatric patients with moyamoya disease have undergone surgical revascularization in the early stages of their illness. Therefore, we can only speculate about the natural history of cognitive function in pediatric patients based on data from the past, when surgical revascularization was less common. Kurokawa et al. (1985) reported that intellectual outcome is very poor in pediatric patients with moyamoya disease, including mild intellectual and/or motor impairment in 26%, requirement for special school or care by parent or institutes after reaching the teen years in 11%, and continuous 24-h care in 7% [1].

Ishii et al. (1984) measured intelligence scores in 20 pediatric patients with moyamoya disease, and reported that the older children had lower intelligence. Thus, full-scale intelligence quotient (FSIQ) was 108.0 ± 12.9, 96.8 ± 22.6, 82.6 ± 16.4 in children at 5–8, 9–12, and 13-16 years of age, respectively [2]. Matsushima et al. (1991) also reported similar results [3]. These findings strongly suggest that a longer duration of disease exposes the developing brain to ischemia or hypoxia for a longer period and finally intellectual deterioration increased with time. In fact, poor intellectual outcome is closely related to an early age at the onset, and cognitive function starts to decline within 5–10 years after the onset [4]. For example, the prevalence of cognitive dysfunction is 1/13 (7.7%), 2/4 (50%), and 6/9 (67.8%) after 0–4, 5–9, and 10–15 years after the onset of moyamoya disease, respectively [1]. However, diagnosis and surgical treatment are much faster than before the 1980s, because moyamoya disease is now widely recognized among pediatricians, physicians, and neurologists. Therefore, it is likely that the number of pediatric patients suffering from cognitive dysfunction is decreasing, and the number of detailed studies is limited since the 2000s [5].

Using ^{133}xenon inhalation method, Ishii et al. (1984) reported a significant correlation between hemispheric cerebral blood flow (CBF) and intelligence score [2]. Bowen et al. (1998) reported two children with cognitive dysfunction due to moyamoya disease. Although plain CT scans detected no parenchymal lesions in the brain, both had a distinct impairment of cerebrovascular reserve in the bilateral hemispheres. Especially, this hemodynamic impairment is most prominent in the frontal lobes, which results in abnormally posterior-dominant distribution of CBF [6].

10.3 Effects of Surgical Revascularization on Intellectual Outcome

Ishii et al. (1984) mainly performed EMS for 20 children with moyamoya disease, and reported that full-scale IQ improved after surgery in 8 of 20 cases [2]. On the other hand, cognitive function did not recover after EDAS [3]. Matsushima et al. (1990) reported that intellectual outcome was poor, especially in children with disease onset at less than 2 years of age even after encephalo-duro-arterio-synangiosis (EDAS) [7]. Bowen et al. (1998) longitudinally monitored cognitive function in two children with moyamoya disease after superficial temporal artery to middle cerebral artery (STA-MCA) anastomosis combined with EDAS on both sides. Cognitive function was still severely impaired when neurophysiological testing was examined 3 months after surgery. However, repeated testing at 1 and 2 years later demonstrated a stepwise improvement of cognitive function in both children [6]. As described in Chap. 18, surgical revascularization is accepted as an effective treatment to prevent further TIA, ischemic stroke, and hemorrhagic stroke in moyamoya disease. However, it should be reminded that about 15 to 30% of children with moyamoya disease still experience some difficulties in social or school life due to residual cognitive dysfunction even after surgery [5, 7–11]. Ishikawa et al. (1997) reported that 7 (30.4%) of 23 patients with moyamoya disease were poorly educated or were on the job of just simple tasks [8]. Collectively, these reports suggest that a history of ischemic stroke, cerebral infarction on CT/MRI, and the onset at younger than 5 years of age are closely associated with poor intellectual outcome.

In recent years, several studies have conducted statistical analyses to extract the factors that determine the intelligence outcome after surgical revascularization in pediatric patients with moyamoya disease. Using a univariate analysis model, Matsushima et al. (1997) reported that only FSIQ before surgery significantly predicted their intellectual outcome after EDAS. However, it should be noted that their study had a non-negligible bias because they excluded patients with an FSIQ lower than 70 from their study. In addition, no multivariate analysis was performed in this study, probably because the sample size was small ($n = 20$) [10]. Subsequently, we conducted a multivariate analysis study using a larger cohort ($n = 52$). Of 52 pediatric patients, 8 (15.4%) were judged as mentally impaired status (FSIQ < 70). As the results, we found two independent predictors for poor intellectual outcome, including a history of completed stroke (odds ratio, 33.4; 95% confidential interval [CI], 2.4–474) and small craniotomy surgery (odds ratio, 19.6; 95%CI, 1.8–215). The majority of pediatric patients with a history of completed stroke already have sequelae such as hemiparesis before surgical revascularization, and motor dysfunction may be closely related to poor intellectual outcome. As the first conclusion, therefore, early diagnosis and surgical revascularization should be performed before they still repeat TIAs or headache attacks and have not progressed to a completed stroke in order to improve the intellectual prognosis of pediatric patients with moyamoya disease.

Furthermore, we classified craniotomies for surgical revascularization into two groups: a small craniotomy group focusing on the temporo-parietal area and a large craniotomy group extending to the frontal area, and investigated the impact of craniotomy location and size on the intellectual outcome. "Small" craniotomy centered on the temporo-parietal area has been used for EDAS and encephalo-myo-synangiosis (EMS) with or without direct bypass procedure. Following EDAS/EMS, TIAs such as hemiparesis easily disappear after surgery, because this surgical technique provides sufficient blood flow to the motor cortex through the surgical collaterals. The disadvantage of this technique, however, is that cerebral ischemia in the frontal lobe persists even after surgery, because the revascularized area is limited to the temporal and parietal regions and is confined to the craniotomy field [12, 13]. We found that both CBF and its reactivity to acetazolamide were significantly lower in small craniotomy group than in large craniotomy group [12, 14]. These findings correlate well with previous data. Thus, Sato et al. (1990) reported that intellectual outcome was poor in 9 of 13 pediatric patients who underwent EDAS or EMS. In fact, CBF improvement was limited around the surgical field, but blood flow reduction was persistent in the frontal lobe [13]. Ohtaki et al. (1998) also reported that STA-MCA anastomosis combined with extensive omental transplantation over the bilateral frontal lobes effectively prevented the worsening of cognitive function in pediatric moyamoya disease [15]. As the second conclusion, therefore, we should plan to perform surgical revascularization through "large" craniotomy covering the frontal lobes in order to improve the intellectual prognosis of pediatric patients with moyamoya disease (Fig. 10.1).

10.4 Pathophysiology

The cognitive function does not originate in a specific region of the brain. Based on above-mentioned knowledge, however, it is at least certain that the frontal lobe is playing a central role in the performance of the cognitive function. Indeed, Nakagawara et al. (2012) performed ^{123}I-iomazenil (IMZ) SPECT in adult moyamoya patients with cognitive dysfunction and found that the neuronal integrity was specifically reduced in the medial frontal lobe and anterior cingulate [16].

On the other hand, it is unclear through which mechanisms cognitive function is impaired in moyamoya patients without parenchymal lesions such as cerebral infarction. In these patients, cognitive function is reported to recover to the normal level after appropriate surgical revascularization. One clue is the speculation that cognitive dysfunction in pediatric moyamoya disease may be related to cerebral ischemia-induced suppression of brain metabolism. Previously, Karasawa and co-workers (1981) conducted a pioneering study and found that oxygen consumption in pediatric moyamoya disease was reduced before surgery, but predominantly increased at 6 months after surgery [17]. Using ^{15}O positron emission tomography, Taki et al. (1988) measured CBF, cerebral blood volume (CBV), cerebral metabolic rate for oxygen ($CMRO_2$), and oxygen extraction fraction (OEF) in five pediatric patients with a mean age of 11 years. They found no significant difference in $CMRO_2$ when compared with healthy adult volunteers with a mean age of 31 years. As described in Chap. 7, however, CBF is much higher in children around 10 years of age than in adults. Therefore, it is probable that oxygen metabolism was lower in the

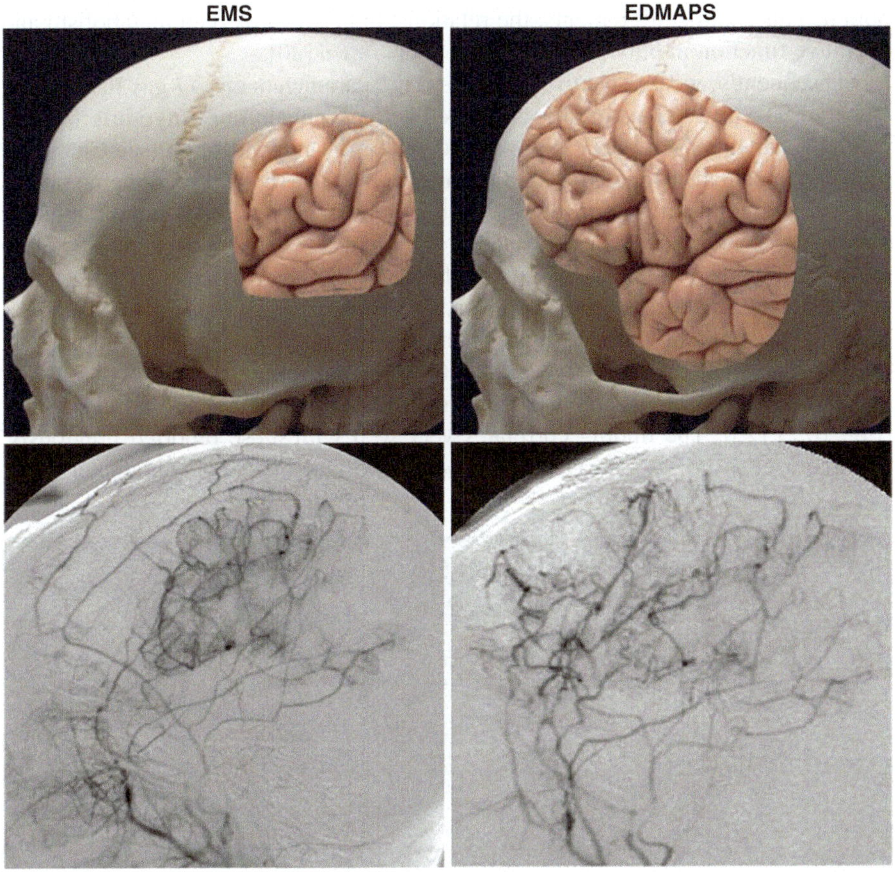

Fig. 10.1 Upper panels show that the location and size of craniotomy largely differ between EMS (small craniotomy group; *left*) and EDMAPS (large craniotomy group; *right*). In the former, craniotomy size is small and is centered on temporo-parietal area, but in the latter, craniotomy is largely extended to the frontal area and its size is also larger. Lower panels demonstrate representative findings on left external carotid angiography 3 to 4 months after EMS (*left*) and EDMAPS (*right*). Note that the extent of surgical collaterals via indirect bypass depends on the location and size of craniotomy

pediatric patients included in this study than in healthy children of the same age, because CBF and $CMRO_2$ are tightly coupled [18]. Indeed, Shirane et al. (1997) measured hemodynamic and metabolic parameters, using ^{15}O PET, and found that $CMRO_2$ was decreased in the frontal and parietal lobes with pronounced ischemia [19]. Hosoda et al. (2010) reported that all intellectual parameters, including Full-Scale Intelligence Quotient (FSIQ), Verbal Intelligence Quotient (VIQ), and Performance Intelligence Quotient (PIQ), were positively associated with $CMRO_2$ in the lower part of the bilateral frontal lobe, the right anterior temporal lobe, and the medial occipital lobe. The VIQ was also positively linked to $CMRO_2$ in the left inferior frontal lobe. Although the findings are very interesting, this study included both pediatric and adult patients, the relationship between oxygen metabolism and cognitive function in only pediatric cases is unknown [20].

Subsequently, we prospectively analyzed the parameters on ^{15}O-gas PET before and after STA-MCA anastomosis combined with encephalo-duro-myo-arterio-pericranial synangiosis (EDMAPS) in patients with moyamoya disease (see Chap. 18) [21, 22]. In pediatric patients, $CMRO_2$ was decreased in 16 of 21 adult hemispheres (76%), but significantly improved in all eight hemispheres without any ischemic or hemorrhagic lesions after surgery. On the other hands, $CMRO_2$ was decreased in 38 of 48 adult hemispheres (79%), but significantly improved in only 13 of 22 lesion-free hemispheres after surgery. Therefore, there was a big discrepancy in postoperative improvement of oxygen metabolism between pediatric and adult patients. Further statistical analysis revealed that postoperative improvement of oxygen metabolism could be observed in pediatric and young (<40 years) adult patients (Fig. 10.2) [23]. The finding correlates very well with those reported previously. Morimoto et al. (1999) measured hemodynamic and metabolic parameters in 5

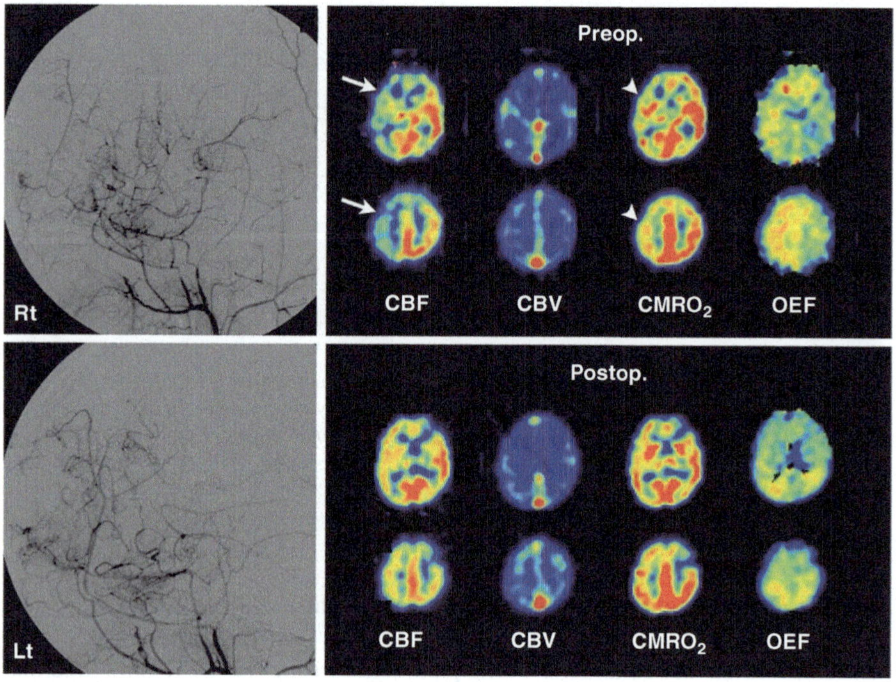

Fig. 10.2 Representative radiological findings of an 8-year-old girl who developed transient weakness of the left extremities due to moyamoya disease and underwent STA-MCA anastomosis and EDMAPS on both sides. Left panels demonstrate the findings on right (*upper*) and left external carotid angiography (*lower*) 4 months after surgery. Note that extensively developed surgical collaterals widely provide blood flow to the bilateral cerebral hemispheres, including the frontal lobes. Right panels show the findings on pre- (*upper*) and postoperative ^{15}O-gas PET (*lower*). Note a marked decrease in CBF (arrows) and $CMRO_2$ (arrowheads) in the right hemisphere followed by postoperative improvement 4 months after surgery

adult patients aged from 19 to 46 years before and after surgery. Following surgery, $CMRO_2$ markedly improved in two of five patients. Age of these two patients was 19 and 20 years, while age of other three patients ranged from 40 to 46 years [24].

These observations on oxygen metabolism in moyamoya disease strongly suggest that cerebral oxygen metabolism may be reversibly depressed in pediatric (and young adult) patients without any parenchymal lesions. In other words, the lesion-free brain of younger humans may have a potential ability to downregulate their oxygen utilization and to protect their brain against chronic ischemia and/or hypoxia by reducing its metabolic demand. This phenomenon is very similar to the condition of reversible brain hibernation [25]. Although the precise mechanism of spontaneous downregulation of oxygen metabolism in the young or immature brain, the author wonders that this phenomenon may be deeply involved in cognitive dysfunction in pediatric moyamoya patients without cerebral infarct [23].

Recently, several MRI studies have reported that impaired white matter microstructure and axon connectivity are involved in cognitive dysfunction in adults with moyamoya disease, but this technique has not been studied in pediatric moyamoya disease until now.

10.5 Conclusion

For a long time, it has been known that cognitive dysfunction in pediatric moyamoya disease is closely related to clinical factors such as infantile onset, completed stroke, and cerebral infarction. However, recent statistical analysis has revealed that in addition to completed stroke, small craniotomy surgery centered on the temporoparietal area is associated with poor intellectual outcome. Therefore, two strategies would be essential to further improve intellectual outcomes in pediatric patients. First, early diagnosis and surgical revascularization should be performed before they still repeat TIAs or headache attacks and have not progressed to a completed stroke. Second, we should perform surgical revascularization through "large" craniotomy covering the frontal lobes that are considered to play a crucial role in cognitive function.

Acknowledgment This work was partly supported by a grant from the Research Committee on Moyamoya Disease, the Japanese Ministry of Health, Labour and Welfare.

References

1. Kurokawa T, Tomita S, Ueda K, Narazaki O, Hanai T, Hasuo K, Matsushima T, Kitamura K. Prognosis of occlusive disease of the circle of Willis (moyamoya disease) in children. Pediatr Neurol. 1985;1:274–7.
2. Ishii R, Takeuchi S, Ibayashi K, Tanaka R. Intelligence in children with moyamoya disease: evaluation after surgical treatments with special reference to changes in cerebral blood flow. Stroke. 1984;15:873–7.
3. Matsushima Y, Aoyagi M, Koumo Y, Takasato Y, Yamaguchi T, Masaoka H, Suzuki R, Ohno K. Effects of encephalo-duro-arterio-synangiosis on childhood moyamoya patients-swift dis-

appearance of ischemic attacks and maintenance of mental capacity. Neurol Med Chir (Tokyo). 1991;31:708–14.
4. Imaizumi C, Imaizumi T, Osawa M, Fukuyama Y, Takeshita M. Serial intelligence test scores in pediatric moyamoya disease. Neuropediatrics. 1999;30:294–9.
5. Lee JY, Phi JH, Wang KC, Cho BK, Shin MS, Kim SK. Neurocognitive profiles of children with moyamoya disease before and after surgical intervention. Cerebrovasc Dis. 2011;31:230–7.
6. Bowen M, Marks MP, Steinberg GK. Neuropsychological recovery from childhood moyamoya disease. Brain Develop. 1998;20:119–23.
7. Matsushima Y, Aoyagi M, Masaoka H, Suzuki R, Ohno K. Mental outcome following encephaloduroarteriosynangiosis in children with moyamoya disease with the onset earlier than 5 years of age. Childs Nerv Syst. 1990;6:440–3.
8. Ishikawa T, Houkin K, Kamiyama H, Abe H. Effects of surgical revascularization on outcome of patients with pediatric moyamoya disease. Stroke. 1997;28:1170–3.
9. Karasawa J, Touho H, Ohnishi H, Miyamoto S, Kikuchi H. Long-term follow-up study after extracranial-intracranial bypass surgery for anterior circulation ischemia in childhood moyamoya disease. J Neurosurg. 1992;77:84–9.
10. Matsushima Y, Aoyagi M, Nariai T, Takada Y, Hirakawa K. Long-term intelligence outcome of post-encephalo-duro-arterio-synangiosis childhood moyamoya patients. Clin Neurol Neurosurg. 1997;99(Suppl 2):S147–50.
11. Miyamoto S, Akiyama Y, Nagata I, Karasawa J, Nozaki K, Hashimoto N, Kikuchi H. Long-term outcome after STA-MCA anastomosis for moyamoya disease. Neurosurg Focus. 1998;5:e5.
12. Kuroda S, Houkin K, Ishikawa T, Nakayama N, Ikeda J, Ishii N, Kamiyama H, Iwasaki Y. Determinants of intellectual outcome after surgical revascularization in pediatric moyamoya disease: a multivariate analysis. Childs Nerv Syst. 2004;20:302–8.
13. Sato H, Sato N, Tamaki N, Matsumoto S. Chronic low-perfusion state in children with moyamoya disease following revascularization. Childs Nerv Syst. 1990;6:166–71.
14. Isobe M, Kuroda S, Kamiyama H, Abe H, Mitumori K. Cerebral blood flow reactivity to hyperventilation in children with spontaneous occlusion of the circle of Willis (moyamoya disease). No Shinkei Geka. 1992;20:399–407.
15. Ohtaki M, Uede T, Morimoto S, Nonaka T, Tanabe S, Hashi K. Intellectual functions and regional cerebral haemodynamics after extensive omental transplantation spread over both frontal lobes in childhood moyamoya disease. Acta Neurochir. 1998;140:1043–53. discussion 1052–1043
16. Nakagawara J, Osato T, Kamiyama K, Honjo K, Sugio H, Fumoto K, Murahashi T, Takada H, Watanabe T, Nakamura H. Diagnostic imaging of higher brain dysfunction in patients with adult moyamoya disease using statistical imaging analysis for [123I]iomazenil single photon emission computed tomography. Neurol Med Chir (Tokyo). 2012;52:318–26.
17. Karasawa J, Kikuchi H, Kuriyama Y, Sawada T, Kuro M, Kobayashi K, Koike T, Mitsugi T. Cerebral hemodynamics in "moyamoya" disease--II. Measurements of cerebral circulation and metabolism by use of the argon desaturation method in pre- and post-neurosurgical procedures (author's transl). Neurol Med Chir (Tokyo). 1981;21:1161–8.
18. Taki W, Yonekawa Y, Kobayashi A, Ishikawa M, Kikuchi H, Nishizawa S, Senda M, Fukuyama H, Harada K, et al. Cerebral circulation and oxygen metabolism in moyamoya disease of ischemic type in children. Childs Nerv Syst. 1988;4:259–62.
19. Shirane R, Yoshida Y, Takahashi T, Yoshimoto T. Assessment of encephalo-galeo-myo-synangiosis with dural pedicle insertion in childhood moyamoya disease: characteristics of cerebral blood flow and oxygen metabolism. Clin Neurol Neurosurg. 1997;99(Suppl 2):S79–85.
20. Hosoda C, Nariai T, Ishiwata K, Ishii K, Matsushima Y, Ohno K. Correlation between focal brain metabolism and higher brain function in patients with Moyamoya disease. Int J Stroke. 2010;5:367–73.

21. Kuroda S, Houkin K, Ishikawa T, Nakayama N, Iwasaki Y. Novel bypass surgery for moyamoya disease using pericranial flap: its impacts on cerebral hemodynamics and long-term outcome. Neurosurgery. 2010;66:1093–101. discussion 1101
22. Kuroda S, Nakayama N, Yamamoto S, Kashiwazaki D, Uchino H, Saito H, Hori E, Akioka N, Kuwayama N, Houkin K. Late (5-20 years) outcomes after STA-MCA anastomosis and encephalo-duro-myo-arterio-pericranial synangiosis in patients with moyamoya disease. J Neurosurg. 2020;1:1–8.
23. Kuroda S, Kashiwazaki D, Hirata K, Shiga T, Houkin K, Tamaki N. Effects of surgical revascularization on cerebral oxygen metabolism in patients with Moyamoya disease: an 15O-gas positron emission tomographic study. Stroke. 2014;45:2717–21.
24. Morimoto M, Iwama T, Hashimoto N, Kojima A, Hayashida K. Efficacy of direct revascularization in adult Moyamoya disease: haemodynamic evaluation by positron emission tomography. Acta Neurochir. 1999;141:377–84.
25. Lutz PL. Mechanisms for anoxic survival in the vertebrate brain. Annu Rev Physiol. 1992;54:601–18.

Cognitive Dysfunction in Adults

11

Yasushi Takagi

Abstract

Moyamoya disease is an occlusive cerebrovascular disease characterized by stenosis or occlusion at the distal ends of bilateral internal arteries. The unusual vascular network (moyamoya vessels) around the circle of Willis with this disease is considered to represent collateral channels formed as a result of progressive brain ischemia. Recently, difficulty with social independence accompanied by cognitive impairment in adult has been recognized as an important unsolved social issue faced by patients with adult moyamoya disease. Several reports published, but the patients with cognitive impairment have difficulty in proving their status because the standard neuroradiological and neuropsychological methods to define cognitive impairment with moyamoya disease are not determined. These patients with cognitive impairment should be supported by social welfare as psychologically handicapped persons. In this chapter, recent reports including our study about cognitive impairment in adult moyamoya disease are summarized.

Keywords

Moyamoya disease · Cognitive dysfunction · IMZ-SPECT · MRI · Neuropsychological study

Y. Takagi (✉)
Department of Neurosurgery, Graduate School of Biomedical Sciences, Tokushima University, Tokushima, Japan
e-mail: ytakagi@tokushima-u.ac.jp

S. Kuroda (ed.), *Moyamoya Disease: Current Knowledge and Future Perspectives*, https://doi.org/10.1007/978-981-33-6404-2_11

Moyamoya disease is an occlusive cerebrovascular disease characterized by progressive stenosis or occlusion at the distal ends of bilateral internal arteries [1]. The etiology of the disease is not fully undefined. The findings that the incidence of the disease is highest in, but not confined to, Japanese and that the condition is frequently familial suggest the involvement of a genetic factor including *RNF213* in its pathogenesis [1]. The unusual vascular network (moyamoya vessels) around the circle of Willis with this disease is considered to represent collateral channels formed as a result of progressive brain ischemia [1–3]. Extracranial–intracranial bypass surgery with or without indirect procedures has been established as an effective neurosurgical intervention that increases cerebral blood flow (CBF) and cerebral vascular reserve (CVR) prevents from ischemic attacks [4, 5]. However, difficulty with social independence accompanied by cognitive impairment in adults has recently been recognized as an important unsolved social issue faced by patients with adult moyamoya disease [6–8].

In our report, it provides a profile of neurocognitive dysfunction in adult patients with moyamoya disease using structured neuropsychologic tasks. A broad range of cognitive functions was disrupted particularly in the patients who had difficulty with social independence. Mean scores of moyamoya patients with cognitive impairment frontal lobe evaluation tasks (Trail Making Test B and Theory of Mind) were significantly lower than healthy patients [9].

These patients with cognitive impairment should be supported by social welfare as psychologically handicapped persons. The characteristics of these patients are physically independent in daily life, but economically dependent. Because it is very difficult for them to obtain vocational skills because of cognitive impairment. But they have difficulty in proving their status because the standard neuroradiological and neuropsychological methods to define cognitive impairment with moyamoya disease are not determined.

Generally, cognitive impairment has been described as a neuropsychological disorder occurring after strokes that shows as disturbances in memory, attention, performance, and social behavioral in mainly pediatric cases [10, 11]. However, recent reports have focused on adult cases with neurocognitive impairment even without neuroradiological evidence of major stroke [8, 9, 12]. It is indicated that even if infarction has not yet occurred, brain dysfunction was associated with persistent hemodynamic compromise in the medial frontal lobes that can be visualized using [^{123}I]iomazenil (IMZ)-single photon emission CT (SPECT) [8]. In addition, a common methodology for neuropsychological evaluation of these patients is yet to be fully determined [6, 12, 13]. As for Japanese neurosurgeons, we want to establish the standard finding of the cognitive impairment in the patients with moyamoya disease. A prospective multicenter trial is on-going in Japan [14]. Our inclusion criteria are described especially included as follows contents: (1) Without a large structural lesions (less than 1 cortical artery region) on neuroradiological studies. (2) No neurological disorder influencing neuropsychological assessment, e.g. aphasia, hemianopsia, and agnosia. (3) Modified Rankin scale ranging from 0 to 4. Without serious cognitive dysfunction assessed by subjective, objective symptoms or daily life situation [14]. As background data of the patients including in this study, institute, sex, age, history of education, history of jobs, familial history, reason for diagnosis, modified Rankin scale, medication, and neurological deficit are recorded.

In our study [14], MRI scans were also performed in all subjects. The scans were acquired on a 1.5 T or a 3 T scanner. T1 structural sequences (3D MPRAGE on Siemens and Philips, 3D IR-SPGR on GE), FLAIR, T2WI (Dual Echo), T2*WI, and TOF-MRA images are obtained in this study [15]. Brain N-isopropyl-p- [^{123}I] iodoamphetamine (*123I*-IMP) SPECT using QSPECT/dual-table autoradiographic (ARG) method with three-dimensional stereotactic surface projection (3D-SSP) is performed to calculate regional cerebral blood flow. To assess regional cerebral vascular reserve, Diamox challenge SPECT is performed. ^{123}I-Iomazenil (IMZ)-SPECT using QSPECT method with 3D-SSP is performed to assess cortical neuronal loss. Cortical neuron loss was analyzed using the stereotactic extraction estimation (SEE) method (level 3: gyrus level) for 3D-SSP Z-score maps as previously reported [8]. These data will clarify the role of neuronal loss and volume of the brain in the cognitive dysfunction of moyamoya disease.

We used the batteries for neuropsychological assessment as follows [14]. Basic cognitive ability was evaluated using the Wechsler Adult Intelligence Scale-Third Edition (WAIS-III) to assess intelligence, the Wechsler Memory Scale-Revised (WMS-R) to assess memory [16, 17], and supplemental subtests for each task. Several frontal-functioning tests were also administered to detect specific neuropsychological deficits associated with adult moyamoya disease that co-occurs with difficulty in social independence. The Frontal Assessment Battery (FAB) tested general frontal cognitive ability. The Trail Making Test Part A (TMT-A) assessed speed of information processing [15, 18] and the Trail Making Test Part B (TMT-B) and the Wisconsin Card Sorting Test assessed executive ability [5]. Word-fluency test and Frontal Systems Behavior Scale (FrSBe) are also used for frontal lobe function [19, 20]. The Beck Depression Inventory—Second Edition (BDI II) and State-Trait Anxiety Inventory (STAI) assess depressive state [21, 22]. In addition, WHOQOL26 assesses quality of life. These batteries are useful to assess neurophysiological functions of moyamoya disease. The item of neuroradiological and neuropsychological study is summarized in Table 11.1. To study the cognitive functions of the patients with moyamoya disease, we emphasize these batteries are important.

This study was named Cognitive Dysfunction Survey of the Japanese Patients with Moyamoya Disease (COSMO Japan study) and the protocol is already published. Inclusion of the patients was already closed, all the data obtained in this study is analyzing now. These data will clear the origin of cognitive impairment in adult moyamoya disease [14].

Illustrative case. 30 year-old, female. MRI (FLAIR) image indicates no major infarction or gross injured area. MRA shows severe stenosis of both internal carotid arteries which is a characteristic of moyamoya disease. She has cognitive dysfunction mainly topographical disorientation. She was dismissed several times by companies (Fig. 11.1).

Patients with moyamoya disease often suffer higher cognitive impairments such as memory, attention, and social behavioral disturbances [9, 12, 13]. However

Table 11.1 Neuroradiological and Neuropsychological studies employed cognitive dysfunction study of moyamoya disease

Neuroradiological study
SPECT
^{123}I-IMP SPECT
^{123}I-IMZ-SPECT
MRI
MPRAGE/IR-SPGR
FLAIR
T2WI (dual echo)
T2*WI TOF-MRA
Neuropsychological study
WAIS-III
WMS-R
FAB
WCST
Stroop test
Word fluency
TMT A/B
BDIII
STAI
FrSBe
WHOQOL26

confirmatory diagnosis of higher cognitive dysfunction in patients with moyamoya disease without obvious brain damages on CT or MRI imaging has not been established and could become social issue [8]. Such cognitive impairments may occur in patients with medial frontal lobe damage including the anterior cingulate cortex.

Karzmark et al. reported that twenty patients (67%) of adult moyamoya disease exhibited small T2 hyperintensities in the cerebral subcortical white matter on brain MRI but no evidence of gray matter damage. Significant cognitive impairment was present in 7 patients (23%). Executive functioning, mental efficiency, and word finding were the ability areas most frequently impaired, whereas memory was relatively intact. Clinically significant emotional distress (depression and/or anxiety) was present in 11 patients (37%). Comparable cognitive findings were also observed in the subset of 10 patients (33%) with completely normal static brain MRI [12].

Kazumata et al. performed neurobehavioral and neuroimaging examinations in 25 adults with MMD prior to and > 12 mo after revascularization surgery. In this study, cognitive function was investigated using the Wechsler Adult Intelligence Scale-III, Trail Making Test, Wisconsin Card Sorting Test, Continuous Performance Test, Stroop test, and Wechsler Memory Scale. They assessed white matter integrity using diffusion tensor imaging, brain morphometry using magnetization-prepared rapid gradient-echo sequences, and brain connectivity using resting-state functional magnetic resonance imaging (MRI). Cognitive examinations revealed significant changes

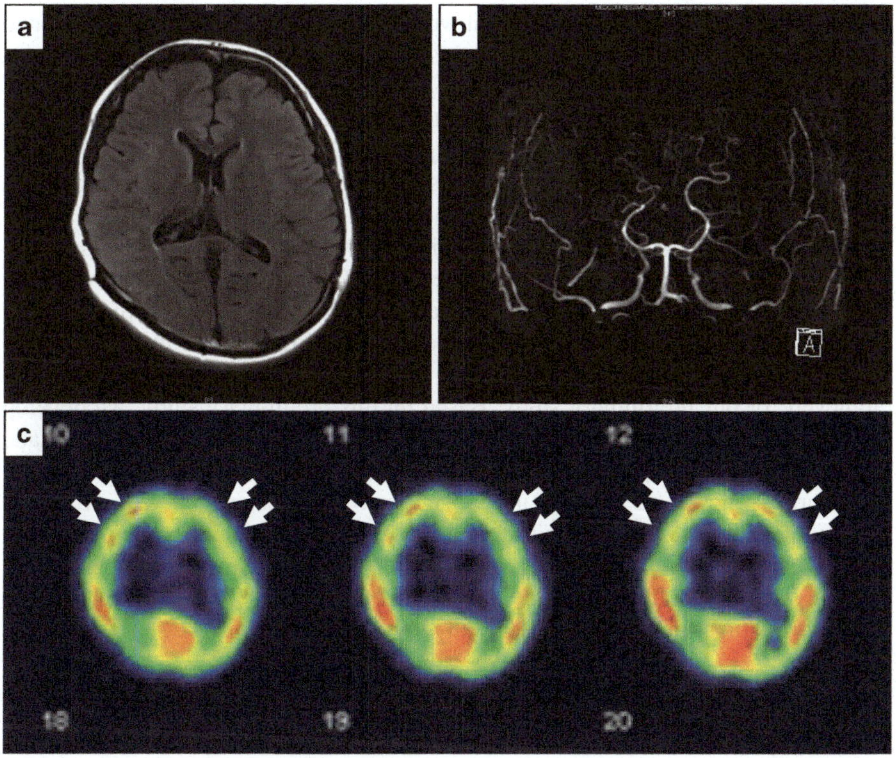

Fig. 11.1 30 y.o. female. (**a**) MRI (FLAIR) axial image. (**b**) MRA anterior-posterior view. (**c**) IMZ-SPECT axial image. Arrows indicated marked low accumulation in both frontal lobes

in the full-scale intelligence quotient (IQ), performance IQ (PIQ), perceptual organization (PO), processing speed, and Stroop test scores after surgery. Enlargement of the lateral ventricle, volume reductions in the corpus callosum and subcortical nuclei, and cortical thinning in the prefrontal cortex were also observed. Fractional anisotropy in the white matter tracts, including the superior longitudinal fasciculus, increased 2 to 4 years after surgery, relative to that observed in the presurgical state. In addition, Resting-state brain connectivity was increased predominantly in the fronto-cerebellar circuit and was positively correlated with improvements in PIQ and PO [23].

In general, higher brain dysfunction associated with adult moyamoya disease could be detected by both neuropsychological findings and obvious medial frontal lobe damage detected by magnetic resonance (MR) imaging [9, 12, 13]. In addition, hemodynamic compromise in this region is analyzed by SPECT at rest and after Diamox challenge [24, 25]. More recently, loss of frontal cortical neuron could be estimated by functional neuroimaging using SPECT, because central benzodiazepine receptor mapping using [123I]iomazenil (IMZ) is available for clinical use [8]. IMZ is a specific radioactive tracer for the central BZ receptor that may be useful as a marker of cortical neuron loss. Recent work using IMZ-SPECT has demonstrated the association between cortical neuron loss in bilateral frontal medial cortices and cognitive dysfunction [8].

Among brain dysfunction, higher cognitive dysfunction has been underestimated in the neurosurgical field. Neuropsychological analysis in the patients with brain damage played an important role in the history of developing the research of brain function [15–18, 24, 26]. This dysfunction is often due to frontal lobe dysfunction. An extensive focus on frontal lobe function has not yet been taken by previous research regarding moyamoya disease. Recent CBF and IMZ studies have shown that antero-medial frontal cortices fed by anterior circulation develop blood insufficiencies [8, 27]. For this reason, several neuropsychological test batteries to evaluate frontal lobe functioning in relation with hemodynamic compromise were employed for our preliminary study. Based on this preliminary study, we develop our study and adopt several tasks to examine frontal lobe functions [9]. To date, several surveys of the patients with moyamoya disease focusing neuroradiological and neuropsychological analysis in association with higher cognitive dysfunction were published. The patients with cognitive impairment should be supported by social welfare as psychologically handicapped persons. The results of neurophysiological studies including our study will play an important role in clarifying higher cognitive dysfunction in the patients with moyamoya disease.

References

1. Suzuki J, Kodama N. Moyamoya disease—a review. Stroke. 1983;14:104–9.
2. Hosoda Y, Ikeda E, Hirose S. Histopathological studies on spontaneous occlusion of the circle of Willis (cerebrovascular moyamoya disease). Clin Neurol Neurosurg. 1997;99(Suppl 2):S203–8.
3. Takekawa Y, Umezawa T, Ueno Y, Sawada T, Kobayashi M. Pathological and immunohistochemical findings of an autopsy case of adult moyamoya disease. Neuropathology. 2004;24:236–42.
4. Houkin K, Kuroda S, Ishikawa T, Abe H. Neovascularization (angiogenesis) after revascularization in moyamoya disease. Which technique is most useful for moyamoya disease? Acta Neurochir. 2000;142:269–76.
5. Karasawa J, Kikuchi H, Furuse S, Kawamura J, Sakaki T. Treatment of moyamoya disease with STA-MCA anastomosis. J Neurosurg. 1978;49:679–88.
6. Festa JR, Schwarz LR, Pliskin N, et al. Neurocognitive dysfunction in adult moyamoya disease. J Neurol. 2010;257:806–15.
7. Miyamoto S, Nagata I, Hashimoto N, Kikuchi H. Direct anastomotic bypass for cerebrovascular moyamoya disease. Neurol Med Chir (Tokyo). 1998;38(Suppl):294–6.
8. Nakagawara J, Osato T, Kamiyama K, et al. Diagnostic imaging of higher brain dysfunction in patients with adult moyamoya disease using statistical imaging analysis for [123I]iomazenil single photon emission computed tomography. Neurol Med Chir (Tokyo). 2012;52:318–26.
9. Araki Y, Takagi Y, Ueda K, Ubukata S, Ishida J, Funaki T, Kikuchi T, Takahashi JC, Murai T, Miyamoto S. Cognitive function of patients with adult moyamoya disease. J Stroke Cerebrovasc. 2014;23:1789–94.
10. Matsushima Y, Aoyagi M, Masaoka H, et al. Mental outcome following encephaloduroarteriosynangiosis in children with moyamoya disease with the onset earlier than 5 years of age. Childs Nerv Syst. 1990;6:440–3.

11. Sato H, Sato N, Tamaki N, et al. Chronic low-perfusion state in children with moyamoya disease following revascularization. Childs Nerv Syst. 1990;6:166–71.
12. Karzmark P, Zeifert PD, Bell-Stephens TE, et al. Neurocognitive impairment in adults with moyamoya disease without stroke. Neurosurgery. 2012;70:634–8.
13. Weinberg DG, Rahme RJ, Aoun SG, et al. Moyamoya disease: functional and neurocognitive outcomes in the pediatric and adult populations. Neurosurg Focus. 2011;30:E21.
14. Takagi Y, Miyamoto S, COSMO-Japan Study Group. Cognitive dysfunction survey of the Japanese patients with Moyamoya disease (COSMO-JAPAN study): study protocol. Neurol Med Chir (Tokyo). 2015;55(3):199–203.
15. Reitan RM. The Halstead-Reitan neuropsychological test battery. Tucson: Neuropsychology Press; 1985.
16. Wechsler D. Wechsler adult intelligence scale-third edition. San Antonio: The Psychological Corporation; 1997.
17. Wechsler D. Wechsler memory scale-revised. San Antonio: The Psychological Corporation; 1987.
18. Dubois B, Slachevsky A, Litvan I, Pillon B. The FAB: a frontal assessment battery at bedside. Neurology. 2000;55:1621–6.
19. Deckel AW, Hesselbrock V, Bauer L. Relationship between alcohol-related expectancies and anterior brain functioning in young men at risk for developing alcoholism. Alcohol Clin Exp Res. 1995;19:476–81.
20. Terada T, Obi T, Yoshizumi M, Murai T, Miyajima H, Mizoguchi K. Frontal lobe-mediated behavioral changes in amyotrophic lateral sclerosis: are they independent of physical disabilities? J Neurol Sci. 2011;309:136–40.
21. Takahashi M, Tanaka K, Miyaoka H. Depression and associated factors of informal caregivers versus professional caregivers of demented patients. Psychiatry Clin Neurosci. 2005;59:473–80.
22. Yamanishi T, Tachibana H, Oguru M, Matsui K, Toda K, Okuda B, Oka N. Anxiety and depression in patients with Parkinson's disease. Intern Med. 2013;52:539–45.
23. Kazumata K, Tha KK, Tokairin K, Ito M, Uchino H, Kawabori M, Sugiyama T. Brain structure, connectivity, and cognitive changes following revascularization surgery in adult Moyamoya disease. Neurosurgery. 2019 Nov 1;85(5):E943–52.
24. Iida H, Nakagawara J, Hayashida K, Fukushima K, Watabe H, Koshino K, Zeniya T, Eberl S. Multicenter evaluation of a standardized protocol for rest and acetazolamide cerebral blood flow assessment using a quantitative SPECT reconstruction program and split-dose 123I-iodoamphetamine. J Nucl Med. 2010;51:1624–31.
25. Yoneda H, Shirao S, Koizumi H, Oka F, Ishihara H, Ichiro K, Kitahara T, Iida H, Suzuki M. Reproducibility of cerebral blood flow assessment using a quantitative SPECT reconstruction program and split-dose 123I-iodoamphetamine in institutions with different γ-cameras and collimators. J Cereb Blood Flow Metab. 2012;32:1757–64.
26. Heaton R, Talley JL, Kay GG, Curtis G. Wisconsin card sorting test manual revised and expanded. Odessa: Psychological Assessment Resources; 1993.
27. Kaku Y, Iihara K, Nakajima N, Kataoka H, Fukuda K, Masuoka J, Fukushima K, Iida H, Hashimoto N. Cerebral blood flow and metabolism of hyperperfusion after cerebral revascularization in patients with moyamoya disease. J Cereb Blood Flow Metab. 2012;32:2066–75.

Asymptomatic Moyamoya Disease

12

Satoshi Kuroda

Abstract

The pathogenesis, prognosis, and treatment strategy of asymptomatic moyamoya disease is still obscure. In this chapter, our knowledge is summarized by reviewing previous articles on asymptomatic moyamoya disease. Then, the results of previous small-volume cohort studies on asymptomatic moyamoya disease are reviewed, and the on-going multicenter observational study in Japan (AMORE Study) is also described.

Keywords

Asymptomatic moyamoya disease · Cerebral infarct · Microbleed · Cerebral blood flow · Outcome · Stroke · Risk · Multicenter observational study

12.1 Introduction

Moyamoya disease (spontaneous occlusion of the circle of Willis) is a disease of unknown etiology that occurs frequently in East Asia, especially in Japan, Korea, and China. This disease was first named as moyamoya disease by Suzuki and Takaku [1]. Recent studies have gradually elucidated the genes involved in the development of moyamoya disease. In addition, advances and widespread use of non-invasive imaging techniques such as MRI have contributed enormously to early diagnosis, understanding of the pathophysiology, prognosis, determination of

S. Kuroda (✉)
Department of Neurosurgery, Graduate School of Medicine and Pharmaceutical Science, University of Toyama, Toyama, Japan
e-mail: skuroda@med.u-toyama.ac.jp

S. Kuroda (ed.), *Moyamoya Disease: Current Knowledge and Future Perspectives*, https://doi.org/10.1007/978-981-33-6404-2_12

treatment strategy, and improved perioperative management [2]. It is widely known that surgical revascularization is effective in preventing future TIAs and cerebral infarctions, and improved surgical techniques and perioperative management have reduced complications and improved long-term outcomes [2]. Recently, the Japan Adult Moyamoya (JAM) Trial, a randomized multicenter trial conducted in Japan, found that surgical revascularization, including direct bypass, significantly reduced rebleeding attacks in adult hemorrhagic moyamoya disease [3, 4].

However, the significance of medical and surgical treatment for incidentally discovered asymptomatic moyamoya disease remains unclear to this day [5]. This section summarizes our knowledge to date on the pathogenesis, prognosis, and treatment strategy of asymptomatic moyamoya disease and reviews the multicenter observational study initiated in January 2012 by the Research Committee on Moyamoya Disease in Japan.

12.2 Definition and Epidemiology

As mentioned above, it is a well-known fact that moyamoya disease can cause cerebral ischemic attacks such as TIA and cerebral infarction or intracranial hemorrhage. In addition, epilepsy, headache, and involuntary movements have also been reported to occur in some patients. Conversely, asymptomatic moyamoya disease is defined as an absence of previous episodes specific to moyamoya disease, such as transient ischemic attack (TIA), cerebral infarction, intracranial hemorrhage (cerebral hemorrhage, intraventricular hemorrhage, or subarachnoid hemorrhage), or involuntary movements [5].

The prevalence of moyamoya disease is reported to range from 3.16 to 10.5 per 100,000 people and has been increasing in recent years due to widespread acceptance of the disease concept and the development of non-invasive diagnostic imaging. However, the prevalence and incidence of asymptomatic moyamoya disease are not known at present. Previously, it was thought that the frequency of asymptomatic moyamoya disease was extremely low because it was mostly detected only in family members of patients with moyamoya disease when they were screened for the disease. However, with the widespread use of non-invasive diagnostic equipment such as MRI and MRA as described above, the detectability of asymptomatic moyamoya disease is increasing. Asymptomatic cases accounted for 1.5% of all cases of moyamoya disease in a nationwide survey conducted by Yamada et al. in 1994 [6], but this figure increased to 17.8% in a 2008 exhaustive survey conducted by Baba et al. in Hokkaido, the most northern island in Japan [7]. Thus, the frequency of asymptomatic moyamoya disease with no prior cerebrovascular events is now considered to be potentially higher than previously thought.

In 2007, the Research Committee on Moyamoya disease in Japan published the results of the first nationwide survey of asymptomatic moyamoya disease in Japan. Totally 40 cases of asymptomatic moyamoya disease were registered in the survey, of which one was in children and 39 in adults. Their age ranged from 13 to 67 years (mean 41.4 years), with a male-to-female ratio of 2.1, and they were found not to be significantly different from the adult symptomatic moyamoya disease. The clue of diagnosis included 14 cases of tension-type headache, 5 cases of non-specific dizziness, 4 cases of head injury, 5 brain check-up, 5 screenings for intra-familial onset, and 7 close examinations for other organ diseases [8].

12.3 Radiological Findings

As mentioned above, the widespread use of MRI and MRA has contributed significantly to the detection of asymptomatic moyamoya disease [5, 7]. There are not so many reports that investigate cerebral angiography in asymptomatic moyamoya disease. Nanba et al. (2003) reported that all 10 cases were bilateral [9], and the first nationwide survey in Japan found that 37 of the 40 cases were bilateral and the other 3 were unilateral [8]. Thus, most moyamoya disease may have already progressed to bilateral form before its onset (Figs. 12.1, 12.2, and 12.3). The former found a tendency for Stage 1–3 to be more common in cases in the

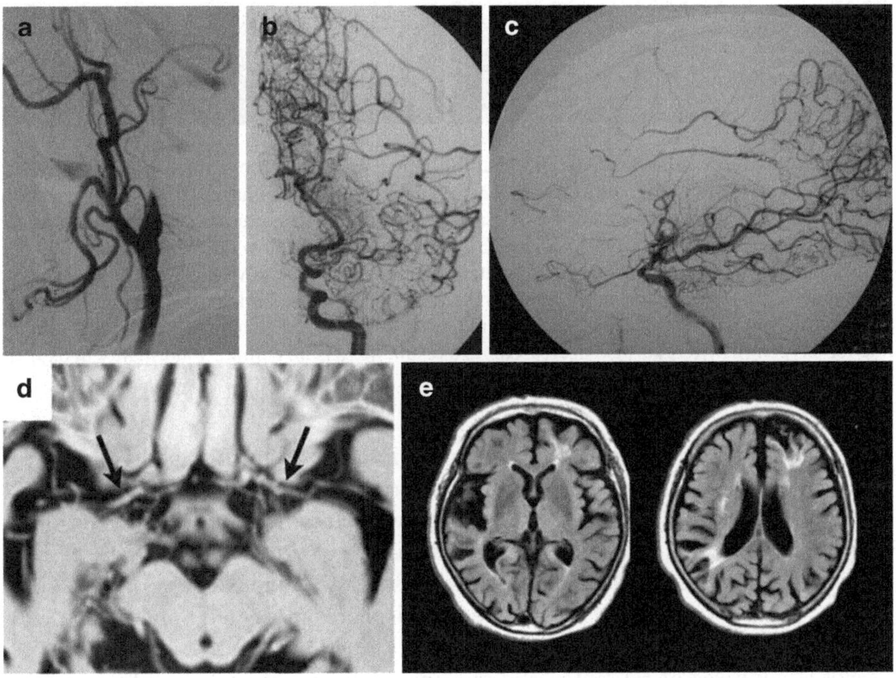

Fig. 12.1 Radiological findings of a 65-year-old female with asymptomatic moyamoya disease. Right carotid angiography (**a**) shows complete occlusion of the internal carotid artery. The Towne's (**b**) and lateral views (**c**) of left internal carotid angiography show an occlusion of supraclinoid portion of the internal carotid artery associated with dilated moyamoya vessels. Inverted image of heavy T2-weighted image (**d**) demonstrates a marked decrease of outer diameter of the middle cerebral artery on both sides (arrows), which is known specific for moyamoya disease (*see Chap.* 14). FLAIR images (**e**) reveal old cerebral infarction in the right deep white matter and parietal lobe and left frontal lobe. All of them correspond to the borderzone areas, suggesting the presence of hemodynamic insufficiency

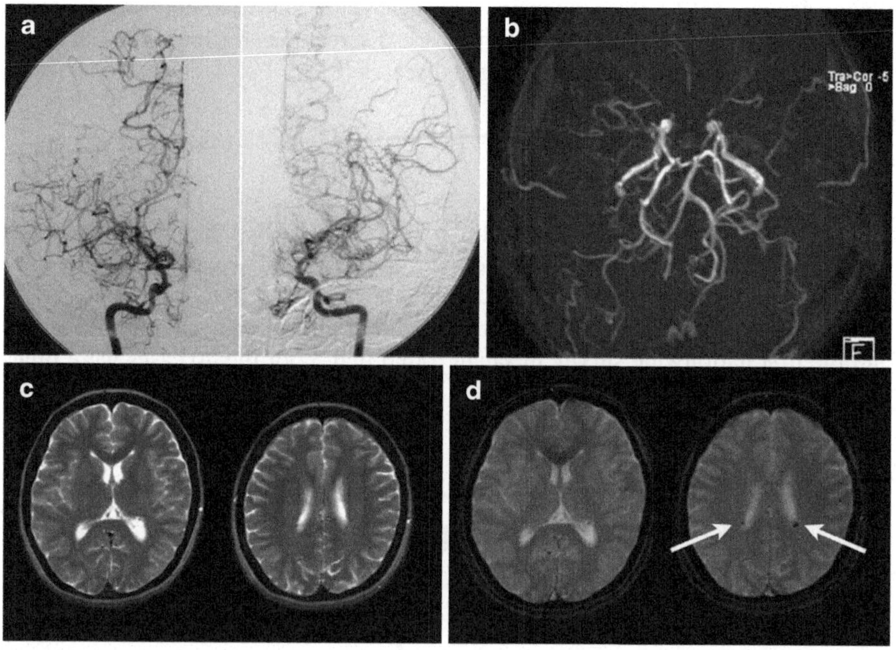

Fig. 12.2 Radiological findings of a 38-year-old female with asymptomatic moyamoya disease. No parenchymal lesions are noted on both T2- (**a**) and T2*-weighted images (**b**). MR angiography (**c**) demonstrated severe stenosis of the supraclinoid portion of the internal carotid artery and its main branches on both sides. On 15O-gas PET (**d**), cerebral blood flow (CBF) is decreased in the right frontal and temporal lobe and left frontal lobe (arrows). Cerebrovascular reactivity to acetazolamide (ACZ) is impaired in the same areas. Cerebral blood volume (CBV) is markedly elevated due to autoregulatory vasodilation in response to prolonged ischemia. Cerebral metabolic rate for oxygen (CMRO2) is also decreased. As a result, there is no definite abnormality in oxygen extraction fraction (OEF)

30s, whereas Stage 4–6 was more common in cases in the 40s and beyond [9]. Conversely, the latter report including a larger cohort showed that of the 72 affected hemispheres, angiographical stage was classified into Stage 1 on the 4 sides (5.6%), Stage 2 on the 10 sides (13.9%), Stage 3 on 33 sides (45.8%), Stage 4 on 21 sides (29.2%), Stage 5 on two sides (2.8%), and Stage 6 on two sides (2.8%). Thus, about 75% of the affected hemispheres presented Stage 3 to 4, with a significant stage progression with age [8].

Not a few cases of asymptomatic moyamoya disease show some abnormalities on brain MRI. According to a report by Nanba et al. (2003), 3 out of 10 cases (30%) had a brain infarction centered in the borderzone area [9]. In a nationwide survey in Japan, cerebral infarction was also found in 16 of 77 affected hemispheres (20.8%) [8]. Thus, cerebral infarction may have already occurred in about 20–30% of cases before the onset of the disease in asymptomatic moyamoya disease (Fig. 12.1). In these two reports, no hemorrhagic lesions have been identified in asymptomatic moyamoya disease, suggesting that a majority of intracranial hemorrhage are symptomatic. However, later, since T2*-weighted images were routinely performed, it

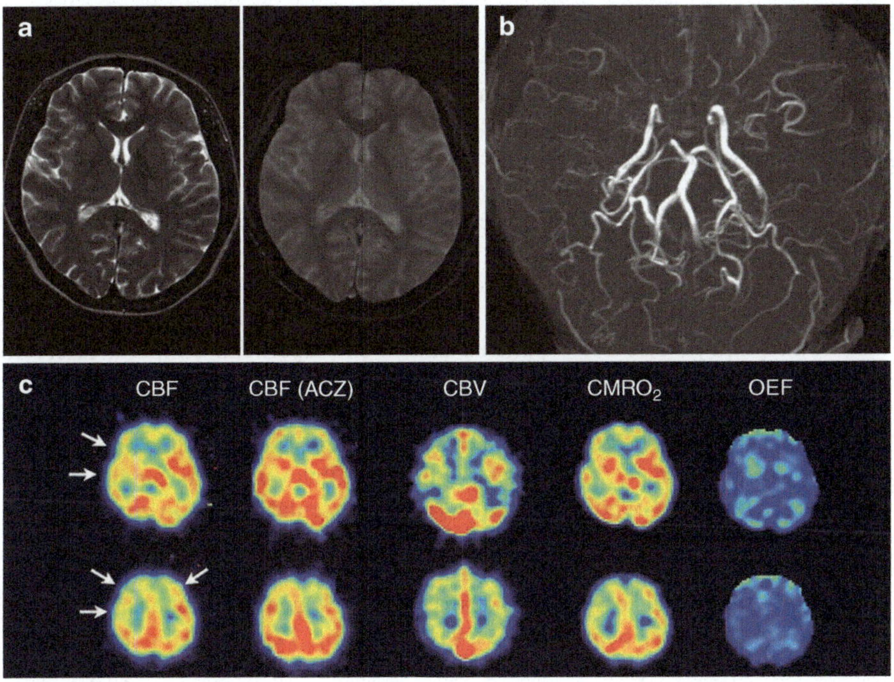

Fig. 12.3 Radiological findings of a 40-year-old female with asymptomatic moyamoya disease. On cerebral angiography (**a**), the supraclinoid portion of the internal carotid artery and its main branches are severely stenotic on both sides, which is associated with typical moyamoya vessels. MR angiography (**b**) demonstrates very similar findings. T2-weighted images (**c**) show no parenchymal lesions, but T2*-weighted images clearly demonstrate the microbleed in the subependymal area of the lateral ventricle on both sides (arrows)

became clear that a certain subgroup of patients with moyamoya disease had microbleeds. Microbleeds in moyamoya disease have been shown to be a risk factor for hemorrhagic stroke [10–12]. Therefore, it remains to be clarified how often patients with asymptomatic moyamoya disease have microbleeds (Fig. 12.2).

Previous reports have shown normal cerebral blood flow (CBF) but reduced cerebrovascular reactivity (CVR) to acetazolamide in 2 of 10 asymptomatic moyamoya disease cases (Type 2), and CBF and CVR were both reduced in a further 2 cases (Type 3) [9]. In a subsequent nationwide survey conducted in 70 hemispheres of asymptomatic moyamoya disease, both CBF and CVR were normal in 39 hemispheres (55.7%), while 24 hemispheres (34.3%) had normal CBF, but decreased CVR, suggesting moderate reduction of cerebral perfusion pressure (CPP). Other 7 hemispheres (10%) showed a decrease in both CBF and CVR, which indicates a marked reduction of CCP because of poorly developed collateral circulation (Fig. 12.3) [8]. Therefore, it is important to keep in mind that the number of cases with potential hemodynamic ischemia is not small even in asymptomatic moyamoya disease. These findings are crucial to addressing the problem of asymptomatic moyamoya disease.

12.4 Natural Course

The natural course of asymptomatic moyamoya disease is also poorly understood. Yamada et al. (2005) reported the outcome in 33 cases of asymptomatic moyamoya disease, of which TIAs occurred in 4 cases and fatal intracranial hemorrhage in two [6]. Nanba et al. (2003) conservatively followed up 10 cases of asymptomatic moyamoya disease for an average of 4.1 years and found that ischemic stroke associated with disease progression occurred in one case. This means that despite the small number of cases, the annual stroke rate was 2.4% [9].

In a subsequent nationwide survey in Japan, of the 40 enrolled cases of asymptomatic moyamoya disease, 6 patients underwent superficial temporal artery to middle cerebral artery anastomosis (STA-MCA) anastomosis and 34 patients were conservatively treated; 11 patients received some kinds of drug therapies, such as anticonvulsants or antiplatelet agents, and 24 patients received no drug therapy. During an average of 43.7 months of follow-up, there were no cerebrovascular events in the 6 patients who underwent surgical revascularization. In contrast, cerebrovascular events occurred in 7 of the 34 patients who were conservatively followed up. This included 3 TIAs, 1 ischemic stroke, and 3 intracranial hemorrhages. That means the annual incidence of stroke was 3.2% and the annual incidence of cerebrovascular events, including TIAs, was 5.7% (Fig. 12.4) [8]. More importantly, hemorrhagic stroke may more readily occur than ischemic stroke in asymptomatic moyamoya disease. The speculation correlates very well with the findings on cerebral angiography in a recent comparative study. In this study, the data set of cerebral angiography were compared between Asymptomatic Moyamoya Registry (AMORE) Study and Japan Adult Moyamoya (JAM) Trial at enrollment. The development of 3 subtypes of collateral vessels, including lenticulostriate, thalamic, and choroidal anastomosis, was evaluated on cerebral angiography. As a result, there were no significant differences in the development of choroidal anastomosis between asymptomatic and hemorrhagic-onset moyamoya disease. Considering an increasing evidence that choroidal channel plays an important role in the occurrence of hemorrhagic stroke, a certain subgroup of cases of asymptomatic moyamoya disease may be at potential risk for hemorrhagic stroke [13].

In addition, there was an association between SPECT/PET findings and prognosis at diagnosis, with a higher rate of ischemic events in patients with reduced cerebral perfusion pressure at diagnosis. On MR imaging and MR angiography, an even higher frequency of imaging changes is identified. That is, various kinds of *de novo* abnormalities were identified in 9 (26.5%) of the 34 patients who did not undergo surgical revascularization. Of these, 3 patients had advanced disease progression and cerebral infarction (2 symptomatic and 1 asymptomatic), 2 had only advanced disease progression (2 asymptomatic), 3 had hemorrhagic attacks, and 1 had new microbleeds (asymptomatic) [8].

These findings strongly suggest that asymptomatic moyamoya disease is not a stable disease, but should be recognized as a preliminary stage to a cerebrovascular event such as TIA, ischemic stroke, or hemorrhagic stroke, with a minor frequency of subclinical progression of the disease or microbleeds or cerebral infarction.

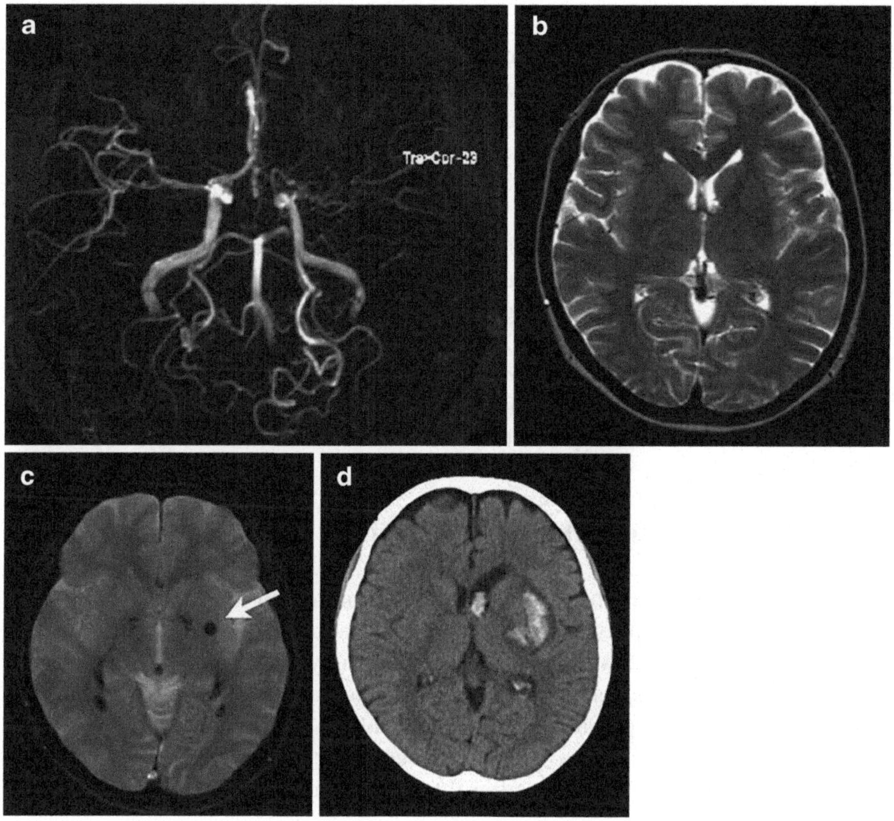

Fig. 12.4 Radiological findings of a 26-year-old female with asymptomatic moyamoya disease. On MR angiography (**a**), the supraclinoid portion of the internal carotid artery and its main branches are severely stenotic on the left sides, which is associated with typical moyamoya vessels. T2-weighted images (**b**) show no parenchymal lesions, but T2*-weighted images (**c**) clearly demonstrate the microbleed in the left putamen (arrow). Plain CT scan (**d**) taken 4 years later shows intracerebral hemorrhage in the left putamen

Therefore, when asymptomatic moyamoya disease is diagnosed, care must be taken to avoid overlooking potential changes, at least through regular MR examinations and imaging checks.

Appropriate surgical revascularization has been widely accepted as a treatment to prevent future TIA, ischemic stroke, and hemorrhagic stroke, but there is very limited information on the efficacy of surgical revascularization for asymptomatic moyamoya disease and no definitive guideline has been established. The "Guidelines for the Diagnosis and Treatment of Moyamoya Disease" published by Japanese group just focuses on the appropriate management of risk factors and lifestyle guidance from a medical perspective. Asymptomatic moyamoya disease does not have a low risk of developing hemorrhagic stroke and therefore the use of antiplatelet agents is not recommended [14]. Recently, Kawai et al. (2010) reported 2 cases of asymptomatic moyamoya disease that presented with a worsening of cerebral hemodynamics due to disease progression during follow-up. Although they had yet experienced no cerebrovascular events, they underwent surgical revascularization, including STA-MCA anastomosis and indirect bypass, and had a good postoperative course [15]. Furthermore, Yamamoto et al. reported a 61-year-old female with asymptomatic moyamoya disease. She had silent microbleeds in the corpus callosum at initial presentation and was conservatively followed up. However, *de novo* microbleeds developed in the right frontal and temporal lobe 6 months later, although she had no cerebrovascular events yet. She underwent STA-MCA anastomosis and indirect bypass on the right side to reduce hemodynamic stress onto the dilated, fragile moyamoya vessels. Postoperative course was uneventful. She is completely free from any cerebrovascular events and repeated MR examinations revealed no further development of *de novo* microbleeds for 7 years after surgery [16]. These data would be important to consider the treatment strategy in the future.

12.5 Asymptomatic Moyamoya Registry (AMORE) Study

Based on these observations, the Research Committee on Moyamoya Disease in Japan have started a prospective multicenter, nation-wide observational study, Asymptomatic Moyamoya Registry (AMORE) study, in January 2012 to further evaluate the epidemiology and outcome in asymptomatic moyamoya disease with a larger cohort [5]. They planned to enroll the eligible cases of asymptomatic moyamoya disease between January 2012 and December 2015 and to follow-up them conservatively for at least 5 years after the enrollment. Totally 20 centers in Japan joined this study.

In this study, the inclusion criteria include age 20–70 years; bilateral or unilateral form of moyamoya disease on cerebral angiography and/or MRA; no episodes that suggest TIA, ischemic stroke, and hemorrhagic stroke; possible to conservatively follow-up; independent in daily life (modified Rankin scale 0 or 1); and written informed consent. Exclusion criteria are previous episodes suggestive of TIA, ischemic stroke, and hemorrhagic stroke, quasi-moyamoya disease (moyamoya syndrome), and non-moyamoya disease. Following data are provided at the enrollment: demographic data, past history, family history, blood pressure, medicine, MRI (FLAIR image, T2-weighted image, and T2*-weighted image), MR angiography or cerebral angiography, and cerebral blood flow data on SPECT or PET.

A follow-up assessment is scheduled every 12 months, including any cerebrovascular event, blood pressure, MRI (T2-weighted images, T2*-weighted images, and FLAIR images), and MR angiography. Primary endpoint is any ischemic and hemorrhagic stroke during a follow-up period of 5 years. In AMORE Study, any ischemic stroke includes fresh cerebral infarction on diffusion-weighted MRI in spite of clinically transient neurological deficits that resolve within 24 hours after the onset. Secondary outcomes are TIA without newly developed cerebral infarction, *de novo* development of silent cerebral infarction and bleeding, disease progression, and any death during a follow-up period of 5 years [5].

The AMORE study is expected to be a clinical study that will provide definitive information for future treatment guidelines for asymptomatic moyamoya disease; by December 2015, 109 cases had been enrolled from participating centers across the country, and a five-year follow-up of all cases will be completed in December 2020. The results are expected to be announced in early 2021.

12.6 Conclusion

The epidemiology, clinical profile, prognosis, and new clinical trial of asymptomatic moyamoya disease are described. As the frequency of asymptomatic moyamoya disease constantly increases, we will face more opportunities to determine a treatment strategy in daily clinical practice in the future; however, the evidence for the outcome and treatment of asymptomatic moyamoya disease has not yet been sufficiently accumulated, and the results of AMORE Study are greatly anticipated.

Acknowledgments This work was partly supported by a grant from the Research Committee on Moyamoya Disease, the Japanese Ministry of Health, Labour and Welfare.

References

1. Suzuki J, Takaku A. Cerebrovascular "moyamoya" disease. Disease showing abnormal net-like vessels in base of brain. Arch Neurol. 1969;20:288–99.
2. Kuroda S, Houkin K. Moyamoya disease: current concepts and future perspectives. Lancet Neurol. 2008;7:1056–66.
3. Miyamoto S, Yoshimoto T, Hashimoto N, Okada Y, Tsuji I, Tominaga T, Nakagawara J, Takahashi JC, Investigators JT. Effects of extracranial-intracranial bypass for patients with hemorrhagic moyamoya disease: results of the Japan adult moyamoya trial. Stroke. 2014;45:1415–21.
4. Takahashi JC, Funaki T, Houkin K, Inoue T, Ogasawara K, Nakagawara J, Kuroda S, Yamada K, Miyamoto S, Investigators JAMT. Significance of the hemorrhagic site for recurrent bleeding: Prespecified analysis in the Japan adult Moyamoya trial. Stroke. 2016;47:37–43.
5. Kuroda S, AMORE Stugy Group. Asymptomatic moyamoya disease: literature review and ongoing AMORE study. Neurol Med Chir (Tokyo). 2015;55:194–8.
6. Yamada M, Fujii K, Fukui M. Clinical features and outcomes in patients with asymptomatic moyamoya disease--from the results of nation-wide questionnaire survey. No Shinkei Geka. 2005;33:337–42.
7. Baba T, Houkin K, Kuroda S. Novel epidemiological features of moyamoya disease. J Neurol Neurosurg Psychiatry. 2008;79:900–4.
8. Kuroda S, Hashimoto N, Yoshimoto T, Iwasaki Y. Radiological findings, clinical course, and outcome in asymptomatic moyamoya disease: results of multicenter survey in Japan. Stroke. 2007;38:1430–5.
9. Nanba R, Kuroda S, Takeda M, Shichinohe H, Nakayama N, Ishikawa T, Houkin K, Iwasaki Y. Clinical features and outcomes of 10 asymptomatic adult patients with moyamoya disease. No Shinkei Geka. 2003;31:1291–5.
10. Ishikawa T, Kuroda S, Nakayama N, Terae S, Kudou K, Iwasaki Y. Prevalence of asymptomatic microbleeds in patients with moyamoya disease. Neurol Med Chir (Tokyo). 2005;45:495–500. discussion 500

11. Kikuta K, Takagi Y, Nozaki K, Sawamoto N, Fukuyama H, Hashimoto N. The presence of multiple microbleeds as a predictor of subsequent cerebral hemorrhage in patients with moyamoya disease. Neurosurgery. 2008;62:104–11. discussion 111-102
12. Kuroda S, Kashiwazaki D, Ishikawa T, Nakayama N, Houkin K. Incidence, locations, and longitudinal course of silent microbleeds in moyamoya disease: a prospective T2*-weighted MRI study. Stroke. 2013;44:516–8.
13. Yamamoto S, Funaki T, Fujimura M, Takahashi JC, Uchino H, Houkin K, Tominaga T, Miyamoto S, Kuroda S, Asymptomatic Moyamoya Registry Investigators, the Japan Adult Moyamoya Trial Investigators. Development of hemorrhage- prone anastomoses in asymptomatic moyamoya disease - a comparative study with Japan adult Moyamoya trial. J Stroke Cerebrovasc Dis. 2019;28:104328.
14. Research Committee on the Pathology and Treatment of Spontaneous Occlusion of the Circle of Willis. Guidelines for diagnosis and treatment of moyamoya disease (spontaneous occlusion of the circle of Willis). Neurol Med Chir (Tokyo). 2012;52:245–66.
15. Kawai K, Kuroda S, Kawabori M, Nakayama N, Terasaka S, Iwasaki Y. Revascularization surgery for asymptomatic adult moyamoya disease presenting silent disease progression: report of two cases. No Shinkei Geka. 2010;38:825–30.
16. Yamamoto S, Kuroda S. Long-term effect of surgical revascularization on silent microbleeds in adult moyamoya disease: a case report. Surg Neurol Int. 2017;8:99.

Part IV

Update on Neuroradiology in Moyamoya Disease

Periventricular Anastomosis 13

Takeshi Funaki and Susumu Miyamoto

Abstract

Periventricular anastomosis is a term used to describe fragile, hemorrhage-prone collateral vessels typical of moyamoya disease. It is defined as pathological anastomoses between the perforating or choroidal arteries and the medullary arteries in the periventricular area. This chapter discusses the anatomic characteristics, the relationship to hemorrhage, and representative radiological findings.

Keywords

Moyamoya disease · Intracranial hemorrhage · Periventricular anastomosis

Periventricular anastomosis is a unique phenomenon occurring in moyamoya disease. It is defined as pathological anastomoses between the perforating or choroidal arteries and the medullary arteries in the periventricular area that serve as collaterals to the cortex via retrograde flow in the medullary arteries (Fig. 13.1). Periventricular anastomosis well explains the mechanism of intracranial hemorrhage in moyamoya disease, given that anastomotic sites are especially fragile because of histologically abnormal connections between vessels. Small pseudoaneurysms indicating bleeding points are commonly observed at the exact site of the anastomoses (Fig. 13.2) (See also Chap. 9).

T. Funaki (✉) · S. Miyamoto
Department of Neurosurgery, Kyoto University Graduate School of Medicine, Kyoto, Japan
e-mail: tfunaki@kuhp.kyoto-u.ac.jp; miy@kuhp.kyoto-u.ac.jp

S. Kuroda (ed.), *Moyamoya Disease: Current Knowledge and Future Perspectives*, https://doi.org/10.1007/978-981-33-6404-2_13

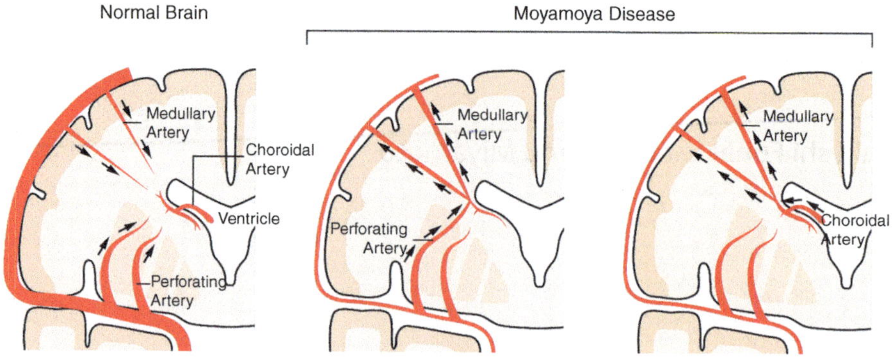

Fig. 13.1 Schematic illustrations showing periventricular anastomosis in coronal planes of the right hemisphere, reprinted with permission from Funaki (Nihon Iji Shimpo 4884: 28–35, 2017)

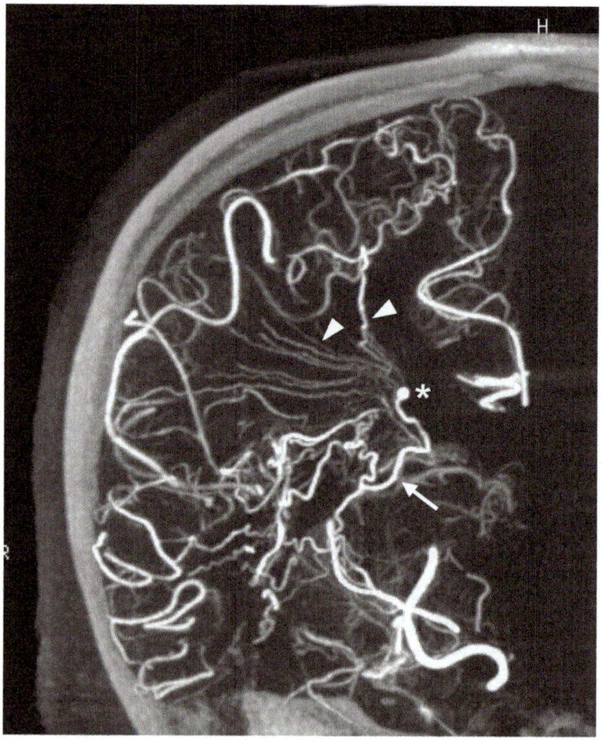

Fig. 13.2 3D rotational internal carotid angiography showing periventricular anastomosis in a coronal plane. Many medullary arteries (arrowheads) radiate from the plexal portion of the anterior choroidal artery (arrow). Note that a pseudoaneurysm is observed at the exact site of the anastomosis (asterisk)

13.1 Anatomy

The traditional theory of vascular supply in the periventricular area provides a clue for understanding the development of periventricular anastomosis. In 1969, Van den Bergh advocated two terminal arteries in the periventricular area, the ventriculofugal and ventriculopetal arteries [1]. According to his original article, ventriculofugal (or centrifugal) arteries originate from subependymal arteries, which consist of the branches from the choroidal or lenticulostriate artery, and diverge "ventriculofugally" (in a direction away from the ventricle). Ventriculopetal (or centripetal) arteries consist of the medullary or lenticulostriate arteries, which are directed toward the ventricle. Van den Bergh's theory became famous because Yasargil introduced the schematic figure in his book [2]. De Reuck classified the patterns of periventricular arterial border zone and considered that the ventriculofugal arteries consist of the choroidal or perforating arteries [3]. According to his description, ventriculofugal arteries originate from the choroidal arteries of the lateral and third ventricles and penetrate into the brain substance from the choroid plexus to meet the ventriculopetal branches at a distance of 3–10 mm from the ventricular walls [3]. Ventriculofugal and ventriculopetal arteries form no anastomosis in the normal brain [1, 3], as the border zone between these arteries is believed to be the cause of periventricular ischemia.

Although the existence of the ventriculofugal artery was once denied in the 1990s [4], Marinkovic and Gibo et al. rediscovered the phenomenon; they showed that tiny vessels arising from all choroidal arteries extended through the subependymal layer of a larger part of the ventricular wall and referred to them as the subependymal artery [5]. The existence of such arteries was confirmed by a clinical study on glioma resection, during which the coagulation of the plexal portion of the choroidal arteries causes infarct in the periventricular white matter [6].

Long-standing cortical ischemia in moyamoya disease might induce an abnormal connection between the perforating or choroidal arteries and the medullary arteries via the ventriculofugal subependymal arteries and result in periventricular anastomosis. Kodama and Suzuki were the first to describe arterial connections between perforating and medullary arteries in fetus brain [7]. In their pioneering work, they considered such connections, which they denoted as "anastomoses," as the rationale of moyamoya vessels. The term "periventricular anastomosis" is named after their contribution. Takahashi was the first to describe angiographic findings showing anastomoses between perforating and medullary arteries in 1980 [8]. Recent angiographic techniques using a microcatheter can more clearly reveal these connections [9, 10], although the procedure is invasive.

The development of high-resolution magnetic resonance (MR) imaging has facilitated non-invasive, meticulous visualization of periventricular anastomosis [11, 12]. Coronal thin-slab maximal-intensity-projection (MIP) reformation of 3 T MR angiography is an especially useful technique for visualizing periventricular anastomosis (Fig. 13.3) [11]. This imaging has also facilitated the systematization of periventricular anastomosis, which is classified into three subtypes according to its origin: lenticulostriate, thalamic, and choroidal (Fig. 13.3; see also Chap. 9). Excellent delineation of periventricular anastomotic channels was reported in a study using 7 T MR angiography [13].

Table 13.1 summarizes the anatomic characteristics of the three subtypes of periventricular anastomosis. The spatial relationship along the anterior-posterior axis helps to understand their anatomic characteristics [14–16].

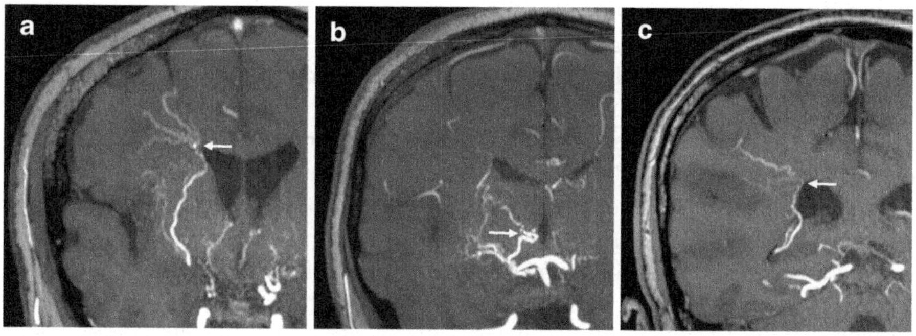

Fig. 13.3 Coronal thin-slab MIP reformation of 3 T MR angiography showing periventricular anastomosis (arrows). (**a**) lenticulostriate anastomosis. (**b**) thalamic anastomosis. (**c**) choroidal anastomosis

Table 13.1 Anatomic characteristics of three subtypes of periventricular anastomosis

	Lenticulostriate Anastomosis	Thalamic Anastomosis	Choroidal Anastomosis
Origin	Lenticulostriate a.	Thalamotuberal a. (from PCoA) Thalamoperforating a. (from P1) Thalamogeniculate a.	Anterior choroidal a. Lateral posterior choroidal a. (medial posterior choroidal a.)
Common site of anastomosis	Subependymal area of the frontal horn or anterior body of LV	Subependymal area of third V	Subependymal area of the atrium of LV
Common type of hemorrhage	ICH in the basal ganglia or frontal lobe IVH at the frontal horn or anterior half of the body of LV	ICH in the thalamus IVH in the third V or LV	IVH in the atrium or posterior part of the lateral ventricle ICH in the temporal or parietal lobe
Common cortical distribution	Anterior to CS Interhemispheric fissure	Insular cortex Around CS	Posterior to CS (occasionally, insular cortex)

a. artery; *CS* central sulcus; *LV* lateral ventricle; *PCoA* posterior communicating artery; *third V* third ventricle

13.2 Relationship between Periventricular Anastomosis and Bleeding

Experts of moyamoya disease have always focused on the choroidal artery in relation to hemorrhage. Kodama and Suzuki described aneurysms occurring in the choroidal arteries in the early days of angiography [17]. They considered the aneurysms as "pseudoaneurysms," indicating the bleeding point. Irikura et al. were perhaps the first to pay special attention to the angiographic finding of choroidal anastomosis; they described "the medullary arteries that were filled from the plexal segment of the choroidal arteries" [18]. They also revealed that this finding was more frequently observed in the hemorrhagic group than in the ischemic group. Morioka et al. revealed in a larger cross-sectional study that "angiographic dilatation and branch extension of the anterior choroidal arteries" was associated with hemorrhagic presentation [19]. Although they did not clearly define the abnormal branches from the choroidal arteries, it is obvious that the medullary arteries represent such branches. The causal relationship between choroidal anastomosis and hemorrhage was proved by longitudinal analyses using the data of a nonsurgical cohort in the Japan Adult Moyamoya Trial (see Chap. 9) [20, 21]. Wang et al. also revealed in a longitudinal study that lateral posterior choroidal anastomosis was an independent predictor of rebleeding [22].

Evidence is being accumulated suggesting that periventricular anastomoses, including choroidal anastomosis, is a potential bleeding source in moyamoya disease. Kazumata et al. demonstrated a topographical correspondence between cerebral microbleeds, which were frequently observed in the periventricular area, and moyamoya vessels detected with source images of time-of-flight MR angiography [23]. They also implied an early concept of periventricular anastomosis. Our cross-sectional study revealed that scoring of periventricular anastomosis with coronal thin-slab MIP MR angiography was highly reliable and that an increase of periventricular anastomosis score was significantly associated with hemorrhagic presentation in a multivariate analysis [11].

While any subtypes of periventricular anastomosis might be associated with hemorrhage, the bleeding risk in a certain period might vary across subtypes [11]. Considering many recent findings, choroidal anastomosis seems to present the highest risk of bleeding among subtypes [14, 20, 24, 25].

Periventricular anastomosis is a common finding not only in adult patients but also in pediatric patients. Although pediatric patients rarely suffer from intracranial hemorrhage, Liu P et al. revealed that the grade of choroidal anastomotic channel in the hemorrhagic group was significantly higher than that in the ischemic group among pediatric patients [26]. Interestingly, Ryu et al. revealed that the periventricular anastomosis score in the child ischemic group was equivalent to that in the adult hemorrhagic group [27]. This suggests the following hypothesis. Pediatric patients with abundant periventricular anastomosis, which moderates ischemic symptoms, could grow up without being diagnosed as moyamoya disease. Such a population might exhibit hemorrhage after they reach adulthood, given that the bleeding risk of periventricular anastomosis might increase with longer duration of its existence.

13.3 Radiological Findings

See also Table 13.1.

13.3.1 Lenticulostriate Anastomosis

This type of periventricular anastomosis arises from the lenticulostriate arteries and connects to the medial end of the medullary arteries at the lateral corner of the

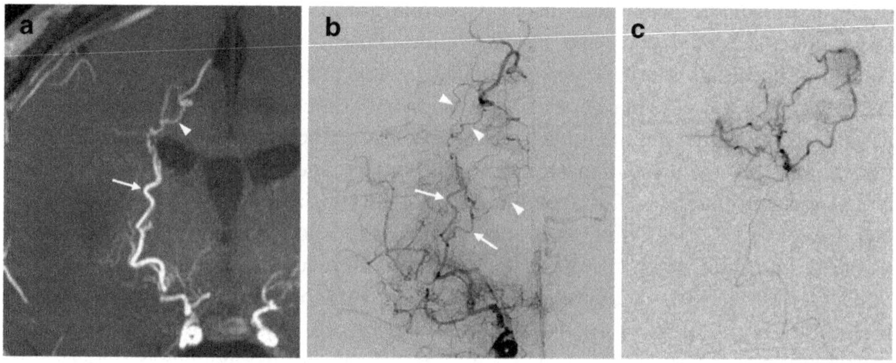

Fig. 13.4 lenticulostriate anastomosis. (**a**) coronal thin-slab MIP MR angiography. (**b**) anterior-posterior view of left internal carotid angiography. (**c**) anterior-posterior view of a superselective injection of one of the lenticulostriate arteries, clearly showing the medullary arteries. Arrows indicate lenticulostriate artery; arrowheads, medullary artery

frontal horn or body of the lateral ventricle (Figs. 13.3a and 13.4) [11]. The medullary arteries from the lenticulostriate anastomosis radiate toward the cortex and reach the cortical arteries located anterior to the central sulcus, mainly to the superior and inferior frontal sulcus [16]. Lenticulostriate anastomosis thus outflows more anteriorly than thalamic or choroidal anastomosis (Fig. 13.5). It should be noted that lenticulostriate anastomosis often shows outflows to the interhemispheric fissure (the cingulate sulcus) (Fig. 13.4) [16, 28]. This might be attributable to the anatomic relationship that lenticulostriate anastomosis is located nearest toward the anterior cerebral artery territory, almost always hemodynamically compromised in moyamoya disease. The characteristic adds an intractable nature to this type [28].

A positive angiographic indicator of lenticulostriate anastomosis is extreme dilation and extension of the lenticulostriate arteries with at least one artery extending beyond the level of the pericallosal artery in the lateral view (Fig. 13.5) [14]. In such a situation, the lenticulostriate arteries are reasonably considered to connect to the medullary arteries at the lateral corner of the lateral ventricle because the position of the pericallosal artery approximates the upper margin of the lateral ventricle.

13.3.2 Thalamic Anastomosis

This type of periventricular anastomosis arises from the thalamotuberal arteries (perforator from the posterior communicating artery) or the thalamoperforating arteries (perforator from the P1 segment of the posterior cerebral artery) and connects to the medullary or insular arteries beneath the ependyma of the third or lateral ventricle (Figs. 13.3b and 13.6) [11]. Thalamic anastomosis can also arise from the thalamogeniculate (or rarely, choroidal) arteries and connect to the insular artery superior to the inferior horn or at the lateral corner of the body of the lateral ventricle. Thalamic anastomosis shows outflows to the sulcus around the central sulcus

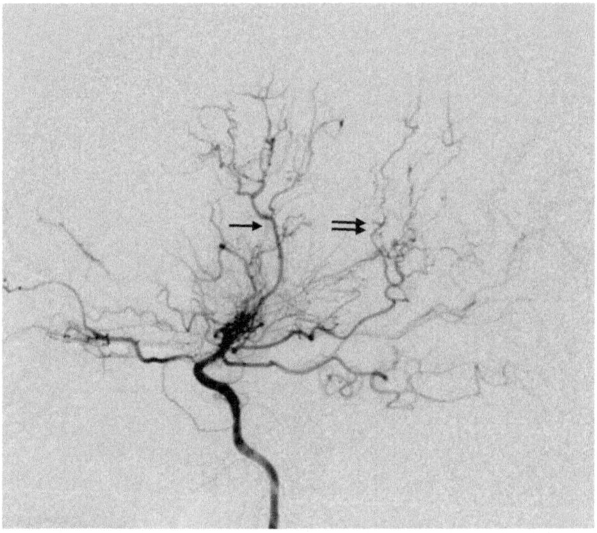

Fig. 13.5 Lateral view of internal carotid angiography showing both lenticulostriate anastomosis (arrow) and choroidal anastomosis (double arrow)

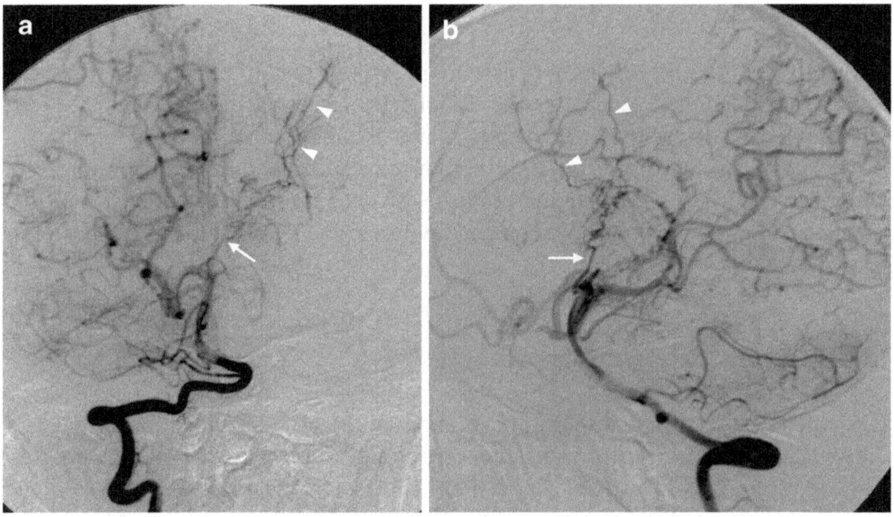

Fig. 13.6 Thalamic anastomosis observed by vertebral angiography. (**a**) anterior-posterior view. (**b**) lateral view. Arrows indicate thalamoperforating artery; arrowheads, medullary artery

via medullary arteries (Fig. 13.6) or to the insular cortex [16]. Unlike lenticulostriate and choroidal anastomoses, however, thalamic anastomosis less commonly outflows to the cortex independently and tends to anastomose with other collateral vessels [16].

A positive angiographic indicator of thalamic anastomosis is extreme dilation and extension of the thalamic perforators with at least one artery extending beyond the position of the medial posterior choroidal artery in the lateral view (Fig. 13.6).

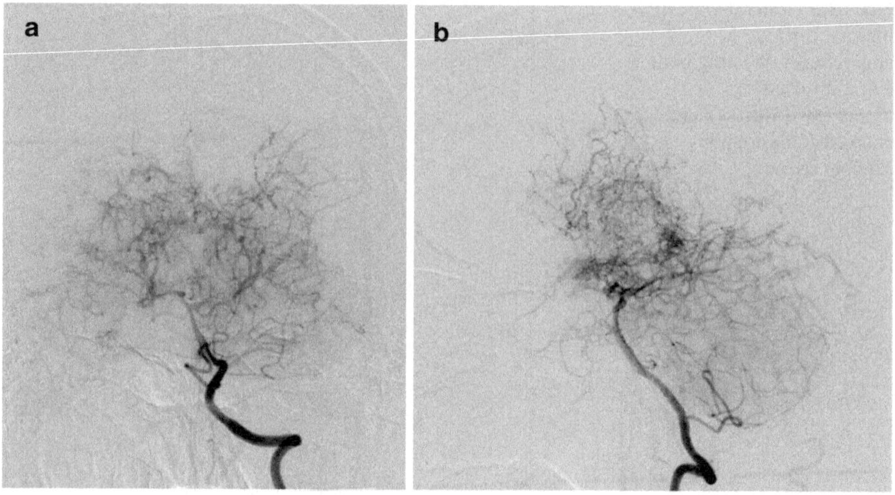

Fig. 13.7 Occlusion of the posterior cerebral artery and cluster of thalamic anastomosis ("posterior basal moyamoya") observed by vertebral angiography. (**a**) anterior-posterior view. (**b**) lateral view

In such a situation, the thalamic perforators are reasonably considered to extend beyond the thalamus to connect to the medullary arteries because the position of the medial posterior choroidal artery approximates the upper margin of the thalamus.

Thalamic anastomosis often develops in relation to occlusion of the posterior cerebral artery (PCA). The senior author (S.M.) has referred to the cluster of thalamic anastomotic channels accompanied with the PCA involvement as "posterior basal moyamoya" [29] (Fig. 13.7).

13.3.3 Choroidal Anastomosis

This type of periventricular anastomosis arises at the plexal segment of the anterior choroidal or lateral posterior choroidal arteries and connects to the medullary arteries beneath the lateral wall of the atrium of the lateral ventricle (Figs. 13.3c and 13.9a) [11]. The medullary arteries typically radiate toward the cortex and reach the cortical arteries located in or posterior to the central sulcus [16]. Choroidal anastomosis thus outflows more posteriorly than lenticulostriate or thalamic anastomosis (Fig. 13.5). Unlike lenticulostriate anastomosis, choroidal anastomosis rarely shows outflows to the interhemispheric fissure, except for one formed by the medial posterior choroidal arteries. Choroidal anastomosis sometimes seems to outflow to the insular cortex. In such cases, however, strictly classifying such collateral channel as either choroidal or thalamic anastomosis might be difficult.

A positive angiographic (lateral view) indicator of choroidal anastomosis is extreme dilation and extension of the choroidal arteries with sudden deviation from the shape of the lateral ventricle at its peripheral portion to connect to the medullary

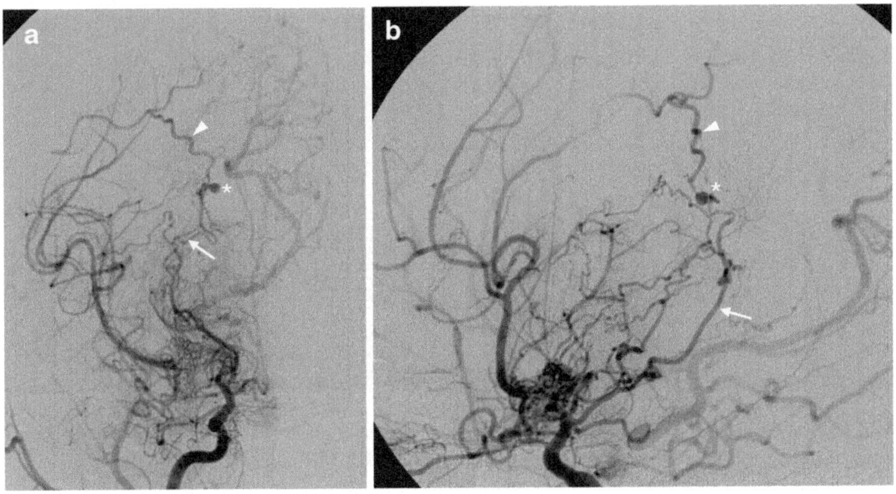

Fig. 13.8 Choroidal anastomosis from the anterior choroidal artery, observed by internal carotid angiography. (**a**) anterior-posterior view. (**b**) lateral view. The plexal portion of the anterior choroidal artery (arrows) connects to the medullary artery (arrowheads), which finally extend to the cortical artery. Note that a pseudoaneurysm is observed at the exact site of the anastomosis (asterisks)

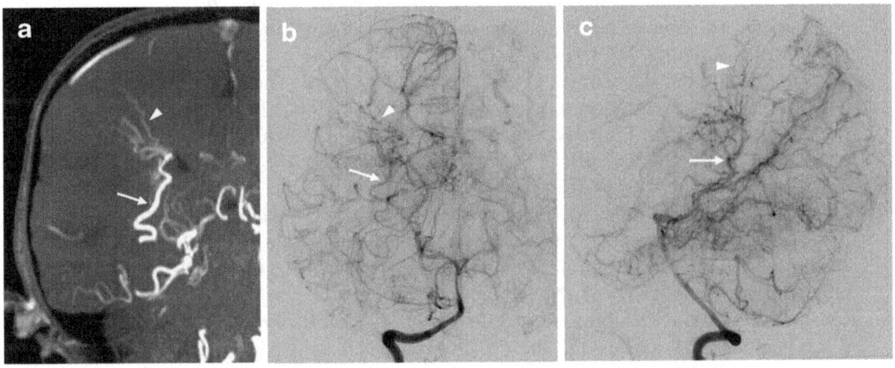

Fig. 13.9 Choroidal anastomosis from the lateral posterior choroidal artery. (**a**) coronal thin-slab MIP MR angiography. (**b**) anterior-posterior view of the right vertebral angiography. (**c**) lateral view of the right vertebral angiography. Arrows indicate the plexal portion of the lateral posterior choroidal artery; arrowheads, medullary artery

arteries (Figs. 13.5 and 13.8); in the anteroposterior view, this collateral has a typical sharp inflection laterally (Fig. 13.8a) [14]. When choroidal anastomosis is formed via the lateral posterior choroidal arteries, careful interpretation of vertebral angiography is required because many overlapping vessels might obscure the anastomotic channel (Fig. 13.9).

Another relatively rare subtype classified as choroidal anastomosis is formed by the medial posterior choroidal arteries, which connects to the pericallosal arteries by penetrating the corpus callosum (Fig. 13.10) [10].

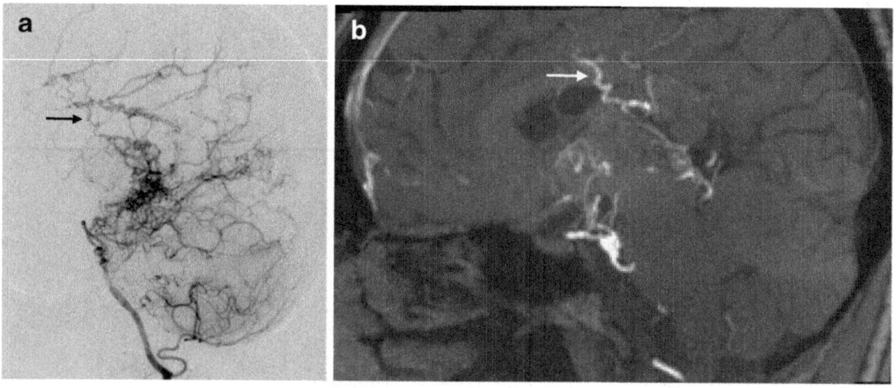

Fig. 13.10 Choroidal anastomosis from the medial posterior choroidal artery (arrows). (**a**) lateral view of the vertebral angiography. (**b**) sagittal thin-slab MIP MR angiography

References

1. Van den Bergh R. Centrifugal elements in the vascular pattern of the deep intracerebral blood supply. Angiology. 1969;20(2):88–94.
2. Yasargil MG. Microneurosurgery. New York: Thieme Medical; 1987. p. 322.
3. De Reuck J. The human periventricular arterial blood supply and the anatomy of cerebral infarctions. Eur Neurol. 1971;5(6):321–34.
4. Nelson MD Jr, Gonzalez-Gomez I, Gilles FH. Dyke award. The search for human telencephalic ventriculofugal arteries. AJNR Am J Neuroradiol. 1991;12(2):215–22.
5. Marinkovic S, Gibo H, Filipovic B, Dulejic V, Piscevic I. Microanatomy of the subependymal arteries of the lateral ventricle. Surg Neurol. 2005;63(5):451–8.; discussion 8. https://doi.org/10.1016/j.surneu.2004.06.013.
6. Saito R, Kumabe T, Sonoda Y, Kanamori M, Mugikura S, Takahashi S, et al. Infarction of the lateral posterior choroidal artery territory after manipulation of the choroid plexus at the atrium: causal association with subependymal artery injury. J Neurosurg. 2013;119(1):158–63. https://doi.org/10.3171/2013.2.JNS121221.
7. Kodama N, Suzuki J. Cerebrovascular Moyamoya disease IIIrd report-the study on the aging of the perforating branches and the possibility of collateral pathway. Neurologia medico-chirurgica Part I. 1974;14(1):55–67. https://doi.org/10.2176/nmc.14pt1.SUPPLEMENT_55.
8. Takahashi M. Magnification angiography in moyamoya disease: new observations on collateral vessels. Radiology. 1980;136(2):379–86. https://doi.org/10.1148/radiology.136.2.7403514.
9. Baltsavias G, Valavanis A, Filipce V, Khan N. Selective and superselective angiography of pediatric moyamoya disease angioarchitecture: the anterior circulation. Interv Neuroradiol. 2014;20(4):391–402. https://doi.org/10.15274/NRJ-2014-10050.
10. Baltsavias G, Khan N, Filipce V, Valavanis A. Selective and superselective angiography of pediatric moyamoya disease angioarchitecture in the posterior circulation. Interv Neuroradiol. 2014;20(4):403–12. https://doi.org/10.15274/NRJ-2014-10041.
11. Funaki T, Takahashi JC, Yoshida K, Takagi Y, Fushimi Y, Kikuchi T, et al. Periventricular anastomosis in moyamoya disease: detecting fragile collateral vessels with MR angiography. J Neurosurg. 2016;124(6):1766–72. https://doi.org/10.3171/2015.6.jns15845.
12. Funaki T, Fushimi Y, Takahashi JC, Takagi Y, Araki Y, Yoshida K, et al. Visualization of periventricular collaterals in Moyamoya disease with flow-sensitive black-blood magnetic reso-

nance angiography: preliminary experience. Neurol Med Chir (Tokyo). 2015;55(3):204–9. https://doi.org/10.2176/nmc.oa.2014-0360.
13. Matsushige T, Kraemer M, Sato T, Berlit P, Forsting M, Ladd ME, et al. Visualization and classification of deeply seated collateral networks in Moyamoya Angiopathy with 7T MRI. AJNR Am J Neuroradiol. 2018;39(7):1248–54. https://doi.org/10.3174/ajnr.A5700.
14. Funaki T, Takahashi JC, Houkin K, Kuroda S, Takeuchi S, Fujimura M, et al. Angiographic features of hemorrhagic moyamoya disease with high recurrence risk: a supplementary analysis of the Japan adult Moyamoya trial. J Neurosurg. 2018;128(3):777–84. https://doi.org/10.3171/2016.11.jns161650.
15. Miyakoshi A, Funaki T, Fushimi Y, Kikuchi T, Kataoka H, Yoshida K, et al. Identification of the bleeding point in hemorrhagic Moyamoya disease using fusion images of susceptibility-weighted imaging and time-of-flight MRA. AJNR Am J Neuroradiol. 2019;40(10):1674–80. https://doi.org/10.3174/ajnr.A6207.
16. Miyakoshi A, Funaki T, Fushimi Y, Nakae T, Okawa M, Kikuchi T, et al. Cortical distribution of fragile periventricular anastomotic collateral vessels in Moyamoya disease: an exploratory cross-sectional study on Japanese moyamoya patients. AJNR. Am J Neuroradiol Epub ahead of print Nov. 2020:5. https://doi.org/10.3174/ajnr.A6861.
17. Kodama N, Suzuki J. Moyamoya disease associated with aneurysm. J Neurosurg. 1978;48(4):565–9. https://doi.org/10.3171/jns.1978.48.4.0565.
18. Irikura K, Miyasaka Y, Kurata A, Tanaka R, Fujii K, Yada K, et al. A source of haemorrhage in adult patients with moyamoya disease: the significance of tributaries from the choroidal artery. Acta Neurochir. 1996;138(11):1282–6.
19. Morioka M, Hamada J, Kawano T, Todaka T, Yano S, Kai Y, et al. Angiographic dilatation and branch extension of the anterior choroidal and posterior communicating arteries are predictors of hemorrhage in adult moyamoya patients. Stroke. 2003;34(1):90–5.
20. Funaki T, Takahashi JC, Houkin K, Kuroda S, Takeuchi S, Fujimura M, et al. High rebleeding risk associated with choroidal collateral vessels in hemorrhagic moyamoya disease: analysis of a nonsurgical cohort in the Japan adult Moyamoya trial. J Neurosurg. 2019;130(2):525–30. https://doi.org/10.3171/2017.9.jns17576.
21. Funaki T, Takahashi JC, Houkin K, Kuroda S, Fujimura M, Tomata Y, et al. Effect of choroidal collateral vessels on de novo hemorrhage in moyamoya disease: analysis of nonhemorrhagic hemispheres in the Japan adult Moyamoya trial. J Neurosurg. 2019:1–7. https://doi.org/10.3171/2018.10.Jns181139.
22. Wang J, Yang Y, Li X, Zhou F, Wu Z, Liang Q, et al. Lateral posterior Choroidal collateral anastomosis predicts recurrent Ipsilateral hemorrhage in adult patients with Moyamoya disease. AJNR Am J Neuroradiol. 2019;40(10):1665–71. https://doi.org/10.3174/ajnr.A6208.
23. Kazumata K, Shinbo D, Ito M, Shichinohe H, Kuroda S, Nakayama N, et al. Spatial relationship between cerebral microbleeds, Moyamoya vessels, and hematoma in Moyamoya disease. Journal of stroke and cerebrovascular diseases: the official journal of National Stroke Association. 2014;23(6):1421–8. https://doi.org/10.1016/j.jstrokecerebrovasdis.2013.12.007.
24. Takahashi JC, Funaki T, Houkin K, Inoue T, Ogasawara K, Nakagawara J, et al. Significance of the hemorrhagic site for recurrent bleeding: Prespecified analysis in the Japan adult Moyamoya trial. Stroke. 2016;47(1):37–43. https://doi.org/10.1161/strokeaha.115.010819.
25. Fujimura M, Funaki T, Houkin K, Takahashi JC, Kuroda S, Tomata Y, et al. Intrinsic development of choroidal and thalamic collaterals in hemorrhagic-onset moyamoya disease: case-control study of the Japan adult Moyamoya trial. J Neurosurg. 2018:1–7. https://doi.org/10.3171/2017.11.Jns171990.
26. Liu P, Han C, Li DS, Lv XL, Li YX, Duan L. Hemorrhagic Moyamoya disease in children: clinical, angiographic features, and long-term surgical outcome. Stroke. 2016;47(1):240–3. https://doi.org/10.1161/strokeaha.115.010512.
27. Ryu J, Hamano E, Nishimura M, Satow T, Takahashi JC. Difference in periventricular anastomosis in child and adult moyamoya disease: a vascular morphology study. Acta Neurochir. 2020;162(6):1333–9. https://doi.org/10.1007/s00701-020-04354-1.

28. Sasagasako T, Funaki T, Tanji M, Arakawa Y, Suzuki H, Miyakoshi A, et al. Intractable medial anastomotic branches from the Lenticulostriate artery causing recurrent hemorrhages in Moyamoya disease: a case report. World Neurosurg. 2019; https://doi.org/10.1016/j.wneu.2019.04.066.
29. Miyamoto S, Kikuchi H, Karasawa J, Nagata I, Ikota T, Takeuchi S. Study of the posterior circulation in moyamoya disease. Clinical and neuroradiological evaluation. J Neurosurg. 1984;61(6):1032–7. https://doi.org/10.3171/jns.1984.61.6.1032.

Arterial Shrinkage 14

Satoshi Kuroda

Abstract

For these 50 years or longer, the diagnosis of moyamoya disease has been based on the information of the lumen of involved arteries, using cerebral angiography and MR angiography. However, this has led to some confusion in the diagnosis of the disease, such as in differentiating it from intracranial arterial stenosis caused by atherosclerosis. On the other hand, studies over the past 10 years have shown that arterial shrinkage appears specifically in affected arteries in moyamoya disease. This phenomenon may not only improve the accuracy of the diagnosis, but may also help to elucidate the still unknown etiology of the disease. In this chapter, I introduce a novel concept of arterial shrinkage specific for moyamoya disease and discuss how we should diagnose moyamoya disease more accurately than before.

Keywords

Moyamoya disease · Outer diameter · Arterial shrinkage · Diagnosis · Pathogenesis · Heavy T2-weighted image · Atherosclerosis

S. Kuroda (✉)
Department of Neurosurgery, Graduate School of Medicine and Pharmaceutical Science, University of Toyama, Toyama, Japan
e-mail: skuroda@med.u-toyama.ac.jp

S. Kuroda (ed.), *Moyamoya Disease: Current Knowledge and Future Perspectives*, https://doi.org/10.1007/978-981-33-6404-2_14

14.1 Introduction

Moyamoya disease is characterized by progressive stenosis of the terminal portion of the internal carotid artery and its main branches such as middle cerebral artery and anterior cerebral artery. In response to disease progression, the perforating arteries, including the lenticulostriate artery, anterior and posterior choroidal arteries, and thalamoperforating artery, start to dilate and function as one of important collateral routes. Almost 50 years have passed since the moyamoya disease was first reported in an English-written journal in 1969 [1]. Since then, the stenosis of the terminal portion of internal carotid artery and its branches has been considered as the essence of the pathogenesis of moyamoya disease. In fact, this finding is an essential part of the diagnostic criteria even now. Pathologically, the affected arteries such as the carotid terminations include fibrocellular thickening of the intima, an irregular undulation (waving) of the internal elastic lamina, and attenuation of the media (*see Chap. 1*). Initially, cerebral angiography was mandatory for diagnosis, but with the development and widespread use of noninvasive MR angiography, MR angiography has been available since 1996 [2]. In pediatric patients, the diagnosis of moyamoya disease is relatively easy because of the paucity of diseases to differentiate. However, adults, especially the relatively elderly, often have difficulty distinguishing whether the stenosis of the affected arteries is due to moyamoya disease or arteriosclerosis, and the diagnosis is often difficult to make. This difficulty in diagnosis may be result from the fact that the diagnosis has been based only on information about the lumen of the affected arteries, regardless of the modalities used.

In this chapter, therefore, we introduce a novel concept of arterial shrinkage specific for moyamoya disease, which has become evident using novel imaging techniques such as heavy T2-weighted images, and discuss how we should diagnose moyamoya disease more accurately than before.

14.2 Arterial Shrinkage in Carotid Fork

As aforementioned, not rarely we encounter cases in which it is difficult to differentiate moyamoya disease from atherosclerotic intracranial artery stenosis. Through these experiences, I have long been eager to develop a different diagnostic method to more accurately diagnose moyamoya disease than ever before. At the same time, I have long remembered the scene of our first direct observation of the carotid fork suffering from moyamoya disease in 1987 when I was in my second year of residency. At that time, my mentor, Prof. Hiroyasu Kamiyama (*see Chap. 18*) performed a craniotomy on an adult male patient with unilateral moyamoya disease on the right side at Hokkaido University Hospital, Sapporo, Japan. The patient had an aneurysm at the bifurcation of the basilar artery and right superior cerebellar artery, so we planned to perform aneurysm clipping and surgical revascularization at the same time. We reached the carotid cistern through the right trans-Sylvian approach. Then, we noticed that the internal carotid artery and the proximal portion of the middle cerebral artery and the anterior cerebral artery were discolored white and had a rough surface. More surprisingly, they significantly reduced in their outer diameters (Fig. 14.1). During surgery, Prof. Kamiyama and I were so surprised and excited by these findings that I still remember it as if it were yesterday. Since that day, my belief that the arteries involved by moyamoya disease would carry the pathophysiology completely different from that of atherosclerosis remains unchanged. Unfortunately, we did not publish the findings during surgery in this case. Therefore, when we published a review article on moyamoya disease in *Lancet Neurology*, we had the opportunity to report the first-ever direct observation of similar findings during clipping and bypass surgery for another case of moyamoya disease complicated by anterior communicating aneurysm [3].

On the other hand, the advances in MRI technology have made it possible to visualize these findings in moyamoya disease non-invasively in the last decade. Most of these findings have been obtained by heavy T2-weighted images in MRI. Typically, T2-weighted images are captured with a repetition time of 3000–5000 msec, echo time of 80–120 msec, and imaging time of 2–4 minutes using the fast spin-echo (fast SE or turbo SE) method. On heavy T2-weighted images, however, the contribution of T2 components is larger and the water signal

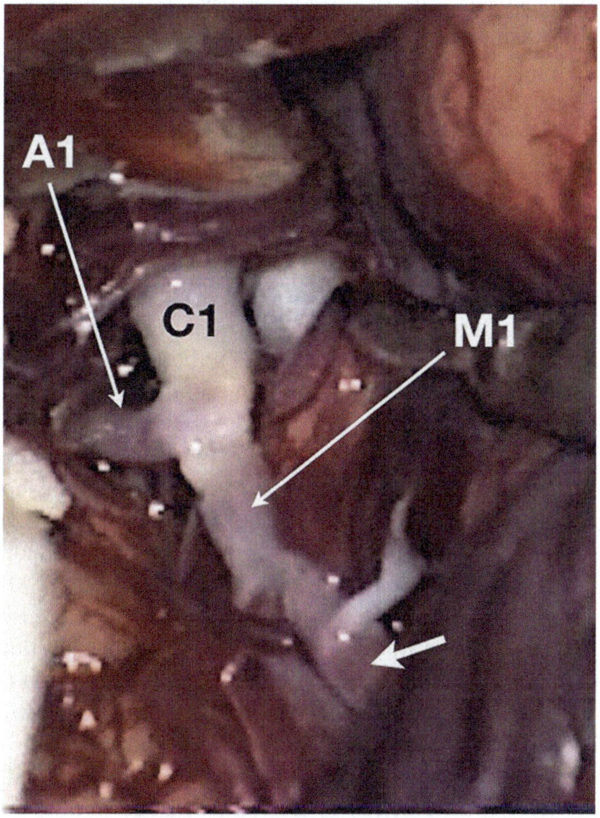

Fig. 14.1 Intraoperative photograph demonstrated that the internal carotid artery (C1) and the proximal portion of the middle cerebral artery (M1) and the anterior cerebral artery (A1) were discolored white and had a rough surface. Their outer diameter was much smaller than usual. Note that the middle cerebral artery distal to the anterior temporal artery showed normal appearance (arrow)

is further enhanced than T2-weighted images, resulting in an image with a good signal-to-noise (S/N) ratio. In contrast, the structures other than water are expressed as low signal intensity, making it extremely suitable to visualize the anatomical relationship between the water and adjacent structures. Therefore, heavy T2-weighted image is recognized suitable to visualize the luminal structures of the cochlea and salivary ducts. In the field of neurosurgery, heavy T2-weighted images have been also proved beneficial in understanding the anatomical relationship between the cranial nerves and offending vessels when performing microvascular decompression surgery for facial spasm, trigeminal neuralgia, and glossopharyngeal neuralgia. As the results, heavy T2-weighted image is also called as "MR hydrography" or "MR cisternography" [4].

Kaku et al. (2012) first reported that the outer diameter of ICA and M1 segment is significantly smaller in moyamoya disease than in the control and in M1 stenosis or occlusion, using 3D-CISS (3-dimensional constructive interference in steady state), one of heavy T2-weighted imaging technique. For example, the outer diameter of the horizontal portion of middle cerebral artery (M1) was 1.9 ± 0.4 mm in moyamoya disease, being significantly smaller than in M1 stenosis/occlusion (3.5 ± 0.6 mm, $P < 0.01$) and the controls (3.3 ± 0.5 mm, $P < 0.01$). This is the first study that denotes arterial shrinkage in moyamoya disease. However, this study included a significant number of pediatric patients, and thus may underestimate the outer diameter in moyamoya disease because the vessel size is smaller in children than in adults [5]. Using high-resolution MRI with a 3.0-Tesla MR apparatus, Kim et al. (2013) compared the outer diameter of the M1 portion between moyamoya disease ($n = 12$) and intracranial atherosclerotic disease (IAD; $n = 20$). They found that the outer diameter was significantly smaller in moyamoya disease (1.6 ± 0.4 mm) than in IAD (3.0 ± 0.5 mm, $P < 0.0001$) [6]. Ryoo et al. (2014) also reported similar results. Thus, they calculated a remodeling index as the ratio of vessel area at MCA to the reference vessel, and found that the value was significantly smaller in moyamoya disease than in IAD (0.19 ± 0.11 vs. 1.00 ± 0.43, $P < 0.001$) [7].

Using 3D-CISS technique, we quantified the outer diameter of the terminal portion of internal carotid artery (C1), the M1 portion, and the horizontal portion of anterior cerebral artery (A1) in 64 adult patients with moyamoya disease. As the results, the outer diameter was 2.3 ± 0.7 mm, 1.3 ± 0.5 mm, 1.0 ± 0.4 mm in the C1, M1, and A1 portions, respectively (Fig. 14.2). All values were significantly smaller than those in both M1 stenosis ($n = 6$) and the healthy controls ($n = 17$). On the other hand, the outer diameter of the basilar artery did not differ among 3 groups (Fig. 14.3). More importantly, there was a negative correlation between their outer diameters and Suzuki's angiographical stage ($P < 0.001$). In other words, the outer diameter of the affected arteries was found to decrease as the stage of the disease progressed. The finding strongly suggests that the outer diameter of carotid fork gradually decreases in parallel to disease progression (Fig. 14.4) [8]. In this study, we also evaluated the ipsilateral-to-contralateral ratio of the outer diameter of carotid fork in 5 children and 15 adults with "unilateral" moyamoya disease, because the values in the contralateral (*normal*) side are useful as the internal standards to prove the phenomenon of arterial shrinkage in moyamoya disease. As the results,

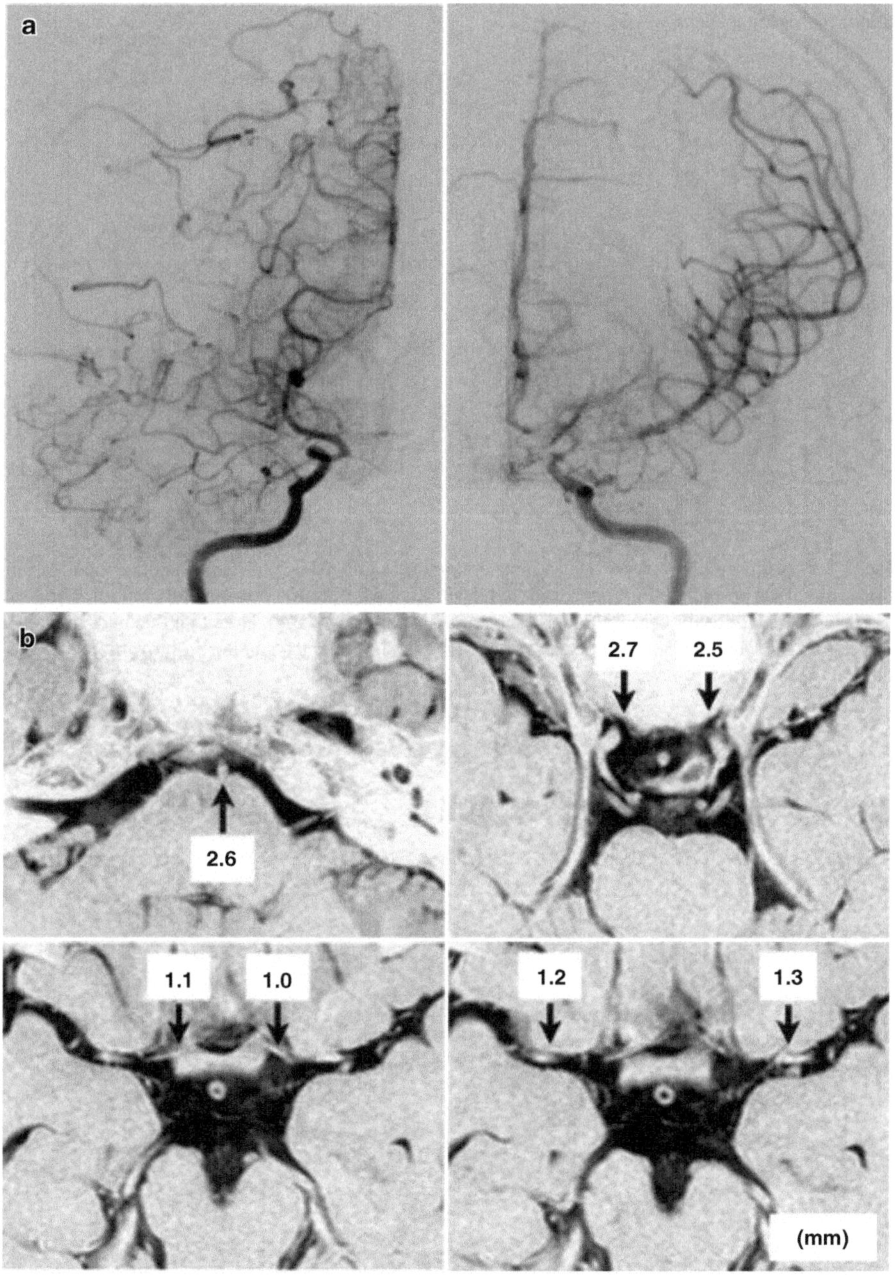

Fig. 14.2 Radiological findings in a 28-year-old female who experienced TIA due to moyamoya disease. Cerebral angiography (**a**) shows typical findings of moyamoya disease. On the other hand, 3D CISS images (**b**) demonstrate a marked reduction of the outer diameter of the terminal portion of the internal carotid artery (2.7 and 2.5 mm), horizontal portion of middle cerebral artery (1.2 and 1.3 mm) and anterior cerebral artery (1.1 and 1.0 mm) on the right and left side, respectively. In contrast, the outer diameter of the basilar artery was within normal limit (2.6 mm)

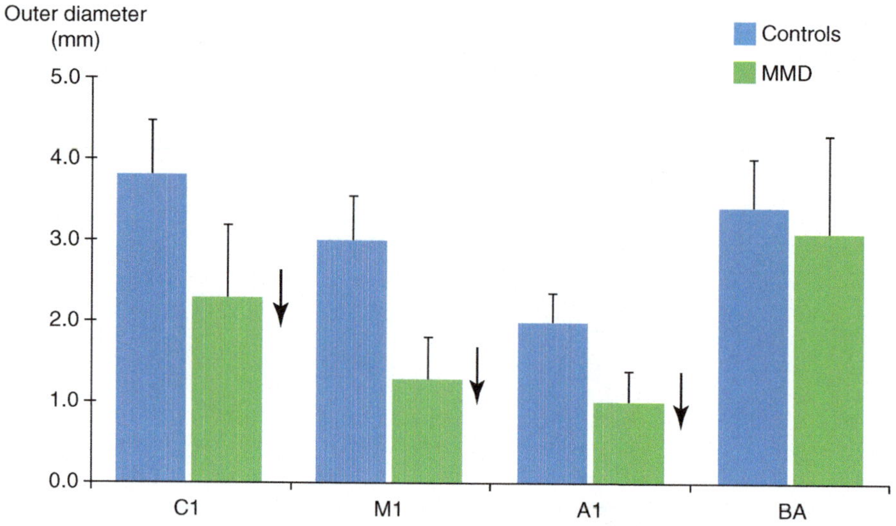

Fig. 14.3 A bar graph demonstrates a mean value and standard deviation of the outer diameter in the terminal portion of the internal carotid artery (C1), the horizontal portion of the middle cerebral artery (M1) and anterior cerebral artery (A1), and basilar artery (BA). Note that the outer diameter of the C1, M1, and A1 portion, but not of the BA, is significantly smaller in moyamoya disease than in the controls

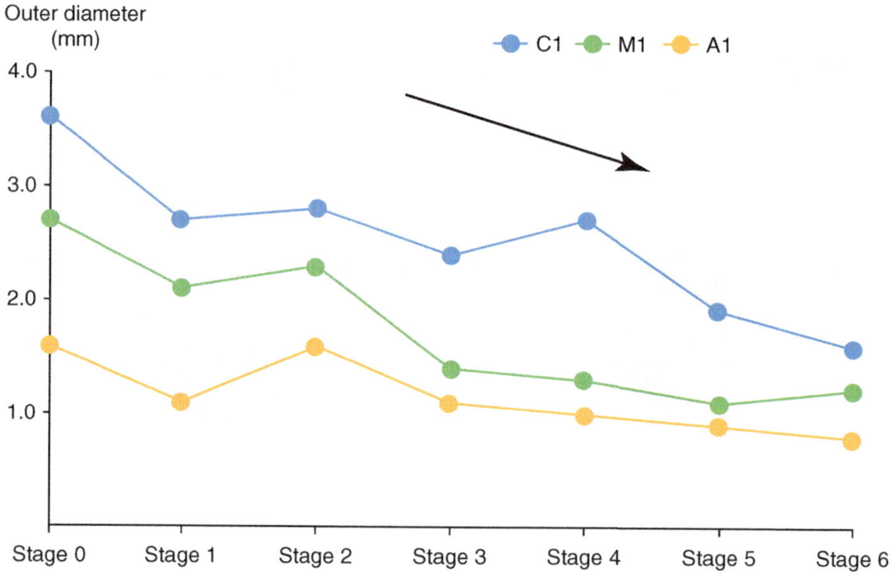

Fig. 14.4 A line graph shows that the mean value of outer diameter of the C1, Ma, and A1 portion gradually decreases in parallel to disease progression

the ratio was 0.68 ± 0.13 and 0.54 ± 0.15 in the C1 and M1 portion, respectively. The values were significantly smaller in unilateral moyamoya disease than in M1 stenosis (1.01 ± 0.09 and 1.06 ± 0.06, respectively) [8].

Subsequently, we also longitudinally evaluated the outer diameter of the involved arteries in non-operated 8 hemispheres that exhibited spontaneous disease progression during follow-up periods. Of these, 7 hemispheres were categorized into Suzuki's Stage 1–3 at initial presentation. In these 7 hemispheres, the outer diameter of the C1, M1, and A1 portion significantly decreased in parallel with subsequent disease progression to Suzuki's Stage 3–6. More interestingly, the outer diameter of the affected arteries was found to decrease with the progression of the disease stage and then continue to shrink progressively over the next 3–12 months. This longitudinal study could first prove that the outer diameter of involved arteries progressively decreases in moyamoya disease [9]. Therefore, progressive shrinkage in parallel with disease progression was confirmed in both cross-sectional study and longitudinal study. Subsequently, several investigators have shown this phenomenon in both Asian and non-Asian patients with moyamoya disease [10–13].

The number of reports on direct observation of the affected arteries during cerebral revascularization surgery for moyamoya disease is very limited, but the findings also support the above-mentioned radiological findings. In addition to the quantification of the outer diameters of C1, M1, and A1 portions using 3D-CISS as described above, we directly observed the affected arteries during surgical revascularization in three cases of adult moyamoya disease [8]. The findings were very similar to our previous observation (*see above*). Thus, the terminal portion of the internal carotid artery, as well as the horizontal portions of the middle cerebral artery and the anterior cerebral artery, was found to be white and their surface was irregular. Most notably, they significantly reduced in diameter in all cases (Fig. 14.5). For example, the outer diameter of C1 portion was 1.2 to 1.7 mm, being much smaller than normal controls (4.2 mm). Likewise, the outer diameter of M1 portion was much smaller in moyamoya disease than in normal controls (0.7–1.4 mm vs. 3.5 mm, respectively) [14].

In summary, the radiological and intraoperative findings over the last several years have revealed that not only does the lumen of the affected arteries narrow, but the outer diameter of the artery gradually shrinks as the disease progresses in moyamoya disease. This phenomenon is not observed in intracranial arterial stenosis due to atherosclerosis, and is believed specific to moyamoya disease at least nowadays. It has long been known that atherosclerosis leads to not only the luminal narrowing but also abnormal dilation of the entire artery, which is called positive or expansive remodeling. Therefore, negative or constrictive remodeling observed in moyamoya disease would be the completely opposite phenomenon. Furthermore, recent high-resolution MRI studies have shown that atherosclerosis causes eccentric lesion in the intracranial arteries, whereas moyamoya disease causes concentric lesions at the site of the stenosis [12, 15]. These observations strongly suggest that intracranial artery stenosis due to atherosclerosis and moyamoya disease is based on completely different pathophysiology (Fig. 14.6).

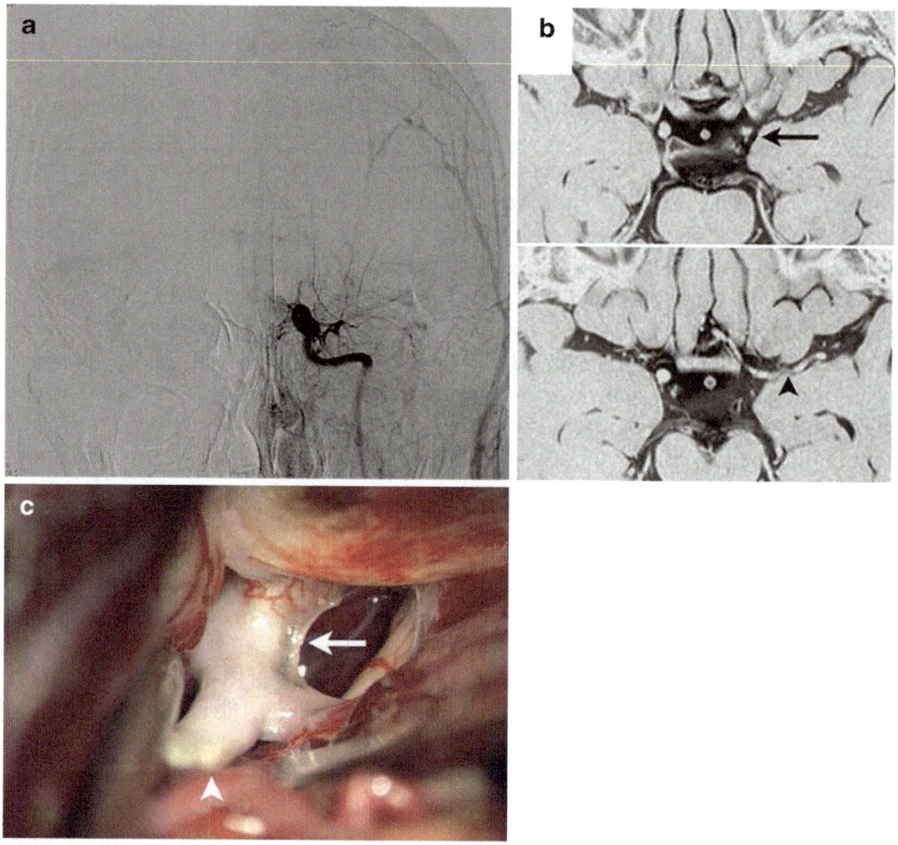

Fig. 14.5 Radiological and intraoperative findings of a 52-year-old patient with unilateral moyamoya disease on the left side. Left carotid angiography (**a**) demonstrates severe stenosis in the supraclinoid portion of the internal carotid artery. 3D CISS images (**b**) show a marked reduction of the outer diameter in the C1 (arrow) and M1 portion (arrowhead) on the left side. Intraoperative photograph during surgical revascularization onto the left hemisphere (**c**) reveals that the C1, M1, and A1 portion are discolored white and are markedly shrinked

It is well known that the intima of the affected arteries becomes thickened, while the tunica media become thinner in moyamoya disease. These pathological observations may be able to explain the mechanism of the reduction of the outer diameter of the affected arteries in moyamoya disease. Unique pathological changes such as duplication and waving are also known to occur in the elastic lamina of the affected arteries in moyamoya disease. However, the underlying mechanism has long been undetermined. If arterial shrinkage occurs in affected arteries of moyamoya disease, it may provide a clear explanation for these pathological changes in the elastic lamina as a secondary effect (*see Chap. 1*). In other words, moyamoya disease *per se* may be pathognomonically defined by both luminal stenosis and arterial shrinkage of the involved carotid forks with a progressive fashion (Fig. 14.6).

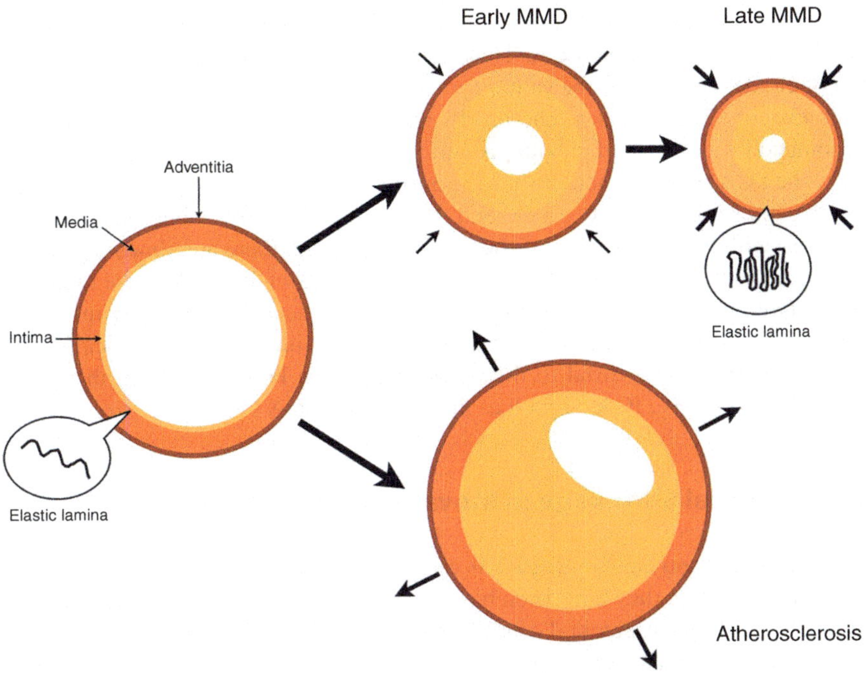

Fig. 14.6 A diagram shows the difference in pathophysiology between moyamoya disease (MMD) and atherosclerosis. Moyamoya disease causes concentric intimal thickening, medial atrophy, and the waving of the elastic lamina, leading to arterial shrinkage (constricting remodeling), but atherosclerosis causes eccentric intimal thickening and expansive remodeling

14.3 Arterial Shrinkage in Posterior Cerebral Artery

The posterior cerebral artery (PCA) is one of the important collateral routes in moyamoya disease. The PCA provides collateral blood flow to the frontal, temporal, and parietal lobes through leptomeningeal anastomosis, posterior pericallosal artery, and posterior choroidal artery. However, the PCA is also known to be involved in about 30% of patients with moyamoya disease. The stenotic lesions usually develop in the P2 or P3 segment of the PCA. Therefore, the occurrence of PCA involvement can easily cause ischemic symptoms not only in the occipital lobe, where the PCA essentially provides blood flow, but also in the parietal and temporal lobes, which receive collateral blood flow from the PCA. Clinical symptoms widely vary, including homonymous hemianopsia, headache attack in the temporal area, sensory aphasia, alexia, agraphia, and numbness of the contralateral extremities. However, there were no studies that denote whether arterial shrinkage occurs in the PCA. Therefore, we analyzed the outer diameter of the P2 portion of PCA in 72 patients with moyamoya disease. In this study, the stenotic lesion of the PCA was divided into 3 grades; Grade 0 (normal), Grade 1 (stenotic), and Grade 2 (occluded) on MR angiography. As the results, we found that the outer diameter of PCA progressively decreased as the stenotic lesion occurred in the PCA. That is, the values for Grade 1 cases fell to about 75% of Grade 0 cases, and the values for Grade 2 cases were even smaller, falling to about 45% of Grade 0 cases. The results were similar for children and adults. The phenomenon was observed in both pediatric and adult patients. In addition, we could follow the PCA outer diameter over time during the progression of PCA disease in 4 hemispheres in 2 pediatric cases, and found that the PCA outer diameter also decreased with the progression of the disease. Although there are almost no studies that denote pathological findings of the stenotic lesions in the PCA, these radiological observations strongly suggest that similar pathological changes occur in stenotic lesions in PCA as in carotid fork. This fact fits well with the embryological knowledge that arteries more distal to the P2 portion of the PCA arise from the cranial ramus of the primitive ICA, as well as the MCA and ACA [16].

14.4 Arterial Shrinkage in Moyamoya Syndrome

The definition of moyamoya disease is rather complicated. The criteria for diagnosis are unique in that they have been based solely on information about the lumen of the affected artery on cerebral angiography and MR angiography for more than 50 years. When the disease was first discovered, moyamoya disease was defined as a disease of unknown etiology, and therefore, the patients with the same radiological findings but concurrent diseases have been diagnosed with moyamoya syndrome or quasi-moyamoya disease in children and adults, bilaterally or unilaterally. Hayashi et al. (2014) reported that about 5% of patients with moyamoya disease are diagnosed as having moyamoya syndrome [17]. Previously reported concurrent diseases are listed in Chap. 2. However, it is unclear from previous studies whether moyamoya syndrome is a completely different disease from moyamoya disease, or whether it is simply a combination of moyamoya disease and concurrent disease. Therefore, we hypothesized that if shrinkage in the affected arteries is specific to moyamoya disease, then it would be very useful to investigate whether this arterial shrinkage also occurs in moyamoya syndrome or not. In this study, we evaluated the outer diameter of the carotid forks in 9 patients with moyamoya syndrome. Concurrent diseases included neurofibromatosis 1 (NF1) in two cases, idiopathic thrombocytopenia (ITP) in one, autoimmune disease such as hyperthyroidism in 3, atherosclerosis in 3. Very interestingly, the outer diameter of the affected arteries markedly differed from the usual moyamoya disease, and there was a great deal of inter-case variability. In 7 of the 9 patients, as in the case of moyamoya disease, the diameter of C1 and M1 decreased as the disease progressed. In these 7 patients, the comorbidities included NF1 ($n = 2$), ITP ($n = 1$), autoimmune disease ($n = 2$), and atherosclerosis ($n = 2$). On the other hand, there was no reduction in the diameter of the affected arteries in the other two patients, both of whom were judged to have Stage 3 disease on cerebral angiography. Their comorbidities were autoimmune disease ($n = 1$) and atherosclerosis ($n = 1$) [18].

These observations strongly suggest that moyamoya syndrome (or quasi-moyamoya disease) is not a uniform disease entity, but can be divided into two pathophysiologically different disorders: the arterial shrinkage group and the non-arterial shrinkage group. The former is considered closely related to definitive moyamoya disease, but the latter may be essentially analogous to atherosclerosis, being divergent from definitive moyamoya disease. In more detail, there may be a significant number of cases that have exactly the same etiology as definitive moyamoya disease but are not diagnosed as moyamoya syndrome because they happen to have comorbidities. On the other hand, there may be some cases that are pathogenetically unrelated to moyamoya disease but are categorized as moyamoya syndrome because of both radiological findings similar to those of moyamoya disease and comorbidities. Anyway, such a distinction would have been highly unlikely when the diagnosis was based solely on information about the lumen of the involved arteries using cerebral angiography and MR angiography. This distinction was first made possible by observing the outer diameter of the involved arteries using heavy T2-weighted images. However, these findings are based on the study with a small sample size. Therefore, multi-center investigations with larger cohorts are warranted to further clarify the pathophysiology and disease entity of moyamoya syndrome [18].

14.5 Clinical Significance of Arterial Shrinkage in Moyamoya Disease

14.5.1 Endovascular Treatment

There are several reports attempting to dilate the stenotic lesions themselves with endovascular techniques for moyamoya disease. Rodruguez et al. (2007) reported that balloon angioplasty in adult patients with early moyamoya disease resulted in effective dilation of stenotic lesions [19]. Several groups of investigators also successfully performed balloon angioplasty and stent placement in children and adults with moyamoya disease or moyamoya syndrome [20–23].

However, Khan et al. (2011) analyzed clinical results of endovascular treatment for 5 patients with moyamoya disease. All of them repeated ischemic attacks after 0–4 months after endovascular treatments. Follow-up angiography revealed severe in-stent restenosis or occlusion in 4 of 5 patients. Finally, all of them underwent surgical revascularization to resolve ischemic attacks [24]. More importantly, Eicker et al. (2011) reported a 18-year-old cases that developed very massive subarachnoid hemorrhage several hours after stent placement of the supraclinoid internal carotid artery [25]. Considering the specific occurrence of arterial shrinkage in moyamoya disease, we should remind that these endovascular procedures may carry the risk of disruption of the affected artery, leading to life-threatening subarachnoid hemorrhage.

14.5.2 Differential Diagnosis of Moyamoya Disease

As aforementioned, it is not rare to encounter the difficulty to distinguish moyamoya disease from atherosclerosis-related intracranial arterial stenosis especially in elder patients. However, heavy T2-weighted image is quite useful to accurately identify moyamoya disease even in very elder patients (Fig. 14.7). This 80-year-old

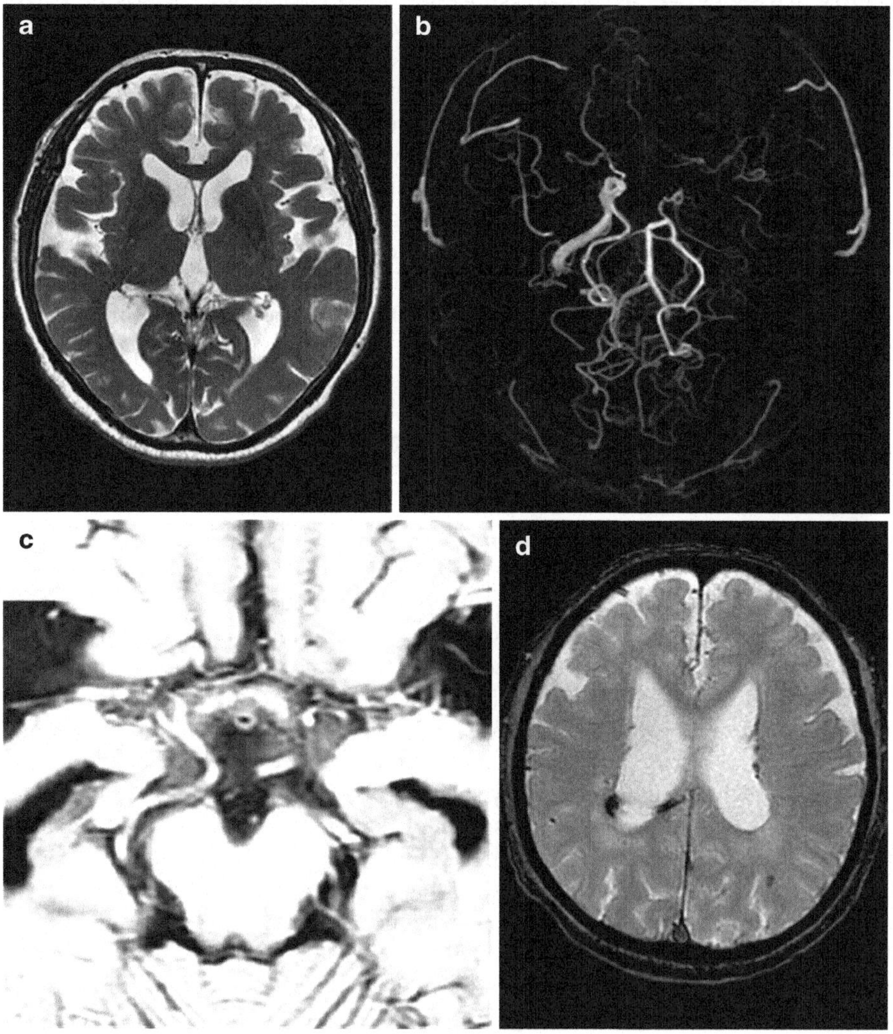

Fig. 14.7 Radiological findings of a 80-year-old male with moyamoya disease. T2-weighted image (**a**) demonstrates no parenchymal lesions, but MR angiography (**b**) reveals complete occlusion of the internal carotid artery at the supraclinoid portion on the right side and at the origin on the left side. 3D CISS image (**c**) reveals a marked arterial shrinkage in the carotid fork on both sides. Therefore, he was diagnosed as moyamoya disease. T2*-weighted image taken 6 months later (**d**) shows multiple bleeding in the subependymal layer of the lateral ventricle on both sides

male suddenly developed syncope and was referred to our hospital. T2-weighted MRI demonstrated no parenchymal lesions, but MR angiography revealed complete occlusion of the internal carotid artery at the supraclinoid portion on the right side and at the origin on the left side. At first, he was diagnosed as atherosclerotic carotid occlusion on both sides, but subsequently performed 3D CISS revealed a marked arterial shrinkage in the carotid fork on both sides. Finally, he was diagnosed as moyamoya disease and was conservatively followed up because of his high age. He was admitted to our hospital again because of sudden consciousness disturbance 6 months after the initial diagnosis. T2*-weighted image showed multiple bleeding in the subependymal layer of the lateral ventricle on both sides, which is the finding that strongly supports previous diagnosis of moyamoya disease.

As this case clearly demonstrates, cerebral angiography and MR angiography, which have been used to diagnose moyamoya disease, only provide information on the lumen of the affected arteries, making it difficult to exclude other diseases such as atherosclerosis. This fact has led to a great deal of confusion in routine clinical practice and research [26]. Therefore, we the Research Committee on Moyamoya Disease in Japan is preparing to revise the diagnostic criteria for moyamoya disease to include heavy T2-weighted image findings in addition to cerebral angiography and MR angiography.

Acknowledgments This work was partly supported by a grant from the Research Committee on Moyamoya Disease, the Japanese Ministry of Health, Labour and Welfare.

References

1. Suzuki J, Takaku A. Cerebrovascular "moyamoya" disease. Disease showing abnormal net-like vessels in base of brain. Arch Neurol. 1969;20:288–99.
2. Fukui M. Guidelines for the diagnosis and treatment of spontaneous occlusion of the circle of Willis ('moyamoya' disease). Research committee on spontaneous occlusion of the circle of Willis (Moyamoya disease) of the Ministry of Health and Welfare, Japan. Clin Neurol Neurosurg. 1997;99(Suppl 2):S238–40.
3. Kuroda S, Houkin K. Moyamoya disease: current concepts and future perspectives. Lancet Neurol. 2008;7:1056–66.
4. Prieto R, Pascual JM, Yus M, Jorquera M. Trigeminal neuralgia: assessment of neurovascular decompression by 3D fast imaging employing steady-state acquisition and 3D time of flight multiple overlapping thin slab acquisition magnetic resonance imaging. Surg Neurol Int. 2012;3:50.
5. Kaku Y, Morioka M, Ohmori Y, Kawano T, Kai Y, Fukuoka H, Hirai T, Yamashita Y, Kuratsu J. Outer-diameter narrowing of the internal carotid and middle cerebral arteries in moyamoya disease detected on 3D constructive interference in steady-state MR image: is arterial constrictive remodeling a major pathogenesis? Acta Neurochir. 2012;154:2151–7.
6. Kim YJ, Lee DH, Kwon JY, Kang DW, Suh DC, Kim JS, Kwon SU. High resolution MRI difference between moyamoya disease and intracranial atherosclerosis. Eur J Neurol. 2013;20:1311–8.
7. Ryoo S, Cha J, Kim SJ, Choi JW, Ki CS, Kim KH, Jeon P, Kim JS, Hong SC, Bang OY. High-resolution magnetic resonance wall imaging findings of Moyamoya disease. Stroke. 2014;45:2457–60.
8. Kuroda S, Kashiwazaki D, Akioka N, Koh M, Hori E, Nishikata M, Umemura K, Horie Y, Noguchi K, Kuwayama N. Specific shrinkage of carotid forks in Moyamoya disease: a novel key finding for diagnosis. Neurol Med Chir (Tokyo). 2015;55:796–804.

9. Yamamoto S, Kashiwazaki D, Akioka N, Kuwayama N, Noguchi K, Kuroda S. Progressive shrinkage of involved arteries in parallel with disease progression in Moyamoya disease. World Neurosurg. 2019;122:e253–61.
10. Cogswell PM, Lants SK, Davis LT, Juttukonda MR, Fusco MR, Donahue MJ. Vessel Wall and lumen features in north American Moyamoya patients. Clin Neuroradiol. 2020;30:545–52.
11. Kathuveetil A, Sylaja PN, Senthilvelan S, Kesavadas C, Banerjee M, Jayanand Sudhir B. Vessel Wall thickening and enhancement in high-resolution intracranial Vessel Wall imaging: a predictor of future ischemic events in Moyamoya disease. AJNR Am J Neuroradiol. 2020;41:100–5.
12. Ya J, Zhou D, Ding J, Ding Y, Ji X, Yang Q, Meng R. High-resolution combined arterial spin labeling MR for identifying cerebral arterial stenosis induced by moyamoya disease or atherosclerosis. Annals of translational medicine. 2020;8:87.
13. Yu LB, He H, Zhao JZ, Wang R, Zhang Q, Shi ZY, Shao JS, Zhang D. More precise imaging analysis and diagnosis of Moyamoya disease and Moyamoya syndrome using high-resolution magnetic resonance imaging. World Neurosurg. 2016;96:252–60.
14. Lang J. Cerebral arterial circle in adults and aneurysms. In: Skull Base and related structures. 2nd ed. Germany: Schattauer GmbH, Stuttgart; 2001. p. 31–48.
15. Mossa-Basha M, de Havenon A, Becker KJ, Hallam DK, Levitt MR, Cohen WA, Hippe DS, Alexander MD, Tirschwell DL, Hatsukami T, Amlie-Lefond C, Yuan C. Added value of Vessel Wall magnetic resonance imaging in the differentiation of Moyamoya Vasculopathies in a non-Asian cohort. Stroke. 2016;47:1782–8.
16. Yamamoto S, Kashiwazaki D, Uchino H, Saito H, Akioka N, Kuwayama N, Noguchi K, Kuroda S (2019) Stenosis severity-dependent shrinkage of posterior cerebral artery in Moyamoya disease. World Neurosurg.
17. Hayashi K, Horie N, Izumo T, Nagata I. Nationwide survey on quasi-moyamoya disease in Japan. Acta Neurochir. 2014;156:935–40.
18. Yamamoto S, Koh M, Kashiwazaki D, Akioka N, Kuwayama N, Noguchi K, Kuroda S. Is quasi-moyamoya disease a uniform disease entity? A three-dimensional constructive interference in steady state imaging study. J Stroke Cerebrovasc Dis. 2016;25:1509–16.
19. Rodriguez GJ, Kirmani JF, Ezzeddine MA, Qureshi AI. Primary percutaneous transluminal angioplasty for early moyamoya disease. J Neuroimaging. 2007;17:48–53.
20. Drazin D, Calayag M, Gifford E, Dalfino J, Yamamoto J, Boulos AS. Endovascular treatment for moyamoya disease in a Caucasian twin with angioplasty and wingspan stent. Clin Neurol Neurosurg. 2009;111:913–7.
21. Kim T, Kwon OK, Oh CW, Bang JS, Hwang G, Lee YJ. Intracranial stenting using a drug-eluting stent for moyamoya disease involving supraclinoid ICA: a case report. Neurol Med Chir (Tokyo). 2014;54:136–8.
22. Kornblihtt LI, Cocorullo S, Miranda C, Lylyk P, Heller PG, Molinas FC. Moyamoya syndrome in an adolescent with essential thrombocythemia: successful intracranial carotid stent placement. Stroke. 2005;36:E71–3.
23. Santirso D, Oliva P, Gonzalez M, Murias E, Vega P, Gil A, Calleja S. Intracranial stent placement in a patient with moyamoya disease. J Neurol. 2012;259:170–1.
24. Khan N, Dodd R, Marks MP, Bell-Stephens T, Vavao J, Steinberg GK. Failure of primary percutaneous angioplasty and stenting in the prevention of ischemia in Moyamoya angiopathy. Cerebrovasc Dis. 2011;31:147–53.
25. Eicker S, Etminan N, Turowski B, Steiger HJ, Hanggi D. Intracranial carotid artery stent placement causes delayed severe intracranial hemorrhage in a patient with moyamoya disease. J Neurointerv Surg. 2011;3:160–2.
26. Miyawaki S, Imai H, Shimizu M, Yagi S, Ono H, Mukasa A, Nakatomi H, Shimizu T, Saito N. Genetic variant RNF213 c.14576G>a in various phenotypes of intracranial major artery stenosis/occlusion. Stroke. 2013;44:2894–7.

Disease Progression

15

Miki Fujimura and Teiji Tominaga

Abstract

Moyamoya disease (MMD) is a chronic occlusive cerebrovascular disease with unknown etiology characterized by progressive stenosis/occlusion at the terminal portion of the internal carotid artery and an abnormal vascular network formation at the base of the brain. MMD has an intrinsic characteristic to represent a gradual conversion of the cortical vascular supply from intra-cranial/internal carotid (*IC*) system to extra-cranial/external carotid (*EC*) system, so-called *IC-EC conversion*. MMD is known to represent bimodal age distribution with a peak each in childhood and young adulthood, and the disease progression in adult patients has been considered to be relatively rare. But recent advances in neuroradiology reveal that MMD patients, either pediatric or adult, have substantial risk for disease progression, although the exact mechanism underlying the progression of MMD is undetermined. The aim of this chapter is to introduce the basic pathology and neuro-radiological characteristic of MMD, especially focusing on its disease progression in adulthood.

Keywords

Moyamoya vasculopathy · Moyamoya disease · Progression · Suzuki's angiographic stage · Basic pathology

---

M. Fujimura (✉)
Department of Neurosurgery, Kohnan Hospital, Sendai, Japan

Division of Advanced Cerebrovascular Surgery, Tohoku University Graduate School of Medicine, Sendai, Japan
e-mail: fujimur@nsg.med.tohoku.ac.jp

T. Tominaga
Department of Neurosurgery, Tohoku University Graduate School of Medicine, Sendai, Japan
e-mail: tomi@nsg.med.tohoku.ac.jp

S. Kuroda (ed.), *Moyamoya Disease: Current Knowledge and Future Perspectives*, https://doi.org/10.1007/978-981-33-6404-2_15

15.1 Introduction

Moyamoya disease (MMD) is characterized by progressive stenosis/occlusion at the terminal portion of the internal carotid artery (ICA) and an abnormal vascular network formation at the base of the brain [1, 2]. The disease progression in adult patients has been considered to be relatively rare [3, 4], but recent advances in neuroradiology reveal that MMD patients, either pediatric or adult, have substantial risk for disease progression [5, 6]. In this chapter, we sought to summarize current understanding of the basic pathology and neuro-radiological characteristic of MMD, focusing on its disease progression in adulthood.

15.2 Suzuki's Angiographic Staging as an Intrinsic Temporal Nature of Physiological Compensatory Reorganization in MMD

MMD has an intrinsic temporal nature to attempt a gradual conversion of the cortical vascular supply from intra-cranial/internal carotid (*IC*) system to extra-cranial/external carotid (*EC*) system, so-called *IC-EC conversion* [7, 8], as initially illustrated by Suzuki's angiographic staging in 1969 [1]. This staging does not represent the severity of patients' clinical condition, but may indicate the natural pathophysiological course of MMD. Insufficiency of this physiological reorganization system occurs at stage 3 or 4 in most patients, when the abnormal vascular networks at the base of the brain are most prominent.

Stage 1: Narrowing of carotid fork.
Stage 2: Initiation of the "moyamoya vessels"; dilatation of the intracerebral main arteries.
Stage 3: Intensification of the "moyamoya vessels"; nonfilling of the anterior and middle cerebral arteries.
Stage 4: Minimization of the "moyamoya vessels"; disappearance of the posterior cerebral artery.
Stage 5: Reduction of the "moyamoya vessels"; the main arteries arising from the internal carotid artery disappear.
Stage 6: Disappearance of the "moyamoya vessels"; the original moyamoya vessels at the base of the brain are completely missing and only the collateral circulation from the external carotid artery is seen.

Malfunction of the "*IC-EC conversion*" system is considered to result in cerebral ischemia and/or hemorrhage from inadequate collateral vascular networks. On the other hand, substantial numbers of MMD patients accomplish "favorable" conversion process without manifesting as deleterious cerebrovascular events [8]. This 47-year-old woman experienced only slight numbness in her left hand while playing woodwind instrument, though her angio-architecture represents stage 6 MMD on the right hemisphere, where all the cortical blood supply is exclusively derived from EC system (Fig. 15.1).

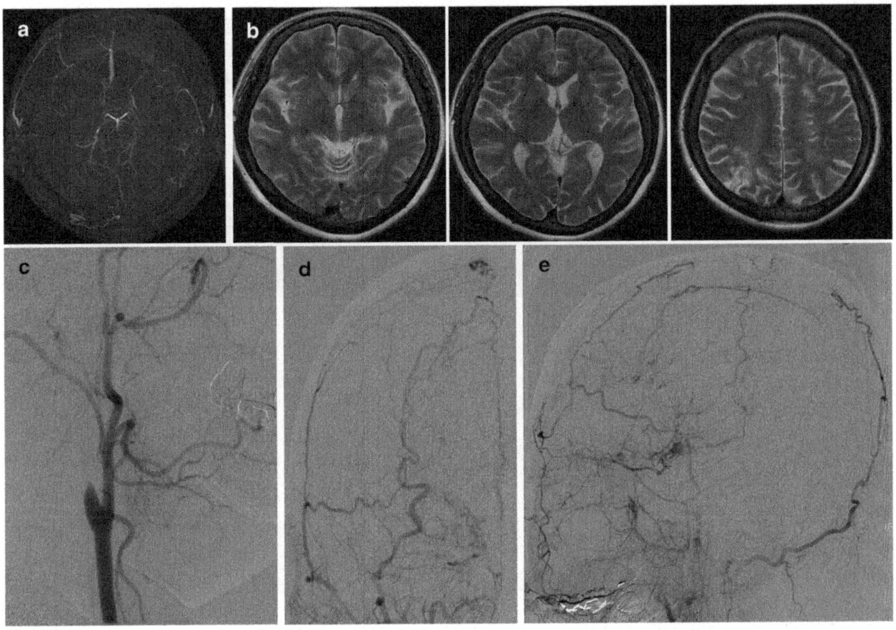

Fig. 15.1 A: Representative findings of stage-6 moyamoya disease (MMD). Magnetic resonance (MR) angiography (**a**), T2-weighted MR imaging (**b**), and right carotid angiogram (**c-e**) of a 47-year-old woman indicating that all the cortical blood supply is derived from external carotid system

15.3 Disease Progression in Adult MMD

The disease progression of MMD had generally been considered to occur exclusively in childhood with angiographic characteristics being completed before adulthood [3, 4]. In contrast to this classic observation, Kuroda et al. first reported in a multicenter observational study on adult MMD that the incidence of disease progression in adult patients was not as rare as previously considered [5] and similar result was reported also by Narisawa and colleagues [6]. In accordance with this observation, there were several reported cases of the de novo development of MMD in adulthood [9–11]. Interestingly, most of them were middle-aged females who generally lacked particular risk factors for atherosclerosis [9–11]. The mechanisms underlying the development and progression of adult MMD are undetermined, but physiological balance between female hormones is considered to be one of the major candidate environmental factors related to the development/progression of adult MMD patients [12]. This 47-year-old woman suffered mild weakness on her left hand and visited neurological service. Initial magnetic resonance (MR) angiography revealed only mild stenosis at the bilateral ICA terminus (Fig. 15.2a), but apparent progression of the steno-occlusive changes was found 1 year later, when she suffered crescendo transient ischemic attack (TIA) (Fig. 15.2b, d, e). In light of the presence of hemodynamic compromise on the

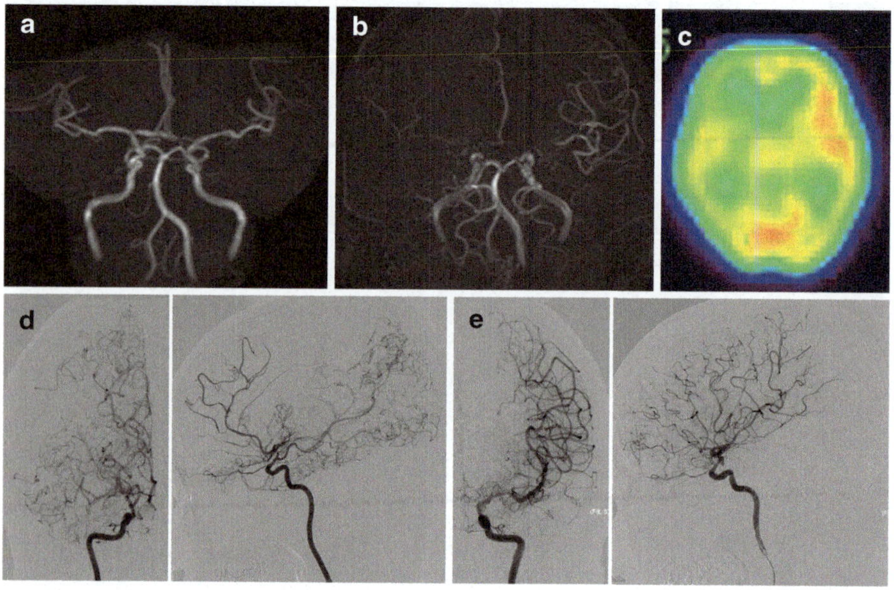

Fig. 15.2 Temporal profile of MR angiography before (**a**) and after the progression (**b**). ^{123}I-IMP SPECT (**c**) and catheter angiography (**d, e**) of this 47-year-old woman after progression demonstrating MMD with hemodynamic compromise on the right hemisphere

symptomatic hemisphere (Fig. 15.2c), she underwent right superficial temporal artery (STA)-middle cerebral artery (MCA) bypass combined with indirect pial synangiosis without complication (Fig. 15.3a-d). The ischemic attack disappeared completely after surgery, and flow study indicated the apparent hemodynamic improvement on the right hemisphere (Fig. 15.3e). Alternatively, possible involvement of the genetic variant of ring finger protein 213 (RNF213), a susceptibility gene for MMD, in the disease progression of MMD has been speculated [13]. In fact, Tashiro and colleagues reported de novo development of MMD in an adult female with a genetic variant of the RNF213 gene [11].

15.4 Significance of Progressive Stenosis in Posterior Cerebral Artery (PCA)

While following up the patients with MMD, it is clinically important not to overlook the progression of PCA stenosis, because the involvement of PCA stenosis has been reported to be significantly associated with the hemodynamic decline and the deterioration of the ischemic condition [14]. This 44-year-old woman was found to have the progression of the steno-occlusive change at the right PCA during her yearly follow-up by MR angiography (Fig. 15.4a, b). One month later, she suffered temporal weakness on her left hand, and catheter angiography confirmed the apparent progression of the right PCA stenosis (asterisk in Fig. 15.4e). Then she underwent right flow augmentation bypass, which resulted in the complete disappearance

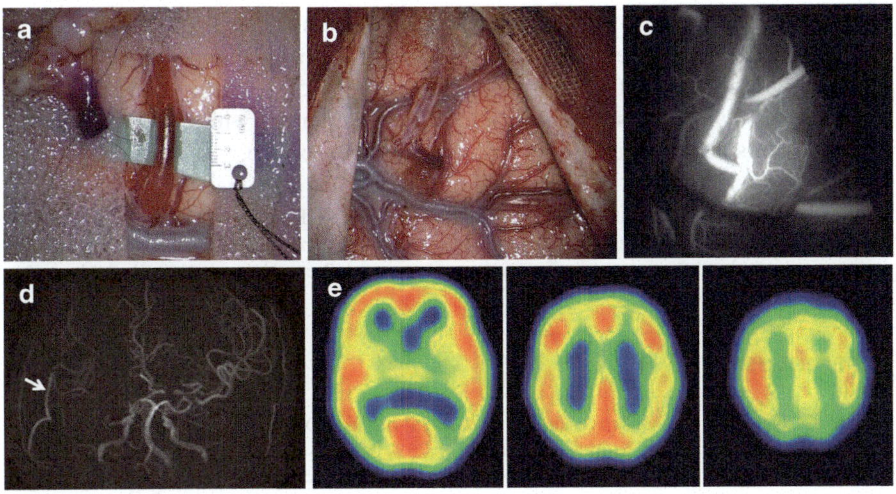

Fig. 15.3 Intra-operative view of direct/indirect combined revascularization. Surgical view before (**a**) and after left superficial temporal artery (STA)-middle cerebral artery (MCA) bypass (**b, c**). Indocyanine green video-angiography demonstrated apparently patent bypass (**c**). Post-operative MR angiography showing patent STA-MCA bypass (arrow in **d**), and hemodynamic improvement by ^{123}I-IMP SPECT (**e**)

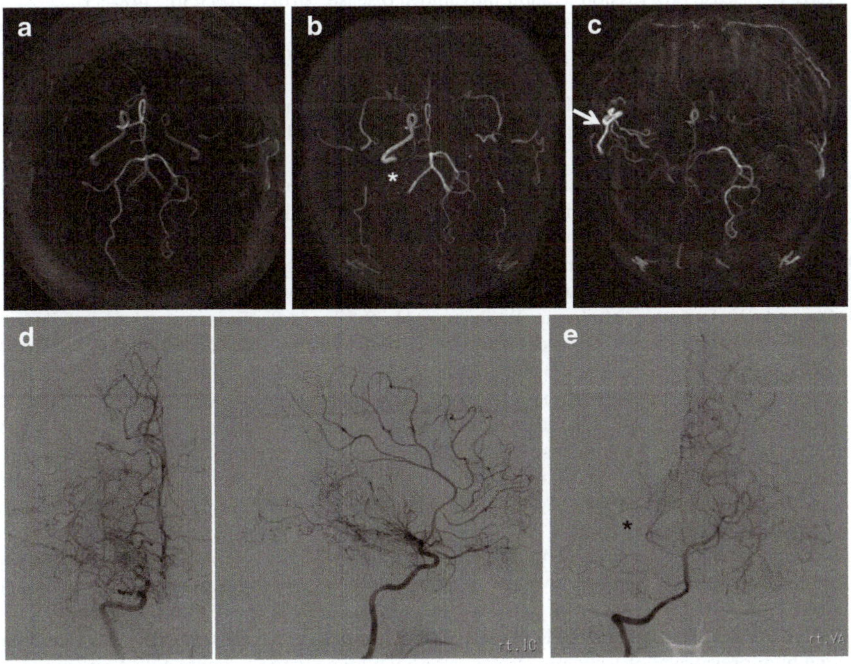

Fig. 15.4 Temporal profile of MR angiography before (**a**) and after the progression of right PCA stenosis (asterisk in **b**). Right carotid (**d**) and vertebral artery angiograms of this 44-year-old woman after progression demonstrating MMD with apparent PCA stenosis (asterisk in **e**). Post-operative MR angiography showing patent STA-MCA bypass (arrow in **c**)

of her TIA. Post-operative MRA indicated the apparently patent bypass (arrow in Fig. 15.4c). PCA involvement is also known to be an independent risk factor of posterior hemorrhage with high risk of re-bleeding [15, 16], thus identification of progressive PCA stenosis/occlusion is clinically important while following up the MMD patients neuro-radiologically at the outpatient service.

Acknowledgement This study was supported by JSPS KAKENHI grant number 20 K09362 (Miki Fujimura). The ethical committee of Kohnan Hospital approved the clinical study of postoperative cerebral blood flow analysis. The authors have no conflict of interest regarding this study.

References

1. Suzuki J, Takaku A. Cerebrovascular 'moyamoya' disease. Disease showing abnormal net-like vessels in base of brain. Arch Neurol. 1969;20:288–99.
2. Fujimura M, Bang OY, Kim JS. Moyamoya disease. Front Neurol Neurosci. 2016;40:204–20.
3. Ezura M, Yoshimoto T, Fujiwara S, Takahashi A, Shirane R, Mizoi K. Clinical and angiographic follow-up of childhood onset moyamoya disease. Childs Nerv Syst. 1995;11:591–4.
4. Houkin K, Yoshimoto T, Kuroda S, Ishikawa T, Takahashi A, Abe H. Angiographic analysis of moyamoya disease—how does moyamoya disease progress? Neurol Med Chir (Tokyo). 1996;36:783–8.
5. Kuroda S, Ishikawa T, Houkin K, Nanba R, Hokari M, Iwasaki Y. Incidence and clinical features of disease progression in adult moyamoya disease. Stroke. 2005;36:2148–53.
6. Narisawa A, Fujimura M, Tominaga T. Efficacy of the revascularization surgery for adult-onset moyamoya disease with the progression of cerebrovascular lesions. Clin Neurol Neurosurg. 2009;111:123–6.
7. Fujimura M, Tominaga T. Lessons learned from moyamoya disease: outcome of direct/indirect revascularization surgery for 150 affected hemispheres. Neurol Med Chir (Tokyo). 2012;52:327–32.
8. Fujimura M, Tominaga T. Current status of revascularization surgery for moyamoya disease: special consideration for its 'internal carotid-external carotid (IC-EC) conversion' as the physiological reorganization system. Tohoku J Exp Med. 2015;236:45–53.
9. Furuya R, Yoshida K, Akiyama T, Kawase T. De novo development of moyamoya disease in an adult female. Case report J Neurosurg. 2009;111:943–6.
10. Shimoda Y, Fujimura M, Inoue T, Shimizu H, Tominaga T. Temporal profile of de novo development of moyamoya vasculopathy in an adult: case report. Neurol Med Chir (Tokyo). 2012;52:339–42.
11. Tashiro R, Fujimura M, Niizuma K, Endo H, Sakata H, Sato-Maeda M, et al. De novo development of Moyamoya disease in an adult female with a genetic variant of the RNF-213 gene: case report. J Stroke Cerebrovasc Dis. 2017;26:e8–e11.
12. Akamatsu Y, Fujimura M, Uenohara H, Shimizu H, Tominaga T. Development of moyamoya disease in pregnancy and puerperium: case report. Neurol Med Chir (Tokyo). 2014;54:824–6.
13. Kamada F, Aoki Y, Narisawa A, Abe Y, Komatsuzaki S, Kikuchi A, et al. A genome-wide association study identifies RNF213 as the first Moyamoya disease gene. J Hum Genet. 2011;56:34–40.
14. Mugikura S, Higano S, Shirane R, Fujimura M, Shimanuki Y, Takahashi S. Posterior circulation and high prevalence of ischemic stroke among young pediatric patients with Moyamoya disease: evidence of angiography-based differences by age at diagnosis. AJNR Am J Neuroradiol. 2011;32:192–8.

15. Funaki T, Takahashi JC, Houkin K, Kuroda S, Takeuchi S, Fujimura M, et al. Angiographic features of hemorrhagic moyamoya disease with high recurrence risk: a supplementary analysis of the Japan Adult Moyamoya Trial. J Neurosurg. 2018;128:777–84.
16. Funaki T, Takahashi JC, Houkin K, Kuroda S, Takeuchi S, Fujimura M, et al. High rebleeding risk associated with choroidal collateral vessels in hemorrhagic moyamoya disease: analysis of a nonsurgical cohort in the Japan Adult Moyamoya Trial. J Neurosurg. 2019;130:525–30.

Postoperative Hyperperfusion 16

Haruto Uchino and Kiyohiro Houkin

Abstract

Cerebral hyperperfusion (HP) syndrome is one of the most serious complications associated with direct bypass surgery for moyamoya disease (MMD), especially in adult patients. Although the mechanisms underlying HP after revascularization surgery in MMD are not fully understood, the unique pathological background of MMD and the process of reperfusion injury represent a key pathogenesis of HP. This chapter focuses on the clinical features, imaging tools, and perioperative management of HP as well as the pathogenesis.

Keywords

Cerebral hyperperfusion · STA-MCA bypass · Transient neurological deficit · Complications · Reperfusion injury

16.1 Introduction

Medical therapy is not generally effective for treating moyamoya disease (MMD), and to date, surgical revascularization is the only prophylactic therapy available for reducing the risk of subsequent stroke. Direct bypasses generate a direct arterial connection from donor arteries to recipient arteries, and then exert their effects immediately after surgery, improving cerebral hemodynamics. Among direct bypass procedures, superficial temporal artery (STA)- middle cerebral artery (MCA) bypass is the most widely used and its effectiveness has been established in both pediatric

H. Uchino (✉) · K. Houkin
Department of Neurosurgery, Hokkaido University, Sapporo, Japan
e-mail: uchino-hok@umin.ac.jp; houkin@med.hokudai.ac.jp

S. Kuroda (ed.), *Moyamoya Disease: Current Knowledge and Future Perspectives*, https://doi.org/10.1007/978-981-33-6404-2_16

and adult patients. Despite its excellent efficacy, several postoperative complications are associated with direct bypass surgery. Although cerebral hyperperfusion (HP) has been well documented as one of the common complications that can occur after direct bypass, the underlying mechanism is not fully understood. This chapter describes postoperative HP in MMD from various aspects.

16.2 Incidence of HP

Historically, Since the 1980s, postoperative HP was identified as one of the serious complications associated with carotid endarterectomy, leading to temporary or permanent neurological deteriorations [1]. HP after STA-MCA bypass for atherosclerotic cerebrovascular diseases has also been reported [2]. Importantly, Uno et al. (1998) first reported HP syndrome in an adult patient with MMD after performing an STA-MCA bypass [3]. At the time, HP after low flow bypass was still considered a rare entity and was not well recognized by most of neurosurgeons especially in MMD until more recently. However, recent studies have found that the incidence of HP syndrome after STA-MCA bypass for the treatment of MMD is not as low as previously believed. For example, Fujimura et al. (2007) reported that HP syndrome occurred in as high as 38.2% of hemispheres in adult MMD patients after STA-MCA bypass [4]. Another study found that symptomatic HP had occurred in 32% of adult patients and 5% of pediatric patients. It was also reported that asymptomatic HP had occurred in 34% of adult patients and 15% of pediatric patients. Taken together, this suggests that radiological (both symptomatic and asymptomatic) HP was observed in >60% of adult patients, and that the incidence of HP is significantly higher in adult patients than in pediatric ones [5]. Therefore, individuals with MMD are at a potentially higher risk for HP syndrome than previously believed, especially adult patients.

16.3 Clinical Features

The clinical features of postoperative HP vary in each case. The onset of HP usually occurs within 7 days of the surgery (Fig. 16.1). A serial SPECT study demonstrated that HP immediately following surgery may easily lead to subsequent neurological symptoms, while the underlying mechanisms that cause early or delayed onset of HP are unclear. Therefore, adult patients with HP immediately following surgery are at significantly higher risk for subsequent neurological symptoms [5]. Typical neurological symptoms due to HP include motor weakness, sensory disturbances, aphasia, dysarthria, and seizures. Among these, aphasia due to HP in the left hemisphere is the most common symptom. This is because the frontal lobe is the area where cerebral hemodynamics is severely impaired in most cases and language functions may be sensitive to HP relative to other areas of the brain. Most HP-related neurological symptoms are transient and disappear within 24 hours, however, in

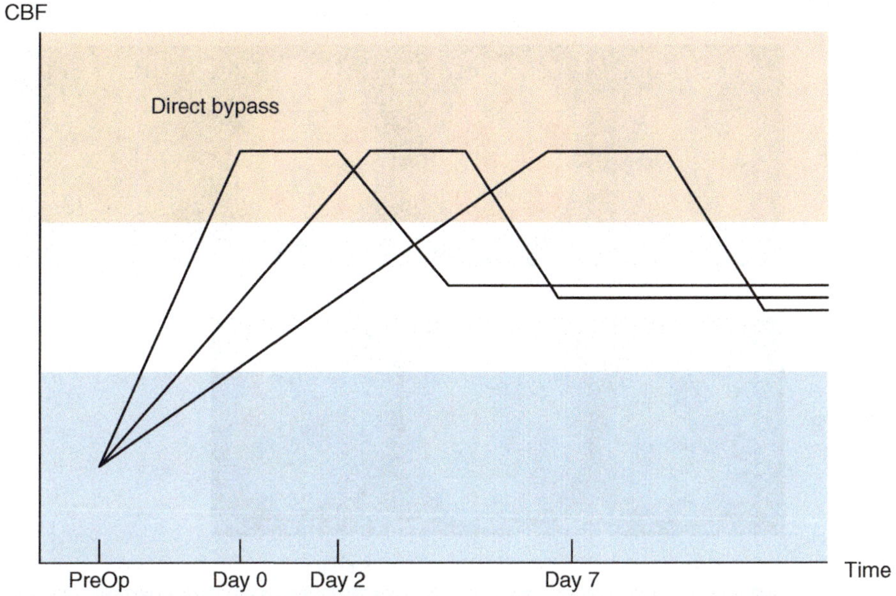

Fig. 16.1 A line graph showing several patterns of CBF changes of postoperative hyperperfusion in moyamoya disease

some cases, the symptoms persist for several days or even weeks. A positron emission tomography (PET) study showed that a preoperative cerebral blood volume (CBV) increase is the independent predictor of both symptomatic and asymptomatic HP in adult MMD (Fig. 16.2) [5]. An increase in CBV suggests the occurrence of autoregulatory vasodilatation in response to the cerebral perfusion pressure reduction. This vasodilation is considered to be one of the key background factors that causes postoperative HP in MMD. Another study found that an increase in patients' preoperative oxygen extraction fraction (OEF) is also a risk factor for HP syndrome [6]. Taken together, these data suggest that patients with an increased OEF and increased preoperative CBV may be at a higher risk for HP syndrome than those with normal CBV. Furthermore, in a recent study, preoperatively reduced cerebrovascular contractile reactivity to hypocapnia under hyperventilation was reported to be an independent predictor of cerebral HP syndrome in adult patients with cerebral misery perfusion [7].

Intracranial hemorrhage is a relatively rare complication after direct bypass in MMD. Although the underlying mechanisms are not fully understood, HP is considered to be one of the factors that causes postoperative hemorrhage. The incidence is reported to be <3% and most of the onset is within 24 hours after surgery [8, 9]. Adult age, hypertension, hemorrhagic presentation, and posterior circulation involvement are reported as independent risk factors for postoperative hemorrhage in MMD [8, 9]. Importantly, hematomas are typically located in the subcortical lesion around the anastomosed site. When the volume of the hematoma is large, immediate hematoma

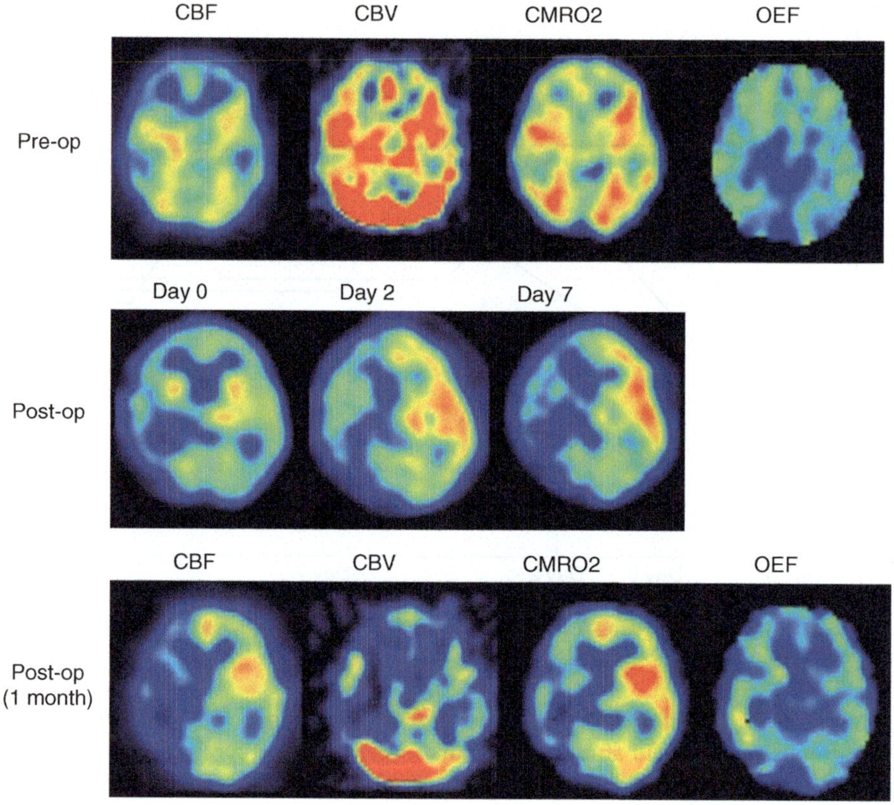

Fig. 16.2 Radiological findings from an MMD patient who underwent STA-MCA bypass on the left hemisphere. **Upper**; Preoperative examinations revealed a marked decrease in cerebral blood flow (CBF) and an increase in cerebral blood volume (CBV) and oxygen extraction fraction (OEF) in the bilateral frontal lobes. **Middle**; Postoperative serial single photon emission CT revealed a significant improvement of CBF just after surgery, but hyperperfusion in the left frontal lobe 2 days and 7 days after surgery. The patient developed motor aphasia 2 days after surgery. **Lower**; 1 month after surgery, positron emission tomography showed a normalization of CBF, CBV, and OEF in the left hemisphere

evacuation is required. According to reported cases, ligation of the STA to prevent worsening of the hemorrhage may not always be necessary. The prognosis of reported cases is generally favorable if appropriate management is performed, but it should be noted that it can potentially result in permanent neurological deficits or mortality.

16.4 Diagnosis

The diagnostic criteria for HP in MMD include all of the following [4]:

1. Presence of a significant focal increase in cerebral blood flow (CBF) at the site of the anastomosis.

2. Visualization of STA-MCA bypass by magnetic resonance angiography (MRA) or other modalities, and the absence of any ischemic changes by diffusion-weighted imaging (DWI).
3. Absence of other causes such as compression of the brain surface by the temporal muscle inserted for indirect synangiosis, ischemic attack, hemorrhage, and seizure.

HP syndrome is diagnosed when a focal CBF increases temporally and spatially corresponds to the existing focal neurological deficits.

Although radiological HP is usually evaluated qualitatively, and there is no consensus regarding the criteria of quantitative CBF values, recent studies aimed to analyze the threshold of the pathological increase in postoperative CBF in MMD. One quantitative CBF study observed that the cutoff increase ratio of CBF change for postoperative HP syndrome was 184.5% (sensitivity = 83.3%, specificity = 94.2%, area under the curve [AUC] value = 0.825) and 241.3% for hemorrhagic HP syndrome [10]. Another PET study found that the peak CBF values during HP syndrome (mean CBF: 218% of preoperative value) were consistent with the traditional concept of post-CEA HP (>100% increase over the baseline) but higher than the predefined CBF threshold values (control+2SD) [6]. Another whole-brain voxel-based perfusion mapping study found that an increase in CBF of more than 115.5% was associated with transient neurologic deficits [11]. Importantly, these cutoff values may change depending on the study design, such as the analyzed postoperative time point and the definition of the regions of interest.

16.5 Intraoperative Evaluations

Intraoperative modalities are useful in evaluating hemodynamic changes immediately after bypass and to predict the occurrence of HP.

16.5.1 Indocyanine Green Videoangiography

Microscope-integrated indocyanine green videoangiography (ICG-VA) has been widely used for intraoperative monitoring of regional cerebral blood flow in cerebrovascular disease. A previous study found that microvascular transit time (MVTT) was prolonged in MMD patients compared to those with atherosclerotic cerebrovascular disease [12]. In the study, MVTT was significantly reduced after bypass surgery, but the ΔMVTT [(post bypass value)—(pre bypass value)] was significantly greater in the HP syndrome group than in the non-HP syndrome group. Furthermore, a ΔMVTT >2.6 seconds was shown to be an independent predictor of HP syndrome. Similarly, a prolonged ICG peak time in the cortical artery is associated with HP [13]. Another useful parameter to evaluate hemodynamic changes after bypass is the blood flow index (BFI), which measures the slope of the ICG intensity-time curve of cortical arteries. A greater increase in the ratio of BFI after bypass has been associated with HP immediately after surgery [14].

16.5.2 Flow Meters

Transit time ultrasonic flow meters and Doppler ultrasonic flow meters can measure intraoperative flow velocity of bypassed arteries. The increase in Vmax ratios of bypassed arteries after bypass is significantly higher in patients with HP [15–17]. Importantly, cortical flow velocity is not directly associated with CBF in normal individuals, who show variable cortical velocities depending on cerebrovascular resistance and diameter. However, in MMD, the vascular network dilates, and cerebrovascular resistance decreases due to chronic ischemia. Under such conditions, cortical flow velocity is likely correlated with regional CBF.

16.5.3 Caliber Mismatch of Donor and Recipient Arteries

Several studies have observed that a mismatch in the size of the donor and recipient arteries has an effect on the occurrence of HP [13, 14, 18]. That is, a higher caliber ratio (donor STA/recipient MCA; mean, approximately 1.7) is associated with postoperative HP in adult patients [13, 14]. One study reported that the incidence of postoperative HP syndrome was 3.66% when donor-recipient vessels were matched during surgery, which was much lower than that in the non-matching group (15.6%) [18].

16.5.4 Hemodynamic Sources of Recipient Arteries

The recipient parasylvian cortical arteries are supplied from anterograde MCA or from non-MCAs of pial collateral circulation in MMD. A recent study revealed that the direct anastomoses of parasylvian arteries with anterograde hemodynamic sources from the MCA were significantly associated with the development of postoperative HP [19]. This is because the anterograde MCA has generally low flow due to more severe stenosis compared to non-MCA collateral flow, and direct bypass to such recipient arteries results in greater postoperative hemodynamic changes. The above-mentioned caliber mismatch of STA and MCA will therefore facilitate the increase in bypass flow in this condition.

Risk factors as well as the predictive factors mentioned are summarized in Table 16.1.

16.6 Postoperative Imaging

The characteristic radiological findings of HP are summarized in Table 16.2.

16.6.1 SPECT/PET

Serial CBF studies are crucial for the evaluation of postoperative hemodynamic changes and appropriate management against postoperative complications. Although

Table 16.1 Risk factors of hyperperfusion syndrome

Adult
Hemorrhagic onset
Left hemisphere
Preoperative OEF increase
Preoperative CBV increase
Reduced cerebrovascular contractile reactivity to hypocapnia
Caliber mismatch of donor and recipient arteries
Prolonged microvascular transit time
High blood flow index
Recipient arteries with anterograde source of middle cerebral arteries

Table 16.2 Radiological findings of hyperperfusion

Modalities	Findings
SPECT	Focal CBF increase, watershed shift phenomenon, crossed cerebellar hypoperfusion
PET	CBV increase
FLAIR	Cortical hyper belt sign (non-specific to HP)
TOF-MRA	Hyper signal intensity and dilation of STA
4D-MRA	Increased flow velocity and focal hyperintense signals on the bypassed arteries

SPECT is widely used, other perfusion imaging modalities, including perfusion CT and perfusion magnetic resonance imaging (MRI), are also effective. A previous PET study observed a prolonged recovery of increased CBV after surgery in patients with HP syndrome [6].

Watershed Shift

A paradoxical decrease in the CBF at the cortex adjacent to the focal CBF increase is observed in some HP cases. This is known as the water shed shift phenomenon and the incidence is reported to be 10.9% after direct bypass for adult MMD [20]. Therefore, the watershed shift phenomenon represents a potential risk for ischemic complications during perioperative management of HP.

Crossed Cerebellar Diaschisis

An association between crossed cerebellar diaschisis (CCD) and HP has also been reported in MMD [21, 22]. Crossed cerebellar hypoperfusion due to HP has been observed in some cases after direct bypass. CCD was first described in the 1980s as an association between a local supratentorial brain lesion and a simultaneous decrease in contralateral cerebellar blood flow and metabolic activity [23]. The underlying mechanisms consist of disruption of the cortico-cerebellar pathway and transneuronal metabolic depression of the contralateral cerebellar hemisphere. Importantly, CCD has not only been reported in cerebral infarction, but also in epilepsy, migraine, glioma, Alzheimer's disease, and cerebral hemorrhage. In general, CCD due to HP following cerebrovascular revascularization was considered to be rare. However, a recent case series reported that CCD was observed in 18.4% of the hemispheres with radiological HP and it was more frequently observed in symptomatic HP than in asymptomatic HP (36.0% vs 11.3%) [24]. Therefore, CCD may represent a radiological marker associated with symptomatic HP or severe neuronal damage due to HP.

16.6.2 MRI

Cortical Hyperintensity Belt Sign

A fluid-attenuated inversion-recovery high-intensity signal in the cortex of the operated hemisphere, known as a cortical hyperintensity belt sign (CHB), is frequently observed after direct bypass in MMD. However, it should be noted that CHB is not a specific sign of HP syndrome. This is quite different from an "ivy sign," which is an extraparenchymal signal that suggests slow arterial flow in the ischemic brain area. The frequency of CHB is reported in 80–90% of cases after direct bypass [25, 26]. While the underlying mechanism(s) are still unclear, CHB is often observed even in the posterior territory of MCA, which is outside of the operative field. Since CHB is usually transient and not associated with a high DWI signal, it is speculated that the pathophysiology of the CHB is vasogenic edemas. A vasogenic edema is the result of cerebral arteriolar dilation, damage of the blood–brain barrier, and extravasation to the brain parenchyma. The association of arteriolar dilation is further supported by the fact that the postoperative increase in CBV is correlated with the CHB [27].

16.7 3 MRA

Time of flight (TOF)-MRA is useful for confirming the postoperative patency of direct bypass in a less invasive manner. During HP syndrome, the postoperative signal increase ratio of STA on TOF-MRA is higher in HP syndrome group than in non-HP syndrome group. The increase ratio of the signal intensity in HP syndrome group is reported to be more than 1.5 times that of the preoperative levels [28]. Four-dimensional magnetic resonance angiography using an arterial spin labeling technique (ASL-4D MRA) is also very useful in evaluating the postoperative dynamic changes in the cerebral blood flow patterns without the need for a contrast enhanced agent. During the occurrence of HP, a ASL-4D MRA can detect congestion of bypass flow at the site of anastomosis and focal hyperintense signals in the bypassed arteries, which TOF-MRA is unable to detect [29].

16.8 Pathogenesis

It is well known that HP syndrome after STA-MCA bypass is much more frequent in MMD patients than those with atherosclerotic occlusive cerebrovascular diseases. This suggests that MMD patients have characteristic pathophysiological conditions that are likely to cause HP. These conditions include maladaptive vasodilation due to chronic cerebral ischemia, a poor network of pial arteries, and blood–brain barrier impairment. After direct bypass, the occurrence of HP is attributed to several hemodynamic factors, including a large pressure gradient from donor to recipient arteries caused by the maladaptive vasodilation. A large STA size relative to the recipient MCA and a prolonged recovery of vascular reserve aggravate the situation. On the other hand, poor distribution of the large amount of bypass flow leads to congestion of the blood flow at the site of anastomosis. In these situations, the excessive arterial blood supply likely leads to oxidative stress that generates free radicals, which then further damage the blood–brain barrier. This would then cause vasogenic edema, disturbing vascular circulation. These processes, in addition to the direct toxic effect of free radicals on neurons, could disrupt the neurovascular unit. As a result, HP-related neurological deficits occur (Fig. 16.3).

Several previous studies have helped advance our understanding of the pathogenesis of HP. For example, during the development of HP syndrome, a decrease in central benzodiazepine receptor binding potential has been reported using iomazenil-SPECT [21]. This data suggests that downregulation of cortical neurotransmitter receptor function due to cerebral HP results in neurological deficits. Furthermore, a serial PET study observed preoperative increases in CBV that persisted during HP, suggesting a prolonged recovery of elevated CBV values despite immediate increases in perfusion pressure after direct bypass [6]. These findings help explain the development of HP and the related neurological symptoms that last for several days.

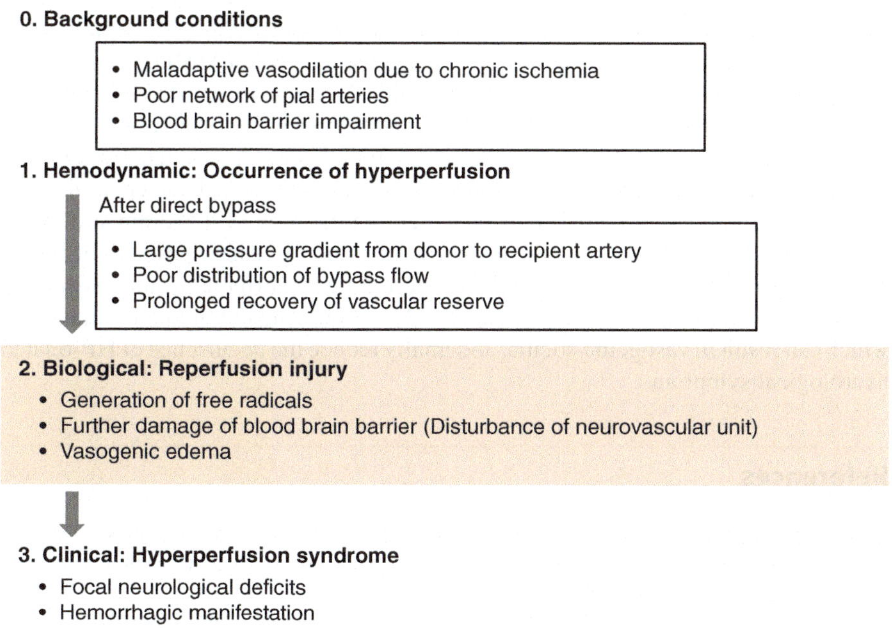

Fig. 16.3 Schema showing pathophysiology of hyperperfusion in moyamoya disease

Although CBV is often elevated in pediatric patients, most of them do not show HP after surgery. This finding strongly suggests that the pathophysiological mechanisms underlying the CBV increase in response to a reduction in cerebral perfusion pressure differ between pediatric and adult MMD patients. An intraoperative ICG-VA analysis also showed that pediatric patients were unlikely to develop HP syndrome despite showing a large ΔMVTT (>2.6 seconds) [12]. These data demonstrate that an abrupt increase in arterial inflow from bypass may be compensated for via mechanisms other than increased peripheral vascular resistance in pediatric patients.

16.9 Perioperative Management of HP

Given that the clinical presentation of postoperative HP syndrome is similar to a transient ischemic attack, CBF analyses and neuroimaging, including MRI/A, are essential for the precise differential diagnosis of postoperative complications. HP-related neurological symptoms are typically evident from the day of surgery up to 7 days post-surgery. Therefore, a CBF analysis is recommended at an early time point (days 0–2) after surgery. Furthermore, bedside monitoring of neurological signs is also crucial for the early detection of HP syndrome especially up until 7 days after surgery.

Postoperative blood pressure control is a mainstay of management for HP syndrome. Mild blood pressure lowering or maintaining normotension has been reported to safely reduce the risk for HP syndrome although excessive blood pressure lowering may increase the risk for ischemic complications [30]. Importantly, sedation is not usually necessary for the management of HP in MMD. Furthermore, perioperative administration of minocycline and edaravone is reported to reduce the incidence of HP syndrome. Minocycline is an antibiotic and anti-inflammatory drug that has neuroprotective effects as an antiapoptotic agent, antioxidant, and matrix metalloproteinase inhibitor [31]. Edaravone, a free radical scavenger, is used to improve neurological prognosis in acute cerebral infarction [32]. Administration of edaravone is believed to protect the neurovascular unit by reducing free radical production during the processes of HP. Thus, these drugs contribute to suppressing the above-mentioned pathological cascade of HP by protecting the blood–brain barrier, which can result in vasogenic edema, and finally reduce the occurrence of HP-related neurological symptoms.

References

1. Reigel MM, Hollier LH, Sundt TM Jr, Piepgras DG, Sharbrough FW, Cherry KJ. Cerebral hyperperfusion syndrome: a cause of neurologic dysfunction after carotid endarterectomy. J Vasc Surg. 1987;5(4):628–34.
2. Heros RC, Scott RM, Kistler JP, Ackerman RH, Conner ES. Temporary neurological deterioration after extracranial-intracranial bypass. Neurosurgery. 1984;15(2):178–85. https://doi.org/10.1227/00006123-198408000-00006.

3. Uno M, Nakajima N, Nishi K, Shinno K, Nagahiro S. Hyperperfusion syndrome after extracranial-intracranial bypass in a patient with moyamoya disease–case report. Neurol Med Chir (Tokyo). 1998;38(7):420–4. https://doi.org/10.2176/nmc.38.420.
4. Fujimura M, Kaneta T, Mugikura S, Shimizu H, Tominaga T. Temporary neurologic deterioration due to cerebral hyperperfusion after superficial temporal artery-middle cerebral artery anastomosis in patients with adult-onset moyamoya disease. Surg Neurol. 2007;67(3):273–82. https://doi.org/10.1016/j.surneu.2006.07.017.
5. Uchino H, Kuroda S, Hirata K, Shiga T, Houkin K, Tamaki N. Predictors and clinical features of postoperative hyperperfusion after surgical revascularization for moyamoya disease: a serial single photon emission CT/positron emission tomography study. Stroke. 2012;43(10):2610–6. https://doi.org/10.1161/STROKEAHA.112.654723.
6. Kaku Y, Iihara K, Nakajima N, Kataoka H, Fukuda K, Masuoka J, et al. Cerebral blood flow and metabolism of hyperperfusion after cerebral revascularization in patients with moyamoya disease. J Cereb Blood Flow Metab. 2012;32(11):2066–75. https://doi.org/10.1038/jcbfm.2012.110.
7. Sato S, Kojima D, Shimada Y, Yoshida J, Fujimato K, Fujiwara S, et al. Preoperatively reduced cerebrovascular contractile reactivity to hypocapnia by hyperventilation is associated with cerebral hyperperfusion syndrome after arterial bypass surgery for adult patients with cerebral misery perfusion due to ischemic moyamoya disease. J Cereb Blood Flow Metab. 2018;38(6):1021–31. https://doi.org/10.1177/0271678X18757621.
8. Tokairin K, Kazumata K, Uchino H, Ito M, Ono K, Tatezawa R, et al. Postoperative Intracerebral hemorrhage after combined revascularization surgery in Moyamoya disease: profiles and clinical associations. World Neurosurg. 2018;120:e593–600. https://doi.org/10.1016/j.wneu.2018.08.132.
9. Chen Y, Ma L, Lu J, Chen X, Ye X, Zhang D, et al. Postoperative hemorrhage during the acute phase after direct or combined revascularization for moyamoya disease: risk factors, prognosis, and literature review. J Neurosurg. 2019:1–10. https://doi.org/10.3171/2019.7.JNS19885.
10. Kameyama M, Fujimura M, Tashiro R, Sato K, Endo H, Niizuma K, et al. Significance of quantitative cerebral blood flow measurement in the acute stage after revascularization surgery for adult Moyamoya disease: implication for the pathological threshold of local cerebral Hyperperfusion. Cerebrovasc Dis. 2019;48(3–6):217–25. https://doi.org/10.1159/000504835.
11. Kazumata K, Uchino H, Tokairin K, Ito M, Shiga T, Osanai T, et al. Cerebral Hyperperfusion syndrome after revascularization surgery in Moyamoya disease: region-symptom mapping and estimating a critical threshold. World Neurosurg. 2018;114:e388–e95. https://doi.org/10.1016/j.wneu.2018.02.190.
12. Yang T, Higashino Y, Kataoka H, Hamano E, Maruyama D, Iihara K, et al. Correlation between reduction in microvascular transit time after superficial temporal artery-middle cerebral artery bypass surgery for moyamoya disease and the development of postoperative hyperperfusion syndrome. J Neurosurg. 2018;128(5):1304–10. https://doi.org/10.3171/2016.11.JNS162403.
13. Horie N, Fukuda Y, Izumo T, Hayashi K, Suyama K, Nagata I. Indocyanine green videoangiography for assessment of postoperative hyperperfusion in moyamoya disease. Acta Neurochir. 2014;156(5):919–26. https://doi.org/10.1007/s00701-014-2054-4.
14. Uchino H, Kazumata K, Ito M, Nakayama N, Kuroda S, Houkin K. Intraoperative assessment of cortical perfusion by indocyanine green videoangiography in surgical revascularization for moyamoya disease. Acta Neurochir. 2014;156(9):1753–60. https://doi.org/10.1007/s00701-014-2161-2.
15. Morisawa H, Kawamata T, Kawashima A, Hayashi M, Yamaguchi K, Yoneyama T, et al. Hemodynamics and changes after STA-MCA anastomosis in moyamoya disease and atherosclerotic cerebrovascular disease measured by micro-Doppler ultrasonography. Neurosurg Rev. 2013;36(3):411–9. https://doi.org/10.1007/s10143-012-0441-y.
16. Kawamata T, Kawashima A, Yamaguchi K, Hori T, Okada Y. Usefulness of intraoperative laser Doppler flowmetry and thermography to predict a risk of postoperative hyperperfusion after

superficial temporal artery-middle cerebral artery bypass for moyamoya disease. Neurosurg Rev. 2011;34(3):355–62. discussion 62. https://doi.org/10.1007/s10143-011-0331-8.
17. Nakayama N, Kuroda S, Houkin K, Takikawa S, Abe H. Intraoperative measurement of arterial blood flow using a transit time flowmeter: monitoring of hemodynamic changes during cerebrovascular surgery. Acta Neurochir. 2001;143(1):17–24. https://doi.org/10.1007/s007010170133.
18. Hu M, Zeng X, Su K, Tian X, Chen J, Zhang J. Matching selection of donor-recipient vessels in revascularization surgery effectively reduce the incidence of postoperative Hyperperfusion syndrome in adult Moyamoya disease: a retrospective comparison study. Cerebrovasc Dis. 2020:1–8. https://doi.org/10.1159/000509138.
19. Zhang J, Li S, Fujimura M, Lau TY, Wu X, Hu M, et al. Hemodynamic analysis of the recipient parasylvian cortical arteries for predicting postoperative hyperperfusion during STA-MCA bypass in adult patients with moyamoya disease. J Neurosurg. 2019:1–8. https://doi.org/10.3171/2019.10.JNS191207.
20. Tashiro R, Fujimura M, Kameyama M, Mugikura S, Endo H, Takeuchi Y, et al. Incidence and risk factors of the watershed shift phenomenon after superficial temporal artery-middle cerebral artery anastomosis for adult Moyamoya disease. Cerebrovasc Dis. 2019;47(3–4):178–87. https://doi.org/10.1159/000500802.
21. Shimada Y, Kojima D, Yoshida J, Kobayashi M, Yoshida K, Fujiwara S, et al. Transient symptomatic Downregulation of cortical neurotransmitter receptor function due to cerebral Hyperperfusion after arterial bypass surgery for a patient with ischemic Moyamoya disease. Neurol Med Chir (Tokyo). 2018;58(11):481–4. https://doi.org/10.2176/nmc.cr.2018-0143.
22. Hokari M, Kuroda S, Simoda Y, Uchino H, Hirata K, Shiga T, et al. Transient crossed cerebellar diaschisis due to cerebral hyperperfusion following surgical revascularization for moyamoya disease: case report. Neurol Med Chir (Tokyo). 2012;52(5):350–3. https://doi.org/10.2176/nmc.52.350.
23. Baron JC, Bousser MG, Comar D, Castaigne P. "Crossed cerebellar diaschisis" in human supratentorial brain infarction. Trans Am Neurol Assoc. 1981;105:459–61.
24. Uchino H, Kazumata K, Ito M, Nakayama N, Kuroda S, Houkin K. Crossed cerebellar diaschisis as an indicator of severe cerebral hyperperfusion after direct bypass for moyamoya disease. Neurosurg Rev. 2020; https://doi.org/10.1007/s10143-020-01265-8.
25. Takemoto Y, Kawano T, Ohmori Y, Kaku Y, Uekawa K, Amadatsu T, et al. Hemodynamic study about cortical hyperintensity belt sign after direct bypass surgery for moyamoya disease. J Clin Neurosci. 2020;74:124–9. https://doi.org/10.1016/j.jocn.2020.02.022.
26. Hamano E, Kataoka H, Morita N, Maruyama D, Satow T, Iihara K, et al. Clinical implications of the cortical hyperintensity belt sign in fluid-attenuated inversion recovery images after bypass surgery for moyamoya disease. J Neurosurg. 2017;126(1):1–7. https://doi.org/10.3171/2015.10.JNS151022.
27. Kaku Y, Iihara K, Nakajima N, Kataoka H, Fukushima K, Iida H, et al. The leptomeningeal ivy sign on fluid-attenuated inversion recovery images in moyamoya disease: positron emission tomography study. Cerebrovasc Dis. 2013;36(1):19–25. https://doi.org/10.1159/000351143.
28. Sato K, Yamada M, Kuroda H, Yamamoto D, Asano Y, Inoue Y, et al. Time-of-flight MR angiography for detection of cerebral Hyperperfusion syndrome after superficial temporal artery-middle cerebral artery anastomosis in Moyamoya disease. AJNR Am J Neuroradiol. 2016;37(7):1244–8. https://doi.org/10.3174/ajnr.A4715.
29. Uchino H, Ito M, Fujima N, Kazumata K, Yamazaki K, Nakayama N, et al. A novel application of four-dimensional magnetic resonance angiography using an arterial spin labeling technique for noninvasive diagnosis of Moyamoya disease. Clin Neurol Neurosurg. 2015;137:105–11. https://doi.org/10.1016/j.clineuro.2015.07.003.
30. Fujimura M, Inoue T, Shimizu H, Saito A, Mugikura S, Tominaga T. Efficacy of prophylactic blood pressure lowering according to a standardized postoperative management protocol to

prevent symptomatic cerebral hyperperfusion after direct revascularization surgery for moyamoya disease. Cerebrovasc Dis. 2012;33(5):436–45. https://doi.org/10.1159/000336765.
31. Fujimura M, Niizuma K, Inoue T, Sato K, Endo H, Shimizu H, et al. Minocycline prevents focal neurological deterioration due to cerebral hyperperfusion after extracranial-intracranial bypass for moyamoya disease. Neurosurgery. 2014;74(2):163–70. discussion 70. https://doi.org/10.1227/NEU.0000000000000238.
32. Uchino H, Nakayama N, Kazumata K, Kuroda S, Houkin K. Edaravone reduces Hyperperfusion-related neurological deficits in adult Moyamoya disease: historical control study. Stroke. 2016;47(7):1930–2. https://doi.org/10.1161/STROKEAHA.116.013304.

Postoperative FLAIR Imaging Changes 17

Daina Kashiwazaki and Satoshi Kuroda

Abstract

Bypass surgery is widely accepted as effective treatment to improve cerebral hemodynamics and to prevent both further ischemic and hemorrhagic stroke in moyamoya disease (MMD). For these 10 years, there is increasing evidence that the hyperintense signal develops in the brain surface on fluid-attenuated inversion recovery (FLAIR) images following bypass surgery. This novel, unique phenomenon is specific for moyamoya disease and does not occur in patients with atherosclerotic carotid artery diseases. This phenomenon can be observed between 3 and 14 days after surgery and completely disappears thereafter. Even now, its pathophysiology and underlying mechanisms are not fully understood. In this chapter, therefore, the authors precisely review recent knowledge on the hyperintense signal on FLAIR image after surgical revascularization for moyamoya disease and discuss future perspective.

Keywords

Bypass surgery · FLAIR · Hyperintense signal · Moyamoya disease · Cerebral blood flow

D. Kashiwazaki · S. Kuroda (✉)
Department of Neurosurgery, Graduate School of Medicine and Pharmaceutical Science, University of Toyama, Toyama, Japan
e-mail: dkashiwa@med.u-toyama.ac.jp; skuroda@med.u-toyama.ac.jp

S. Kuroda (ed.), *Moyamoya Disease: Current Knowledge and Future Perspectives*, https://doi.org/10.1007/978-981-33-6404-2_17

17.1 Introduction

Moyamoya disease (MMD) is an uncommon cerebrovascular disease characterized by progressive occlusion of the terminal portion of the internal carotid artery and its main branches [1]. Bypass surgery is a widely accepted treatment for MMD to prevent further ischemic and hemorrhagic events [1, 2]. Various procedures for surgical revascularization have been developed and are divided into indirect bypass, direct bypass, and combined bypass. It is well-known that hemodynamic status drastically changes after bypass surgery, leading to various pathophysiological changes in and around the operative field [3–5]. Of these, recent studies have shown that MMD patients often develop a hyperintense signal in the ipsilateral cortex on fluid-attenuated inversion recovery (FLAIR) images following bypass surgery. An illustrative case is presented in Fig. 17.1. The hyperintense signal on postoperative FLAIR images is located along the cerebral sulci and is clearly different in

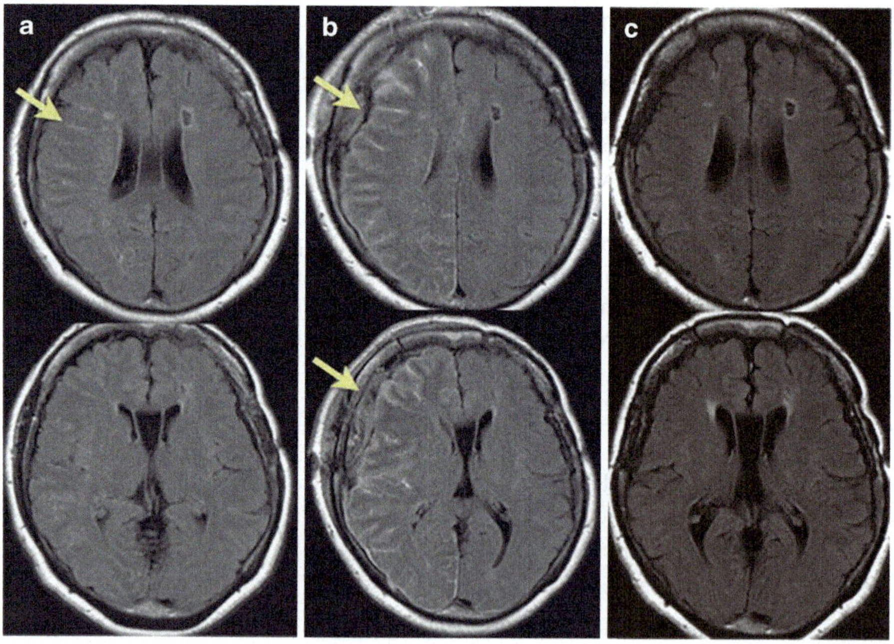

Fig. 17.1 Serial FLAIR images at the level of the basal ganglia (*lower*) and the body of the lateral ventricle (*upper*) before surgery (**a**) and 7 days (**b**) and 30 days after STA-MCA anastomosis and indirect bypass on the right side (**c**). Prior to surgery, the increased signal can be observed in the arteries within the cortical sulci or on the surface of the brain (arrow, **a**). This finding is called as "ivy" sign. Note that the hyperintense signal is widely distributed in the operated right hemisphere at 7 days post-surgery (arrows, **b**) and completely disappears at 30 days post-surgery. The appearance of the transient hyperintense signal after surgery is completely different from that of "ivy sign" before surgery

appearance from the hyperintense signal of the superficial arteries observed prior to surgery, which is called as "ivy sign." However, the underlying mechanisms and clinical significance of this MMD-specific signal change are poorly understood.

FLAIR imaging has mostly replaced proton density-weighted imaging for the evaluation of supra-tentorial brain disease due to its increased lesion contrast, suppression of normal cerebrospinal fluid (CSF) signal intensity, and ability to acquire images within a relatively short acquisition time owing to fast imaging techniques [6–9]. Compared to T2-weighted and proton density-weighted imaging, FLAIR imaging is known superior for evaluating parenchymal lesions near the CSF.

This section aims to review the extant literature regarding this hyperintense sign on FLAIR imaging after bypass surgery for MMD, focusing on its clinical features and mechanisms and identifying any unresolved issues. Understanding the underlying pathophysiology of this hyperintense sign may lead to valuable improvements in the perioperative management for MMD patients.

17.2 Radiological Features of the Hyperintense Signal

Nowadays, it is known that a newly developed hyperintense signal in the ipsilateral hemisphere can be observed on FLAIR images after bypass surgery [10–12]. This radiological finding presents several unique features; first, the sign is only temporally observed and disappears within 30 days after surgery. Second, its intensity substantially increases immediately after surgery and reaches a peak within 7 days post-surgery followed by a gradual recovery to original levels (Fig. 17.1). Furthermore, the extension of the hyperintense sign varies widely among patients. Its location is also varied and often exceeds the extent of the craniotomy. Illustrative cases are presented in Fig. 17.2. While this hyperintense signal may appear similar to blood in the subarachnoid space following the surgical procedure, other sequences

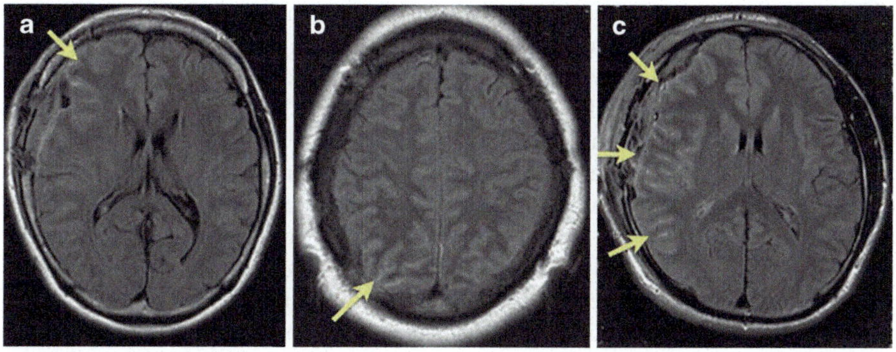

Fig. 17.2 FLAIR images at 7 days after STA-MCA anastomosis and indirect bypass in 3 patients with moyamoya disease. Note that the distribution of the hyperintense signal after surgery largely differs among 3 patients even after the same surgical procedure (arrows)

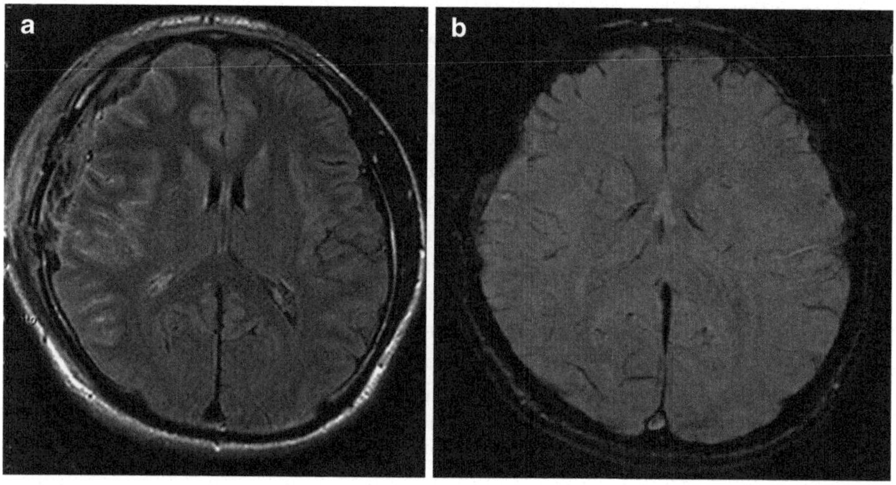

Fig. 17.3 FLAIR (**a**) and susceptibility-weighted MRI (**b**) at 7 days after STA-MCA anastomosis and indirect bypass in the patients with moyamoya disease. Susceptibility-weighted MRI clearly demonstrates that the hyperintense signal in the cortical sulci on FLAIR image does not represent the blood clots after surgery

sensitive to blood clots such as T2* or susceptibility-weighted imaging clearly reveal no existence of blood clots in the subarachnoid space (Fig. 17.3) [13, 14]. Therefore, we can conclude that this hyperintense signal does not indicate the blood clots in the CSF space resulting from the surgical procedure.

It should be noted that this hyperintense sign is only evident in patients with MMD and not in patients with arteriosclerosis after standard STA-MCA anastomosis. A key characteristic of this sign is its occurrence in both adult and pediatric MMD patients. Furthermore, this hyperintense signal is present regardless of the type of clinical onset. Shiba et al. (2018) also found that there were not significant differences in the occurrence of hyperintense signs on surgically treated hemispheres between single and double bypass procedures [15].

The frequency of this hyperintense sign has been examined in several reports, although its incidence widely varies from 58% to 93% [10–12, 15]. Based on our experiences, this hyperintense sign can be observed in all MMD patients (100%) after bypass surgery. The reason of the differences remains unknown. At least, however, all patients included in these reports underwent a combined bypass and there are no reports regarding the incidence of this phenomenon following direct or indirect bypass only. Indirect bypass induces neovascularization from donner tissues such as the temporal muscle and dura mater, but it requires 2 to 3 months to complete the formation of arterial connection between the donor tissues and the arteries on the brain surface. Therefore, the main driving force to develop the hyperintense sign after bypass surgery may result from direct bypass.

Horie et al. (2014) first reported this hyperintense signal on FLAIR imaging after bypass surgery for MMD and called it a "*de novo*" ivy sign [11]. The ivy sign is well-known as an increased blood signal within the artery due to slow flow-related enhancement and has been defined as a continuous linear leptomeningeal high-signal intensity along the cortex and subarachnoid spaces [16, 17]. In their report, Horie et al. (2014) speculated that this newly-observed phenomenon after surgery represented a signal change in the operated hemispheres' vasculatures [11]. However, it is less likely that the hyperintense sign similarly reflects the vasculature changes in the subarachnoid space, because it does not contain a continuous tube-like structure. Previous study suggested that the ivy sign might reflect the slow flow of developed leptomeningeal collaterals in patients with MMD and disappear after hemodynamic alternation due to bypass surgery [18]. From this view point, therefore, we consider that the postoperative hyperintense sign would be inconsistent with ivy sign.

Subsequently, Hamano et al. (2017) reported the same phenomenon in MMD and concluded that this belt-like hyperintense sign after surgery on the brain surface might reflect the signal changes in the cerebral cortex on FLAIR image [10]. Takemoto et al. (2020) presented a case with the hyperintense sign following bypass surgery and speculated that this hyperintense signal may occur from the congested blood in the cerebral cortex. They suggested the possibility that STA-MCA anastomosis may cause pial vessel dilation and venous stasis in the subcortical white matter, leading to the appearance of the hyperintense signal after surgery [12].

17.3 The Role of Cerebral Hemodynamics

17.3.1 Preoperative Cerebral Hemodynamics

There are several reports evaluating the impact of preoperative hemodynamic parameters on the development of the hyperintense sign after surgery. Horie et al. (2014) found no significant differences in onset pattern, preoperative cerebral hemodynamics in the MCA area, and preoperative ivy sign scores between patients with postoperative hyperintense sign and those without [11]. Hamano et al. (2017) also observed no significant relationship between qualitative hyperintense sign scores and regional cerebral blood flow increase ratios [10]. However, they acknowledged the difficulty to determine the difference in the degree of cerebral ischemia before surgery between patients with postoperative hyperintense signal and those without because of the lack of quantitative CBF measurement in their study. On the other hands, they found that this phenomenon was closely related to postoperative transient neurological deficits with undetermined pathophysiology, and hypothesized that the hyperintense sign developed through vasogenic edema of the cerebral cortex. Postoperative neurological deficits were observed in 61% of surgically treated cases. The symptoms included numbness (35.5%), aphasia (25.5%), motor weakness (12.1%), dysarthria (10.6%), and other symptoms (3.5%). These patients had significantly higher qualitative hyperintense sign scores than others. Furthermore, the total qualitative hyperintense sign score was linked to the duration of neurological deficits. They speculated that autoregulatory vasodilation occurred in response to cerebral ischemia before surgery and induced excessive inflow of blood flow through direct bypass, leading to extravasation of fluid in the cerebral cortex [10].

Takemoto et al. (2020) hypothesized that the pathophysiology of the hyperintense sign is vasogenic edema, because the postoperative cerebral blood volume (CBV) increase correlated with the hyperintense sign [12]. The CBV increased ratio was significantly higher in the profound hyperintense sign group than in the subtle hyperintense sign group. They also found that preoperative CBF and the mean transit time (MTT) values did not differ between patients with postoperative hyperintense sign and those without [12].

According to our experiences, the hyperintense sign on FLAIR imaging occurs in all MMD patients after surgery to varying degree as described above, but the intensity and extent of the phenomenon largely differ among them. Statistical analysis has demonstrated that the degree of cerebral ischemia before surgery is closely related to the intensity of the hyperintense sign after surgery (unpublished data). As shown in Fig. 17.4, the hyperintense sign occurs in the area where cerebral hemodynamics is markedly impaired before surgery, including outside the extent of craniotomy or in the contralateral ACA territory.

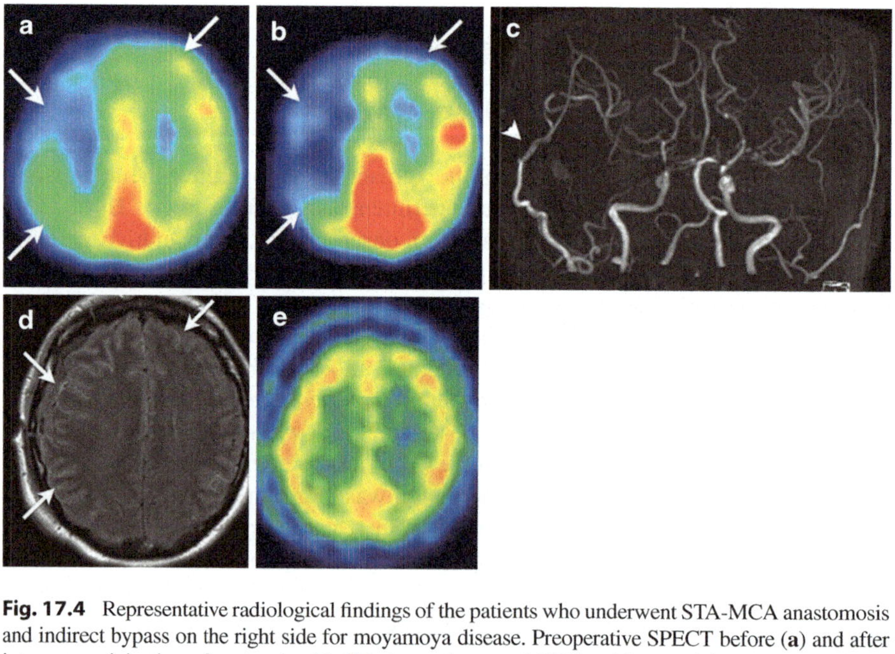

Fig. 17.4 Representative radiological findings of the patients who underwent STA-MCA anastomosis and indirect bypass on the right side for moyamoya disease. Preoperative SPECT before (**a**) and after intravenous injection of acetazolamide (**b**) shows decreased CBF and its reactivity to acetazolamide stress in the right ACA and MCA territories and the left ACA territory (arrows). MR angiography performed 3 days after surgery (**c**) demonstrates good patency of STA-MCA double anastomosis on the right side (arrowhead). Simultaneous FLAIR image (**d**) clearly demonstrates that the hyperintense signal is observed in the areas where both CBF and its reactivity to acetazolamide decreased before surgery (arrows). On postoperative SPECT (**e**), CBF completely recovers to the normal level

17.3.2 Postoperative Hyperperfusion

Several reports have proposed the possible mechanisms through which the hyperintense sign on FLAIR imaging may develop after surgery in MMD. Of these, Horie et al. (2014) first speculated the relationship between postoperative increase in cerebral blood flow (CBF) and the hyperintense sign, because the hyperintense sign is closely related to postoperative hyperperfusion (odds ratio, 7.75; 95% confidence interval [CI], 1.08–55.75; $P = 0.04$). Likewise, they found that the hyperintense sign preferably occurred in the territory of STA-MCA anastomosis, which suggested that drastic hemodynamic changes after bypass surgery contributed to the unique phenomenon. They have also speculated that the hyperintense sign on FLAIR imaging may be specific for MMD, because the focal CBF increase in the pial vessels is much higher in MMD than in atherosclerotic carotid artery diseases. Finally, they concluded that the postoperative hyperintense sign could be a marker of postoperative hyperperfusion in MMD [11]. As described above, Hamano et al. (2017) suggested that the hyperintense sign is completely different from the ivy sign before surgery and is confined to the intraparenchymal signal change in the cerebral cortex. They also concluded that there were no significant relationships between the hyperintense sign and postoperative hyperperfusion, because the hyperintense sign was not linked with the postoperative CBF increase [10]. Takemoto et al. (2020) also found that CBF increase ratio was not related to their hyperintense sign scores. Tanioka et al. (2016) reported a MMD case with the hyperintense sign following STA-MCA anastomosis and encephalo–duro–myo-synangiosis in spite of normal CBF after surgery [19]. These observations strongly suggest that postoperative hyperintense sign in MMD does not reflect hyperperfusion phenomenon after surgery, which correlates very well with our personal experience (unpublished data).

17.4 Future Perspective

We are still in front of unresolved mysteries regarding the hyperintense sign on FLAIR images after bypass surgery for MMD. The exact mechanisms through which this unique phenomenon occurs is poorly understood. Moreover, it is still unclear where this phenomenon is occurring; in the vasculature, in the cerebral cortex, or in somewhere else. The contradictory speculations among the investigators indicate the need for additional, more detailed studies on this issue.

References

1. Kuroda S, Houkin K. Moyamoya disease: current concepts and future perspectives. Lancet Neurol. 2008;7:1056–66. https://doi.org/10.1016/S1474-4422(08)70240-0.
2. Miyamoto S, Yoshimoto T, Hashimoto N, Okada Y, Tsuji I, Tominaga T, Nakagawara J, Takahashi JC, Investigators JAMT. Effects of extracranial-intracranial bypass for patients with hemorrhagic moyamoya disease: results of the Japan adult Moyamoya trial. Stroke. 2014;45:1415–21. https://doi.org/10.1161/STROKEAHA.113.004386.

3. Fujimura M, Shimizu H, Inoue T, Mugikura S, Saito A, Tominaga T. Significance of focal cerebral hyperperfusion as a cause of transient neurologic deterioration after extracranial-intracranial bypass for moyamoya disease: comparative study with non-moyamoya patients using N-isopropyl-p-[(123)I]iodoamphetamine single-photon emission computed tomography. Neurosurgery. 2011;68:957–64. discussion 964-955. https://doi.org/10.1227/NEU.0b013e318208f1da.
4. Kim SH, Choi JU, Yang KH, Kim TG, Kim DS. Risk factors for postoperative ischemic complications in patients with moyamoya disease. J Neurosurg. 2005;103:433–8. https://doi.org/10.3171/ped.2005.103.5.0433.
5. Uchino H, Kuroda S, Hirata K, Shiga T, Houkin K, Tamaki N. Predictors and clinical features of postoperative hyperperfusion after surgical revascularization for moyamoya disease: a serial single photon emission CT/positron emission tomography study. Stroke. 2012;43:2610–6. https://doi.org/10.1161/STROKEAHA.112.654723.
6. Alexander JA, Sheppard S, Davis PC, Salverda P. Adult cerebrovascular disease: role of modified rapid fluid-attenuated inversion-recovery sequences. AJNR Am J Neuroradiol. 1996;17:1507–13.
7. Brant-Zawadzki M, Atkinson D, Detrick M, Bradley WG, Scidmore G. Fluid-attenuated inversion recovery (FLAIR) for assessment of cerebral infarction. Initial clinical experience in 50 patients. Stroke. 1996;27:1187–91. https://doi.org/10.1161/01.str.27.7.1187.
8. Kates R, Atkinson D, Brant-Zawadzki M. Fluid-attenuated inversion recovery (FLAIR): clinical prospectus of current and future applications. Topics in magnetic resonance imaging: TMRI. 1996;8:389–96.
9. Tourbah A, Deschamps R, Stievenart JL, Lopez A, Iba-Zizen MT, Lyon-Caen O, Cabanis EA. Magnetic resonance imaging using FLAIR pulse sequence in white matter diseases. J Neuroradiol. 1996;23:217–22.
10. Hamano E, Kataoka H, Morita N, Maruyama D, Satow T, Iihara K, Takahashi JC. Clinical implications of the cortical hyperintensity belt sign in fluid-attenuated inversion recovery images after bypass surgery for moyamoya disease. J Neurosurg. 2017;126:1–7. https://doi.org/10.3171/2015.10.JNS151022.
11. Horie N, Morikawa M, Morofuji Y, Hiu T, Izumo T, Hayashi K, Nagata I. De novo ivy sign indicates postoperative hyperperfusion in moyamoya disease. Stroke. 2014;45:1488–91. https://doi.org/10.1161/STROKEAHA.114.004755.
12. Takemoto Y, Kawano T, Ohmori Y, Kaku Y, Uekawa K, Amadatsu T, Hayashi K, Kitajima M, Mukasa A. Hemodynamic study about cortical hyperintensity belt sign after direct bypass surgery for moyamoya disease. J Clin Neurosci. 2020;74:124–9. https://doi.org/10.1016/j.jocn.2020.02.022.
13. Noguchi K, Ogawa T, Inugami A, Toyoshima H, Sugawara S, Hatazawa J, Fujita H, Shimosegawa E, Kanno I, Okudera T, et al. Acute subarachnoid hemorrhage: MR imaging with fluid-attenuated inversion recovery pulse sequences. Radiology. 1995;196:773–7. https://doi.org/10.1148/radiology.196.3.7644642.
14. Noguchi K, Seto H, Kamisaki Y, Tomizawa G, Toyoshima S, Watanabe N. Comparison of fluid-attenuated inversion-recovery MR imaging with CT in a simulated model of acute subarachnoid hemorrhage. AJNR Am J Neuroradiol. 2000;21:923–7.
15. Shiba M, Toma N, Tanioka S, Yasuda R, Sakaida H, Suzuki H. Significance of novel subcortical low intensity score on transient neurological events after revascularization surgery for moyamoya disease. Clin Neurol Neurosurg. 2018;167:70–5. https://doi.org/10.1016/j.clineuro.2018.02.019.
16. Kaku Y, Iihara K, Nakajima N, Kataoka H, Fukushima K, Iida H, Hashimoto N. The leptomeningeal ivy sign on fluid-attenuated inversion recovery images in moyamoya disease: positron emission tomography study. Cerebrovasc Dis. 2013;36:19–25. https://doi.org/10.1159/000351143.
17. Nam KW, Cho WS, Kwon HM, Kim JE, Lee YS, Park SW, Rhim JH, Son YJ. Ivy sign predicts ischemic stroke recurrence in adult Moyamoya patients without revascularization surgery. Cerebrovasc Dis. 2019;47:223–30. https://doi.org/10.1159/000500610.

18. Kawashima M, Noguchi T, Takase Y, Nakahara Y, Matsushima T. Decrease in leptomeningeal ivy sign on fluid-attenuated inversion recovery images after cerebral revascularization in patients with Moyamoya disease. AJNR Am J Neuroradiol. 2010;31:1713–8. https://doi.org/10.3174/ajnr.A2124.
19. Tanioka S, Shiba M, Umeda Y, Sano T, Maeda M, Suzuki H. A case of Moyamoya disease with a transient neurologic deterioration associated with subcortical low intensity on fluid-attenuated inversion recovery magnetic resonance images after bypass surgery. World Neurosurg. 2016;88:688 e617–21. https://doi.org/10.1016/j.wneu.2015.11.063.

Part V

Real World of Surgical Revascularization for Moyamoya Disease

Overview of Surgical Revascularization and Long-Term Outcome in Japan

18

Satoshi Kuroda

Abstract

Surgical revascularization is now accepted as an effective treatment to reduce the incidence of subsequent cerebrovascular events, including ischemic and hemorrhagic stroke, although precise analysis of long-term outcome after surgery is required. In this Part V "Real World of Surgical Revascularization for Moyamoya Disease," very skillful and experienced neurosurgeons around the world would discuss their surgical technique and long-term outcome in patients with moyamoya disease. It also includes special topics on perioperative complications, indirect bypass, combined bypass, and unique clinical features in infantile and elderly patients. In this chapter, I briefly overview surgical techniques for moyamoya disease and describe recent data on postoperative, long-term (>10 years) outcome in Japan.

Keywords

Moyamoya disease · Surgical revascularization · Indirect bypass · Direct bypass Long-term outcome

S. Kuroda (✉)
Department of Neurosurgery, Graduate School of Medicine and Pharmaceutical Science, University of Toyama, Toyama, Japan
e-mail: skuroda@med.u-toyama.ac.jp

S. Kuroda (ed.), *Moyamoya Disease: Current Knowledge and Future Perspectives*, https://doi.org/10.1007/978-981-33-6404-2_18

18.1 Introduction

Even now, there is no effective strategy to medically treat moyamoya disease itself. Medication with anticonvulsants and antiplatelets does not fundamentally solve the disease and is merely a symptomatic treatment, although the use of antiplatelets for moyamoya disease is still controversial [1, 2]. Only surgical revascularization is accepted effective treatment to resolve persistent cerebral ischemia and thus to erase or reduce ischemia-related events such as headache attacks, TIA, and ischemic stroke. These therapeutic benefits of surgical revascularization have been established in much earlier studies such as case series analysis, and thus it is accepted unnecessary to conduct randomized clinical trials (RCTs) again to verify the beneficial effects of surgical revascularization on the outcome in patients with ischemic-type moyamoya disease [3]. On the other hand, until the 1990s, the effect of surgical revascularization on adult patients with moyamoya disease suffering from hemorrhagic stroke was controversial. Japanese group (2014) conducted a randomized clinical trial in 2000 and finally reached a conclusion that direct or combined bypass procedure significantly reduced the incidence of rebleeding (*see Chap. 9*) [4, 5]. Based on these observations, surgical revascularization has established itself as an effective treatment to reduce the incidence of subsequent cerebrovascular events, including ischemic and hemorrhagic stroke. However, we should remind that surgical revascularization still carries a risk of about 5–10% of perioperative complications [6–13]. Furthermore, although surgical treatment is targeted at children and young adults, most of previously published studies have reported outcomes of around 3 to 5 years after surgery, with very limited reports of long-term postoperative outcomes over 10 years [3]. In the future, therefore, it is quite important to develop safer methods and strategies of surgical revascularization for moyamoya disease than ever before. Furthermore, it is essential to evaluate the prognosis of patients with moyamoya disease over a period of longer than 10 to 30 years.

Based on these considerations, I decided to focus on "Real World of Surgical Revascularization for Moyamoya Disease" in this Part V. Very skillful and experienced neurosurgeons around the world would discuss their surgical technique and long-term outcome in patients with moyamoya disease. This Part V. also includes special topics on perioperative complications, indirect bypass, combined bypass, and unique clinical features in infantile and elderly patients. In this chapter, I briefly overview surgical techniques for moyamoya disease and describe recent data on long-term (>10 years) outcome in Japan.

18.2 Surgical Procedures

The prevalence of moyamoya disease is not so high over the world, but surgical procedures very widely varied among neurosurgeons. Roughly speaking, surgical procedures can be classified into three categories; indirect bypass, direct bypass, and combined bypass [3]. I also recommend the readers to refer to an English-written review article on the history of the development of surgical revascularization for moyamoya disease by Matsushima [14].

18.2.1 Indirect Bypass Surgery

Indirect bypass procedures are based on the unexpected fact that gradual angiogenesis occurs between the vascularized donor tissues attached to the surface of the brain and the brain, starting to provide collateral blood flow to the operated hemispheres several months post-surgery [3]. Such spontaneous angiogenesis would be the phenomenon very specific for moyamoya disease, because indirect bypass does not function in patients with atherosclerotic intracranial carotid artery diseases [15]. Several pioneering works have contributed to the development of indirect bypass procedures; Henschen (1950) performed bilateral encephalo-myo-synangiosis (EMS) in patients with bilateral internal carotid artery occlusion that caused epilepsy and named it "Encephalo-Myo-Synagiose." Unfortunately, their paper does not describe whether angiogenesis occurred through EMS or not, but they did invent the term "encephalo-xxxxx-synangiosis," which is still in use today, and this is a significant achievement [16]. In 1964, Tsubokawa et al. performed a procedure in which a dural flap containing the meningeal artery was placed onto the surface of the brain in a child with moyamoya disease; 2 months later, cerebral angiography showed the formation of collateral vessels through the meningeal artery. They named this procedure "durapexia" [17]. Then, Karasawa et al. (1977) reported their experience of EMS in 10 cases of moyamoya disease. In their paper, they described "*Since in most of the cases the postoperative angiography revealed spontaneous transdural anastomoses between the drainage area of the middle cerebral and external carotid arteries, the temporal muscles were placed over the cortex where no host vessel for anastomosis was found, in an attempt to facilitate these spontaneous anastomoses.*" Therefore, it would not be an overstatement to say that the indirect bypass procedure is a product of their detailed reading of cerebral angiography, novel ideas, and deep insight (*see Chap. 24*) [18]. Subsequently, Matsushima et al. started to perform encephalo-duro-arterio-synangiosis (EDAS) in 1980 [19]. The donor tissues used for indirect bypass procedures include the dura mater, temporal muscle, pericranium, and galea aponeurotica. The arteries providing blood flow to each donor tissues are the middle meningeal artery (MMA), deep temporal artery (DTA), ophthalmic artery, and superficial temporal artery (STA), respectively. In addition to these, angiogenesis directly from the STA to the arterioles on the brain's surface occurs when the superficial temporal artery itself is attached to the brain surface (Fig. 18.1). In some cases, the omentum has been also used as a donor tissue to widely cover the brain surface, although an end-to-end anastomosis of the related arteries and veins is required to restore blood flow of the donor [20, 21]. A number of designations have been reported, depending on the donor tissue used (*see Chap. 24*).

The molecular mechanism of angiogenesis through indirect bypass in moyamoya disease remains unclear. However, an interesting finding has been reported very recently. Thus, Hayashi and colleagues (2020) created a mouse model of bilateral carotid artery stenosis and performed EMS on the right side. After EMS, the deposition of collagen occurred between the temporal muscle and neocortex, and CD31-positive vessels significantly increased in both tissues, leading to the improvement of cerebral blood flow on the EMS side, but not on the non-EMS side. Collagen is

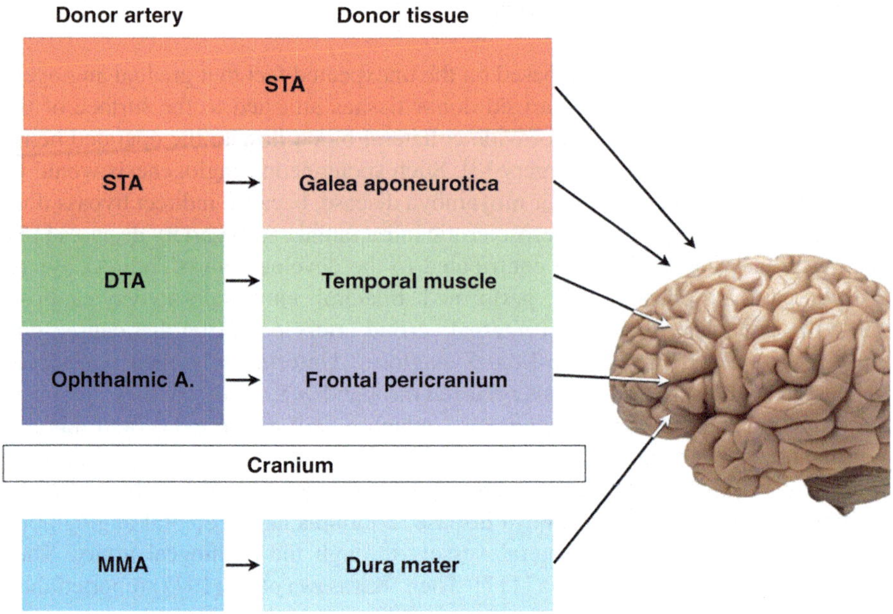

Fig. 18.1 A diagram showing the relationship between the donor tissues for indirect bypass surgery and their feeding arteries. *STA* superficial temporal artery, *DTA* deep temporal artery, *MMA* middle meningeal artery

known to highly support the proliferation, survival, and migration of endothelial cells and thus is essential for angiogenesis by forming the matrix framework for new vessel sprouting. Therefore, it is quite natural that the collagen deposition induced angiogenesis between the temporal muscle and ischemic neocortex [22]. More interestingly, systemic inactivation of the gene for platelet-derived growth factor receptor (PDGFR)–α almost canceled the angiogenesis between the temporal muscle and brain. These findings strongly suggest that the cascade of PDGF-α is playing a critical role in angiogenesis after indirect bypass surgery in moyamoya disease [22]. This speculation is supported by several reports. First, Kang et al. (2010) found that the plasma concentration of PDGF was higher in moyamoya patients than in the controls [23]. Second, Marushima et al. (2020) reported that EMS-induced angiogenesis was enhanced when the gene for PDGF-BB was transfected in a murine chronic ischemia model [24].

For experienced neurosurgeons, indirect bypass procedures are very simple and easy. Collateral channels can be established in almost 100% of pediatric patients. However, it should be reminded that indirect bypass only works in about 50–80% of adult patients with moyamoya disease [25, 26]. In contrast to direct bypass, indirect bypass requires several months to create adequate collateral blood circulation, and therefore carries a higher risk of ischemic complications such as ischemic stroke during perioperative period, especially immediately after surgery [27]. More importantly, the design of the surgery is quite important. Because indirect bypass basically creates collateral blood circulation around the area where donor tissue is attached through craniotomy, it is important to select the location and extent of craniotomy that can sufficiently cover the area with cerebral ischemia for indirect bypass surgery. In particular, moyamoya disease is characterized by a high degree of cerebral ischemia in the frontal region, so the surgical design of indirect bypass should be determined to cover a wide area in the frontal region. In fact, previous studies have shown that indirect or combined bypass surgery that widely covers the frontal region can improve intellectual prognosis in pediatric patients (*see Chap. 10*) [28].

During craniotomy, great care must be taken to avoid damaging the middle meningeal artery (MMA), which travels over the dura mater of convexity and then provides blood flow to the ACA territory via the anterior falcian artery, an important collateral route. However, it is known that in many cases the MMA runs within the sphenoid bone, as evidenced by the fact that fractures of the temporal bone frequently result in acute epidural hematoma. Therefore, normal fronto-temporal craniotomy can damage the MMA. Therefore, an alternative type of fronto-temporal craniotomy, which does not include the sphenoid bone, has been proposed in order to preserve the MMA. After craniotomy, the sphenoid bone can be removed separately using a rongeur or high-speed drill to preserve the MMA. Through this surgical procedure, it was shown that the anatomical relationship between the MMA and the sphenoid bone can be classified into bridge, monorail, and tunnel types, and that children have fewer tunnel types than adults [29, 30].

18.2.2 Direct Bypass Surgery

According to a review article by Prof. Yonekawa, superficial temporal artery to middle cerebral artery (STA-MCA) anastomosis was first performed in June 1972 by Prof. Yasargil in Switzerland and Prof. Reichman in the USA independently [31, 32]. Subsequently, this surgical procedure has been started by Kikuchi, Karasawa, and their colleagues in Japan since 1974 [33, 34].

Direct bypass procedures are almost always performed by STA-MCA anastomosis [3]. In contrast to indirect bypass procedures, direct bypass procedures have several advantages as follows: it can quickly improve cerebral hemodynamics after surgery, and thus can significantly lower the incidence of perioperative ischemic events, including transient ischemic attack (TIA) and ischemic stroke [27]. Furthermore, TIA and/or headache attack quickly decreases in the frequency or disappears after surgery. These clinical results of direct bypass are supported by immediate blood flow improvement just after surgery. In cases of carotid occlusion due to atherosclerosis, the cortical artery of the MCA is less difficult to anastomose because the diameter of the MCA cortical artery is around 1 mm and the arterial wall is of such a thickness that the arterial anastomosis is not very difficult to perform. However, in cases of moyamoya disease, the diameter of the cortical artery in the MCA is often as small as 0.3 to 0.8 mm, and more importantly the arterial wall is very thin, making the arterial anastomosis technique much more difficult. This phenomenon strongly suggests that the pathophysiology of moyamoya disease extends not only to the terminal portion of the internal carotid artery but also to the periphery of the MCA [35]. When the cortical arteries of the MCA are clamped and opened for anastomosis, the blood drains out of the arteries and the vessel becomes almost transparent, making it difficult to visualize the anastomosis site, even with a high-powered microscope. Until the 1980s, therefore, this surgical technique was quite challenging, but the procedure was greatly facilitated by a method pioneered by Kamiyama et al. in 1993 [36]. They succeeded to clearly visualize the ostium of an arteriotomy by staining it blue with methylrosaniline chloride (pyoctaninum blue). In addition, while a majority of neurosurgeons previously inserted a piece of white, transparent surgical glove underneath the cortical artery of the MCA for direct bypass, Kamiyama and colleagues started to place a green silicone sheet, a complementary color to the red, to dramatically increase the visibility of the anastomotic vessels [36]. Today, this technique is used worldwide, with minor differences, and has been applied to a variety of bypass procedures (Fig. 18.2).

The author usually prefers STA-MCA double anastomosis for anterior circulation, in which two branches of the STA are anastomosed to the frontal and temporal

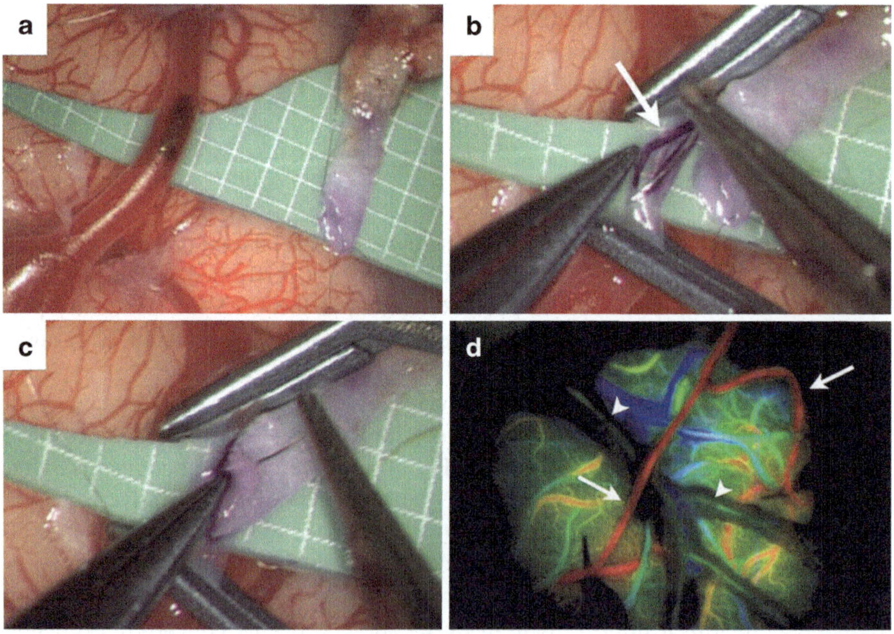

Fig. 18.2 Intraoperative photographs during STA-MCA anastomosis for pediatric patients with moyamoya disease. (**a-c**) Note that the sites of arteriotomy is stained blue with methylrosaniline chloride (pyoctaninum blue) to clearly visualize the anastomosis site (arrow). A green silicone sheet is also placed underneath the cortical artery of the MCA to dramatically increase the visibility of the anastomotic vessels. (**d**) Indocyanine green (ICG) videoangiography demonstrates a good patency of double STA-MCA anastomosis (arrows). Note that the main branches of the middle meningeal artery are also patent on ICG videoangiography (arrowheads)

branches of the MCA, respectively. This procedure would be reasonable when we aim to provide sufficient blood flow to both the frontal and temporal lobes. It is because moyamoya disease often involves a stenotic lesion in the proximal portion of the MCA, so that when the STA is anastomosed to the frontal branch of the MCA, the temporal lobe does not always receive adequate blood flow from the STA. Alternatively, STA-MCA single anastomosis is indicated in patients who have only one branch of the STA or MCA appropriate for direct bypass procedure. In such cases, the STA should be anastomosed to the frontal branch of the MCA, because cerebral ischemia is most dense in the frontal lobe in a majority of patients with moyamoya disease.

The procedures can flexibly be modified as STA-anterior cerebral artery (ACA) or STA-posterior cerebral artery (PCA) anastomosis according to patients' conditions such as dense ischemia in the territory of the ACA or PCA [37–40].

In addition, it should be reminded that direct bypass procedure would carry the risk for postoperative hyperperfusion, which sometime causes severe neurological sequelae and/or mortality unless appropriate managements are indicated. Precise information on postoperative hyperperfusion should be referred to Chap. 16.

18.2.3 Combined Bypass Surgery

Combined bypass procedure is a combination of direct and indirect bypass procedures performed simultaneously. Combined bypass procedure may also carry a risk for postoperative hyperperfusion, but has the advantage to immediately improve cerebral hemodynamics followed by further improvement of cerebral hemodynamics through indirect bypass-mediated angiogenesis. A reciprocal and synergistic relationship exists between the direct and indirect bypass in the development of collateral circulation after the combined bypass procedure [26, 41].

The formation of collateral blood vessels via indirect bypass is usually evaluated a few months after surgery. In the past, cerebral angiography was primarily used, but in recent years, MR angiography has proven to be useful. More recently, Uchino et al. (2019) quantitatively analyzed postoperative changes in STA and DTA diameter using 3-dimensional time-of-flight source images and found that the postoperative changes in their diameters are useful to predict the degree of development of collateral circulation through direct and indirect bypass procedures, respectively [42].

18.3 Long-Term Outcome in Japan

In 2019, 50 years have passed since this disease was first named as moyamoya disease in an English-written journal by Suzuki and Takaku in 1969 [43]. As mentioned above, STA-MCA anastomosis was performed soon afterwards in the early 1970s, followed by indirect bypass in the mid-1970s, so surgical revascularization for moyamoya disease is believed to have a history of nearly 50 years. However, as mentioned above, there are not so many reports of long-term results after surgical revascularization of moyamoya disease for more than 10 years, even in Japan where surgical treatment is considered the earliest to be started.

Karasawa et al. (1992) reported a long-term prognosis of a mean of 9.6 years (4.8 to 16 years) in 104 children who underwent STA-MCA anastomosis and/or EMS between 1974 and 1991. This case series analysis demonstrated that patients aged 7 years and older had better functional outcomes, and about 35% of patients aged 3 years or younger had poor intellectual outcomes, and there was a strong correlation between functional and intellectual outcomes [34]. Imaizumi et al. (1998) evaluated a long-term outcome in 25 pediatric patients who were treated medically or surgically. Of these, one patient developed TIA and successfully underwent STA-MCA anastomosis and EMS. This patient never experienced TIA after surgery, but died of hemorrhagic stroke about 12 years after surgery [44]. Recently, two Japanese groups from Tokyo and Kyoto have published long-term (>10 year) outcome in a significant number of pediatric patients after surgery. Mukawa et al. (2012) followed up 172 pediatric patients for a mean of 14.3 years after EDAS, one of indirect bypass procedures. They reported that the incidence of late cerebrovascular events occurred in 6 patients 8 or more years after EDAS. Of these, 3 patients developed ischemic stroke 13 to 22 years after EDAS. Other 3 patients experienced hemorrhagic stroke 8 to 21 years after EDAS, all of whom repeated hemorrhagic stroke later. As the results, the 10-year, 20-year, and 30-year cumulative incidences of late cerebrovascular events were 0.8%, 6.3%, and 10%, respectively (0.24% per year) [45]. On the other hand, Funaki et al. (2014) analyzed the incidence of late cerebrovascular events in 56 pediatric patients who underwent STA-MCA anastomosis and EMS between 1978 and 2003. A mean follow-up period was 18.1 years. They found that 4 patients (7.1%) developed late cerebrovascular events. As the results, the 10-year, 20-year, and 30-year cumulative incidences of late cerebrovascular events were 1.8%, 7.3%, and 13.1%, respectively (0.85% per year). Of the 4 patients, one developed ischemic stroke 2 years after surgery due to disruption of surgical collaterals in a traffic accident. More importantly, the remaining 3 patients developed hemorrhagic stroke 14 to 20 years after surgery, although the bypasses were still working at the time of hemorrhagic stroke [46]. These observations strongly suggest that a certain subgroup of pediatric patients may be at a risk for hemorrhagic stroke even 10 to 20 years after surgical revascularization. Therefore, I would like to emphasize that we should carefully follow up the moyamoya patients for longer than 10 to 20 years after surgery, even if their clinical condition is stable.

On the other hand, there are almost no reports that denote a long-term (>10 years) outcome in adult patients with moyamoya disease. As noted above, almost all investigators report only 5 to 6 years of follow-up results at best. Only Bao et al. (2018) reported a 12-year results after EDAS in 145 adult patients. They reported that 1-, 5-, and 10-year cumulative stroke rates were 2.1%, 6.8%, and 8.9%, respectively. According to their data, bilateral involvement and hypertension may be risk factors for ischemic stroke during follow-up periods [47].

Very recently, therefore, we conducted a long-term (>10 year) follow-up study of moyamoya disease after combined bypass surgery. In this study, we enrolled a total of 93 patients who underwent STA-MCA anastomosis and

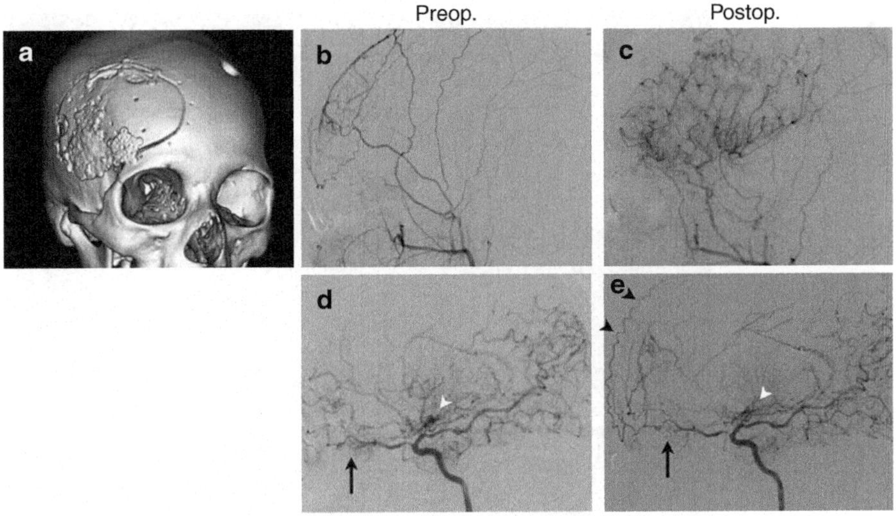

Fig. 18.3 Representative radiological findings in a 14-year-old girl before and after STA-MCA anastomosis and EDMAPS. (**a**) Postoperative 3D skull CT demonstrates a large fronto-temporal craniotomy extending to the frontal area. (**b**) Preoperative external carotid angiography shows spontaneous collateral routes to the ACA via the middle meningeal artery. (**c**) Postoperative external carotid angiography demonstrates an extensive development of surgical collaterals via the STA, DTA, and MMA. (**d**) Preoperative internal carotid angiography reveals a marked development of basal moyamoya (white arrowhead) and ethmoidal moyamoya (arrow). (**e**) Postoperative internal carotid angiography demonstrates the diminishment of basal moyamoya (white arrowhead) and ethmoidal moyamoya (arrow). Note an extensive development of the branches arising from the ophthalmic artery within the frontal pericranium (arrowheads)

encephalo-duro-myo-arterio-pericranial synangiosis (EDMAPS) between 1998 and 2014, and were followed up for 5 to 20 years (mean, 10.5 years). This study included 35 pediatric and 58 adult patients. In this case series, we performed STA-MCA anastomosis and EDMAPS, in which the frontal pericranium was used as a novel donor tissue in addition to traditional donor tissues such as the dura mater, temporal muscle, and STA. We used the frontal pericranium to cover a wider area of the frontal lobe, enabling us to perform indirect bypass in a single operation more safely and extensively than either of the conventional procedures (Fig. 18.3a). STA-MCA anastomosis and EDMAPS induce rich collateral circulations through the external carotid arteries, including the STA, DTA, and MMA (Fig. 18.3b, c). In addition, the ophthalmic artery starts to provide collateral blood flow through the frontal pericranium (Fig. 18.3d, e). As the results, abnormal collateral channels such as basal moyamoya and ethmoidal moyamoya diminish or disappear after surgery (Fig. 18.3d, e). The findings on cerebral blood flow (CBF) measurement also correlate very well with those on cerebral angiography. For example, the follow-up SPECT demonstrates that CBF and its reactivity to acetazolamide significantly improve in the ACA territory as well as the MCA territory 3 to 4 months after surgery (Fig. 18.4). Subsequently, only one adult with hemorrhagic

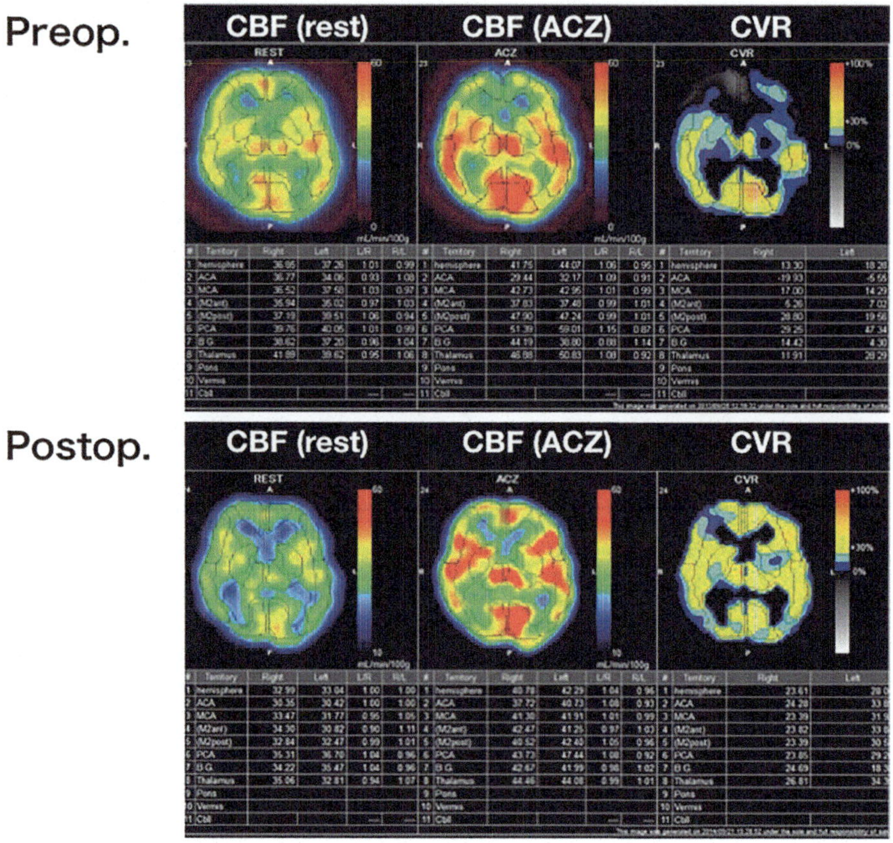

Fig. 18.4 Representative SPECT findings in a 28-years-old female before and after STA-MCA anastomosis and EDMAPS. Before surgery, CBF before and after an intravenous injection of 10 mg/kg acetazolamide (ACZ) was reduced in the frontal lobe on both sides. Cerebrovascular reactivity to ACZ was impaired in the same area. These abnormalities completely resolved after surgery in both the MCA and ACA territories

onset recurred hemorrhagic stroke 9.5 years after surgery. Other 92 patients were free from late cerebrovascular events. Therefore, annual risk of late cerebrovascular events was 0.1% per patient-year. The results are better for both children and adults than the previous reports mentioned above. We believe this is because the use of the frontal pericranium allows for a wider coverage of the frontal lobe and improves cerebral hemodynamics not only in the MCA territory but also in the ACA territory. However, we believe that another 20 to 30 years of postoperative follow-up will be warranted to further evaluate the long-term therapeutic effect of this surgical procedure [12]. On the other hand, this study led us to another conclusion. Thus, repeated MR angiography every 6 to 12 months during follow-up periods revealed that disease progression occurred in 19 hemispheres of 15 patients in the contralateral internal carotid artery and posterior cerebral artery.

Such disease progression occurred in both children and adults. The timing of disease progression was found to be very late, ranging from 6 months to 15 years after surgery. In some cases, TIAs developed and required repeat bypass surgery [40]. Therefore, it is our responsibility to carefully monitor patients with moyamoya disease for as long as 10 to 20 years after surgery to prevent late cerebrovascular events [12].

Acknowledgments This work was partly supported by a grant from the Research Committee on Moyamoya Disease, the Japanese Ministry of Health, Labour and Welfare.

References

1. Kraemer M, Berlit P, Diesner F, Khan N. What is the expert's option on antiplatelet therapy in moyamoya disease? Results of a worldwide survey. European journal of neurology: the official journal of the European Federation of Neurological Societies. 2012;19:163–7.
2. Yamada S, Oki K, Itoh Y, Kuroda S, Houkin K, Tominaga T, Miyamoto S, Hashimoto N, Suzuki N, Research Committee on Spontaneous Occlusion of Circle of W. Effects of surgery and antiplatelet therapy in ten-year follow-up from the registry study of research committee on Moyamoya disease in Japan. J Stroke Cerebrovasc Dis. 2016;25:340–9.
3. Kuroda S, Houkin K. Moyamoya disease: current concepts and future perspectives. Lancet Neurol. 2008;7:1056–66.
4. Miyamoto S, Yoshimoto T, Hashimoto N, Okada Y, Tsuji I, Tominaga T, Nakagawara J, Takahashi JC, Investigators JT. Effects of extracranial-intracranial bypass for patients with hemorrhagic moyamoya disease: results of the Japan adult moyamoya trial. Stroke. 2014;45:1415–21.
5. Takahashi JC, Funaki T, Houkin K, Inoue T, Ogasawara K, Nakagawara J, Kuroda S, Yamada K, Miyamoto S, Investigators JAMT. Significance of the hemorrhagic site for recurrent bleeding: Prespecified analysis in the Japan adult Moyamoya trial. Stroke. 2016;47:37–43.
6. Funaki T, Takahashi JC, Takagi Y, Kikuchi T, Yoshida K, Mitsuhara T, Kataoka H, Okada T, Fushimi Y, Miyamoto S. Unstable moyamoya disease: clinical features and impact on perioperative ischemic complications. J Neurosurg. 2015;122:400–7.
7. Houkin K, Ishikawa T, Yoshimoto T, Abe H. Direct and indirect revascularization for moyamoya disease surgical techniques and peri-operative complications. Clin Neurol Neurosurg. 1997;99(Suppl 2):S142–5.
8. Iwama T, Hashimoto N, Tsukahara T, Murai B. Peri-operative complications in adult moyamoya disease. Acta Neurochir. 1995;132:26–31.
9. Kazumata K, Ito M, Tokairin K, Ito Y, Houkin K, Nakayama N, Kuroda S, Ishikawa T, Kamiyama H. The frequency of postoperative stroke in moyamoya disease following combined revascularization: a single-university series and systematic review. J Neurosurg. 2014;121:432–40.
10. Kim SH, Choi JU, Yang KH, Kim TG, Kim DS. Risk factors for postoperative ischemic complications in patients with moyamoya disease. J Neurosurg. 2005;103:433–8.
11. Kuroda S, Houkin K, Ishikawa T, Nakayama N, Iwasaki Y. Novel bypass surgery for moyamoya disease using pericranial flap: its impacts on cerebral hemodynamics and long-term outcome. Neurosurgery. 2010;66:1093–101. discussion 1101
12. Kuroda S, Nakayama N, Yamamoto S, Kashiwazaki D, Uchino H, Saito H, Hori E, Akioka N, Kuwayama N, Houkin K. Late (5-20 years) outcomes after STA-MCA anastomosis and encephalo-duro-myo-arterio-pericranial synangiosis in patients with moyamoya disease. J Neurosurg. 2020:1–8.
13. Sato K, Shirane R, Yoshimoto T. Perioperative factors related to the development of ischemic complications in patients with moyamoya disease. Childs Nerv Syst. 1997;13:68–72.

14. Matsushima T, Inoue K, Kawashima M, Inoue T. History of the development of surgical treatments for moyamoya disease. Neurol Med Chir (Tokyo). 2012;52:278–86.
15. Komotar RJ, Starke RM, Otten ML, Merkow MB, Garrett MC, Marshall RS, Elkind MS, Connolly ES. The role of indirect extracranial-intracranial bypass in the treatment of symptomatic intracranial atheroocclusive disease. J Neurosurg. 2009;110:896–904.
16. Henschen C. Surgical revascularization of cerebral injury of circulatory origin by means of stratification of pedunculated muscle flaps. Langenbecks Arch Klin Chir Ver Dtsch Z Chir. 1950;264:392–401.
17. Tsubokawa T, Kikuchi M, Asano S, Ito H, Urabe M. Surgical treatment for intracranial thrombosis - case report of "durapexia". Neurol Med Chir (Tokyo). 1964;6:48–9.
18. Karasawa J, Kikuchi H, Furuse S, Sakaki T, Yoshida Y. A surgical treatment of "moyamoya" disease "encephalo-myo synangiosis". Neurol Med Chir (Tokyo). 1977;17:29–37.
19. Matsushima Y, Fukai N, Tanaka K, Tsuruoka S, Inaba Y, Aoyagi M, Ohno K. A new surgical treatment of moyamoya disease in children: a preliminary report. Surg Neurol. 1981;15:313–20.
20. Karasawa J, Kikuchi H, Kawamura J, Sakai T. Intracranial transplantation of the omentum for cerebrovascular moyamoya disease: a two-year follow-up study. Surg Neurol. 1980;14:444–9.
21. Yoshioka N, Tominaga S, Suzuki Y, Yamazato K, Hirano S, Nonaka K, Inui T, Matuoka N. Cerebral revascularization using omentum and muscle free flap for ischemic cerebrovascular disease. Surg Neurol. 1998;49:58–65. discussion 65-56
22. Hayashi T, Yamamoto S, Hamashima T, Mori H, Sasahara M, Kuroda S. Critical role of platelet-derived growth factor-alpha in angiogenesis after indirect bypass in a murine moyamoya disease model. J Neurosurg. 2020:1–9.
23. Kang HS, Kim JH, Phi JH, Kim YY, Kim JE, Wang KC, Cho BK, Kim SK. Plasma matrix metalloproteinases, cytokines and angiogenic factors in moyamoya disease. J Neurol Neurosurg Psychiatry. 2010;81:673–8.
24. Marushima A, Nieminen M, Kremenetskaia I, Gianni-Barrera R, Woitzik J, von Degenfeld G, Banfi A, Vajkoczy P, Hecht N. Balanced single-vector co-delivery of VEGF/PDGF-BB improves functional collateralization in chronic cerebral ischemia. J Cereb Blood Flow Metab. 2020;40:404–19.
25. Mizoi K, Kayama T, Yoshimoto T, Nagamine Y. Indirect revascularization for moyamoya disease: is there a beneficial effect for adult patients? Surg Neurol. 1996;45:541–8. discussion 548–549
26. Uchino H, Kim JH, Fujima N, Kazumata K, Ito M, Nakayama N, Kuroda S, Houkin K. Synergistic interactions between direct and indirect bypasses in combined procedures: the significance of indirect bypasses in Moyamoya disease. Neurosurgery. 2017;80:201–9.
27. Ishikawa T, Houkin K, Kamiyama H, Abe H. Effects of surgical revascularization on outcome of patients with pediatric moyamoya disease. Stroke. 1997;28:1170–3.
28. Kuroda S, Houkin K, Ishikawa T, Nakayama N, Ikeda J, Ishii N, Kamiyama H, Iwasaki Y. Determinants of intellectual outcome after surgical revascularization in pediatric moyamoya disease: a multivariate analysis. Childs Nerv Syst. 2004;20:302–8.
29. Hori S, Kashiwazaki D, Akioka N, Hayashi T, Hori E, Umemura K, Horie Y, Kuroda S. Surgical anatomy and preservation of the middle meningeal artery during bypass surgery for moyamoya disease. Acta Neurochir. 2015;157:29–36.
30. Tanabe N, Yamamoto S, Kashiwazaki D, Akioka N, Kuwayama N, Noguchi K, Kuroda S. Indocyanine green visualization of middle meningeal artery before craniotomy during surgical revascularization for moyamoya disease. Acta Neurochir. 2017;159:567–75.
31. Krayenbuhl HA. The Moyamoya syndrome and the neurosurgeon. Surg Neurol. 1975;4:353–60.
32. Yonekawa Y. Operative neurosurgery: personal view and historical backgrounds (9) Moyamoya Angiopathy (MMA): past history and status Presens. No Shinkei Geka. 2012;40:67–87.
33. Karasawa J, Kikuchi H, Furuse S, Kawamura J, Sakaki T. Treatment of moyamoya disease with STA-MCA anastomosis. J Neurosurg. 1978;49:679–88.

34. Karasawa J, Touho H, Ohnishi H, Miyamoto S, Kikuchi H. Long-term follow-up study after extracranial-intracranial bypass surgery for anterior circulation ischemia in childhood moyamoya disease. J Neurosurg. 1992;77:84–9.
35. Takagi Y, Hermanto Y, Takahashi JC, Funaki T, Kikuchi T, Mineharu Y, Yoshida K, Miyamoto S. Histopathological characteristics of distal middle cerebral artery in adult and pediatric patients with Moyamoya disease. Neurol Med Chir (Tokyo). 2016;56:345–9.
36. Kamiyama H, Takahashi A, Houkin K, Mabuchi S, Abe H. Visualization of the ostium of an arteriotomy in bypass surgery. Neurosurgery. 1993;33:1109–10.
37. Hayashi T, Shirane R, Tominaga T. Additional surgery for postoperative ischemic symptoms in patients with moyamoya disease: the effectiveness of occipital artery-posterior cerebral artery bypass with an indirect procedure: technical case report. Neurosurgery. 2009;64:E195–6. discussion E196
38. Iwama T, Hashimoto N, Miyake H, Yonekawa Y. Direct revascularization to the anterior cerebral artery territory in patients with moyamoya disease: report of five cases. Neurosurgery. 1998;42:1157–61. discussion 1161–1152
39. Teo M, Johnson J, Steinberg GK. Strategies for and outcome of repeat revascularization surgery for Moyamoya disease: an American institutional series. Neurosurgery. 2017;81:852–9.
40. Uchino H, Kashiwazaki D, Akioka N, Koh M, Kuwayama N, Houkin K, Kuroda S. Strategy and effect of repeat bypass surgery for anterior/posterior circulation in refractory moyamoya disease. J Neurosurg. 2019:1–11.
41. Amin-Hanjani S, Singh A, Rifai H, Thulborn KR, Alaraj A, Aletich V, Charbel FT. Combined direct and indirect bypass for moyamoya: quantitative assessment of direct bypass flow over time. Neurosurgery. 2013;73:962–7. discussion 967–968
42. Uchino H, Yamamoto S, Kashiwazaki D, Akioka N, Kuwayama N, Noguchi K, Kuroda S. Using postoperative remodeling of donor arteries on MR angiography to predict the development of surgical collaterals in moyamoya disease. J Neurosurg. 2019:1–9.
43. Suzuki J, Takaku A. Cerebrovascular "moyamoya" disease. Disease showing abnormal net-like vessels in base of brain. Arch Neurol. 1969;20:288–99.
44. Imaizumi T, Hayashi K, Saito K, Osawa M, Fukuyama Y. Long-term outcomes of pediatric moyamoya disease monitored to adulthood. Pediatr Neurol. 1998;18:321–5.
45. Mukawa M, Nariai T, Matsushima Y, Tanaka Y, Inaji M, Maehara T, Aoyagi M, Ohno K. Long-term follow-up of surgically treated juvenile patients with Moyamoya disease. J Neurosurg Pediatr. 2012;10:451–6.
46. Funaki T, Takahashi JC, Takagi Y, Yoshida K, Araki Y, Kikuchi T, Kataoka H, Iihara K, Sano N, Miyamoto S. Incidence of late cerebrovascular events after direct bypass among children with moyamoya disease: a descriptive longitudinal study at a single center. Acta Neurochir. 2014;156:551–9. discussion 559
47. Bao XY, Zhang Y, Wang QN, Zhang Q, Wang H, Zhang ZS, Li DS, Duan L. Long-term outcomes after Encephaloduroarteriosynangiosis in adult patients with Moyamoya disease presenting with ischemia. World Neurosurg. 2018;115:e482–9.

Perioperative Complications

19

Ken Kazumata and Kiyohiro Houkin

Abstract

Although revascularization surgery in patients with moyamoya disease improves cerebral hemodynamics and symptoms, its benefits are reduced by perioperative complications through either transient or permanent neurological deficits. Apart from hyperperfusion syndrome, perioperative complications associated with revascularization surgery have been described in the literature and our clinical experience. Typical perioperative complications include ischemic stroke caused by hemodynamic insufficiency, which characteristically occurs in the advanced stages of moyamoya disease. Moreover, the progression of the main cerebral artery occlusion induces cerebral ischemia far from the surgery site. Intracranial hemorrhage associated with postoperative hyperperfusion is the most severe adverse effect after direct anastomosis. Other known and critical postoperative complications include skin necrosis, anastomotic site aneurysm, and arteriovenous shunt formation. Understanding the various complications and their risk factors could contribute toward lowering the perioperative complication rate in revascularization surgery, as well as improving the long-term outcomes.

Keywords

Moyamoya disease · Revascularization · Complications · Cerebral infarction
Intracranial hemorrhage · Skin trouble

K. Kazumata (✉) · K. Houkin
Department of Neurosurgery, Hokkaido University Graduate School of Medicine, Sapporo, Japan
e-mail: kazumata@med.hokudai.ac.jp; houkin@med.hokudai.ac.jp

S. Kuroda (ed.), *Moyamoya Disease: Current Knowledge and Future Perspectives*, https://doi.org/10.1007/978-981-33-6404-2_19

19.1 Background

Moyamoya disease is a progressive steno-occlusive cerebrovascular disease that is characterized by collateral vascular networks that resemble “a puff of smoke” (moyamoya vessels) at the brain base [1, 2]. Various revascularization procedures can improve cerebral hemodynamics and decrease the ischemic stroke risk. However, hemodynamic compromises and fragile collateral arteries increase the risk of postoperative neurological morbidity. Furthermore, revascularization-specific surgical procedures for moyamoya disease are associated with rare but critical complications. It is important to understand the various perioperative complications and the underlying mechanisms in order to improve patient management and maximize the benefit of revascularization surgery in stroke prevention.

19.2 Frequency and Pathophysiology of Perioperative Complications

19.2.1 Classification

Perioperative complications result from a combination of surgical procedures and hemodynamic insufficiency, as well as the fragility of collateral arteries at the brain base. Based on the main underlying mechanisms, complications were characterized as disease- or procedure-related complications. Typical disease-related complications are perioperative ischemic/hemorrhagic stroke, while typical procedure-related complications include skin trouble, hyperperfusion, graft spasm/occlusion, and postoperative intracranial hematoma.

19.3 Perioperative Stroke

Perioperative stroke is generally indicative of either infarction or intracranial hemorrhage (ICH), intraventricular hemorrhage, and subarachnoid hemorrhage, which develop intraoperatively or within 4 postoperative weeks. Hyperperfusion is mostly observed in adult moyamoya disease and can cause intracerebral hemorrhage or seizures. Hyperperfusion diagnosis largely depends on the definition and frequency of radiological studies.

19.3.1 Ischemic Complications

In anesthetic management, intraoperative hypocapnia induces a critical decrease in cerebral blood flow (CBF). Moreover, crying is known to induce hyperventilation and stroke during the perioperative period in children [3, 4]. Furthermore, hemodynamic compromise is aggravated by blood loss, decreased circulating volume, and low blood pressure [5, 6].

Previous study reported angiographic outcome of direct/combined bypass as excellent in 57.5% (95% CI; 13.2–100%), good in 35.8% (95% CI; 12.5–70.3%), and poor in 6.7% (95%CI; 0–17.7%), respectively [7]. In indirect bypass, angiographic outcome was excellent in 37.9% (95% CI; 16.4–59.4%), good in 38.0% (95% CI; 23.5–50.8%), and poor in 24.1% (95%CI; 5.8–42.8%). Complication rate was reported as 5.4% (ischemic; 4.1%, hemorrhagic 1.3%) in combined direct/indirect surgery, whereas it was 5.5% (ischemic 5.2%, hemorrhagic; 0.27%) in indirect surgery. In a single university study, the reported postoperative stroke frequency is 4.7% per surgery (95% confidence interval [CI], 2.5–7.0) in direct/combined bypass [7]. Compared with indirect procedures, surgery involving direct anastomosis is technically demanding. However, performing direct anastomosis in both pediatric and adult patients may not increase ischemic complications. In adult patients, there was no significant difference in postoperative stroke between direct/combined bypass (7.6%) and indirect bypass (5.1%). Furthermore, in pediatric patients, perioperative stroke was significantly more frequent in indirect bypass (6.0%) than in direct/combined bypass (2.5%) (odds ratio [OR], 2.36; 95% CI, 1.48–3.76). Additionally, ischemic complications in indirect surgery have been reported in pediatric patients (7.1%) [8]. In combined direct/indirect surgery, postoperative stroke was more frequent (8.5%) in adults than in pediatric patients (1.1%) (OR, 8.29; 95% CI, 1.87–36.79) [7]. However, there is a need for special caution in children aged under 3 years and in surgery within 6 weeks of the most recent stroke [8].

Postoperative cerebral infarction can occur remotely to craniotomy and in the contralateral hemisphere [9, 10]. Progressive occlusion in the main cerebral arteries following revascularization surgery could cause remote cerebral infarction [5, 11]. Since collateral vessel development (i.e., moyamoya vessels) is generally unremarkable in adults and moyamoya syndrome, the acute progression of main cerebral artery occlusion could induce severe consequences [12]. Specifically, in a combined direct/indirect procedure, acute occlusive changes in major cerebral arteries have been reported in approximately half of all postoperative ischemic strokes [7]. Out of 358 procedures, rapid progression (<1 postoperative month) has been observed in the anterior cerebral artery ($n = 3$), middle cerebral artery ($n = 1$), and posterior cerebral artery ($n = 2$)(Fig. 19.1 a-c) [7]. TIA for several postoperative months could be the underlying thromboembolic mechanism when radiological examination reveals the normalization of regional CBF.

Risk factors for ischemic stroke include anemia, preoperative frequent TIA, history of minor completed stroke, PCA involvement, and diabetes [6, 13, 14]. Fatal stroke can occur during the postoperative period [9]. A history of cerebral infarction is considered a risk factor for adverse outcomes. Furthermore, spontaneous/iatrogenic intracranial hemorrhage can increase intracranial pressure at a critical level, which causes severe low perfusion in the cerebral tissue and subsequently fatal stroke.

Moreover, ischemic stroke can occur during diagnostic procedures. The acetazolamide test for determining the perfusion reserve could result in critical adverse effects. In patients with severe hemodynamic compromise, the acetazolamide test

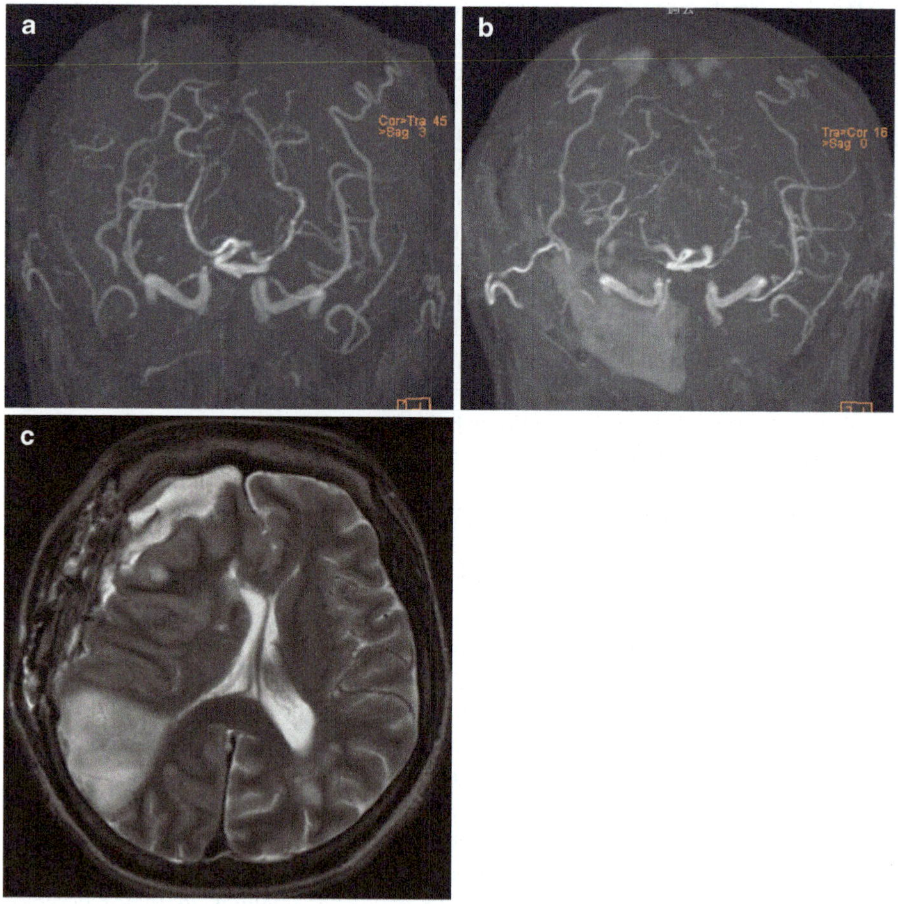

Fig. 19.1 Postoperative ischemic stroke in a 31-year-old patient with moyamoya syndrome after combined direct/indirect anastomosis. The bilateral posterior cerebral artery became diminutive after right revascularization surgery (**a**; preoperative MRA, **b**; postoperative MRA). Cerebral infarction appeared in the right temporo-occipital region (**c**)

further reduces CBF in the affected area (steal phenomenon). Therefore, especially in pediatric patients, this test should be avoided when there is a significant reduction in the resting-state CBF.

19.4 Hemorrhagic Complications

The frequency of postoperative ICH is 1.7–3.0% in revascularization surgery involving direct anastomosis [7, 9, 15]. Previous studies have reported postoperative hemorrhage at 4 hours and 10 days postoperatively [9]. The most frequent ICH onset timing was reported to be within 7 days or within 24 hours postoperatively [15, 16]. Hemorrhage can either occur at the subcortical lesion beneath the anastomosed cortex or as a subarachnoid hemorrhage. A previous study reported that half of the postoperative hemorrhage cases required hematoma evacuation. Untreated cerebral aneurysms can bleed during the postoperative acute phase. Moreover, ICH can occur far from the surgical site [15, 17]. Remote cerebral hemorrhage could involve postoperative hyperperfusion beyond the revascularization area, which is remarkable both in the medial frontal lobe and caudate head [18].

There is an association of postoperative ICH with older age [15]. Furthermore, hemorrhagic presentation at onset and increased blood pressure from the pre- to the postoperative stage are significantly associated with postoperative ICH [15].

19.4.1 Postoperative Hyperperfusion

Hyperperfusion is a frequent complication mostly observed in adult moyamoya disease that can cause intracerebral hemorrhage or seizures. Recent studies have reported frequent postoperative hyperperfusion [19, 20]. Details regarding hyperperfusion syndrome have been described in part IV, Chap. 16.

19.5 Procedure-Related Complications

Revascularization surgery involves the several steps of the indirect procedure (inverting the dura matter, suturing the temporalis muscle to the dura, and placing the pericranial flap), as well as harvesting of the scalp arteries. Skin necrosis, temporal muscle swelling, and subdural hematoma are the three most critical procedure-related complications.

(a) Subdural hematoma

An acute subdural hematoma is the most critical complication after direct/combined and indirect surgery. In adults, brain atrophy and the preoperative administration of antiplatelet medication may increase the subdural hematoma risk. Previous studies have reported chronic subdural hematoma [21]; however, it is a rather rare complication of revascularization for moyamoya disease.

(b) Temporal muscle swelling

Temporal muscle swelling causes brain compression [22, 23]. Increased intracranial pressure resulting from the inserted extracranial tissue can cause headache and ischemic brain injury (Fig. 19.2a–d). Temporal muscle swelling is observed when the drainage vein is sacrificed during extracranial work. Moreover, bleeding from the muscle undersurface is critical due to acute subdural hematoma.

(c) Wound break down due to skin necrosis

Wound complications have been reported in 2%, 17.6%, and 21.4% of cases of revascularization surgery [17, 24]. They are more common when the superficial

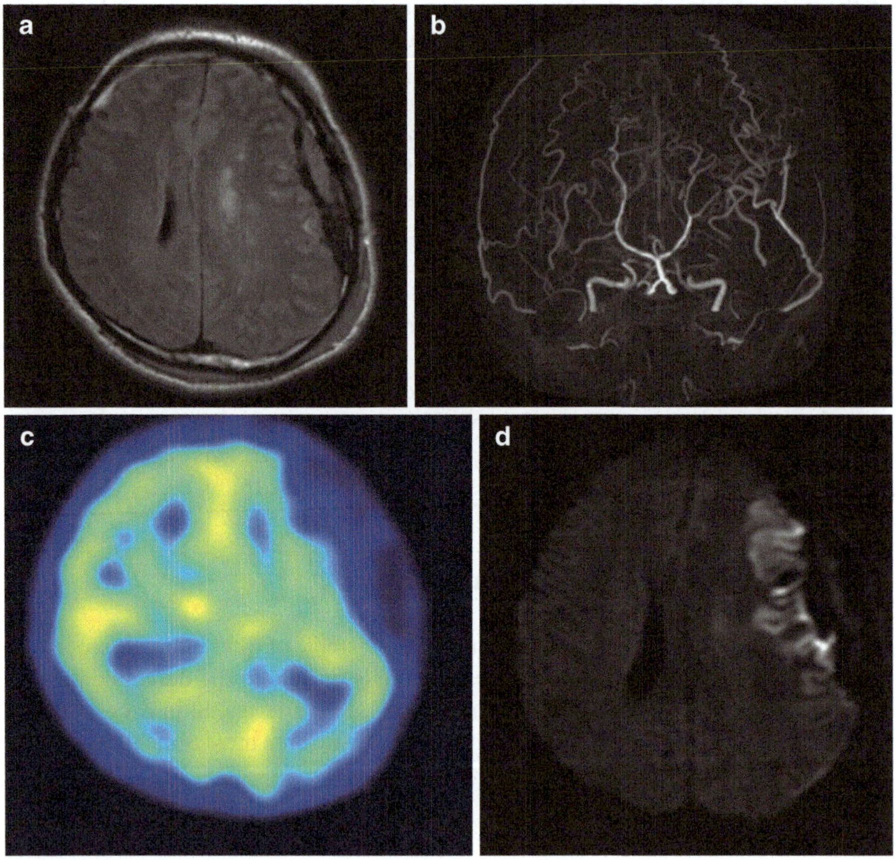

Fig. 19.2 Postoperative MRI shows temporal muscle swelling in the left frontal region (**a**). Postoperative magnetic resonance angiography revealed patency of the left superficial temporal artery—middle cerebral artery bypass (**b**). Moderate reduction of the regional cerebral blood flow was observed on 123I- N-isopropyl-p-[123I]iodoamphetamine/single-photon emission computed tomography (**c**). Ischemic brain damage was observed along with cortical laminar on diffusion-weighted imaging (**d**)

temporal artery (STA) is peripherally harvested and/or both the frontal and parietal branches of the STA are harvested [24]. Diabetes may increase the risk of skin trouble [24]. Major skin complications have been reported in 21.4% of 98 revascularization surgeries [24]; however, the risk of skin trouble largely depends on the skin incision design and the harvesting procedures. Mild wound ulceration commonly occurs at the hemicoronal incision corner (Fig. 19.3). Mild wound ulceration can be treated using hydroxyproline, antibiotic ointment, and prostaglandin E1 ointment. Severe skin erosion can progress to osteomyelitis in the bone flap. Treatment for severe skin erosion and infection requires bone flap removal and necrotic skin tissue debridement. Once the wound infection subsides, tissue expansion in the midline area can be performed for scalp flap advancement. Cranioplasty using an artificial bone flap was performed after 3–6 months later with scalp defect reconstruction.

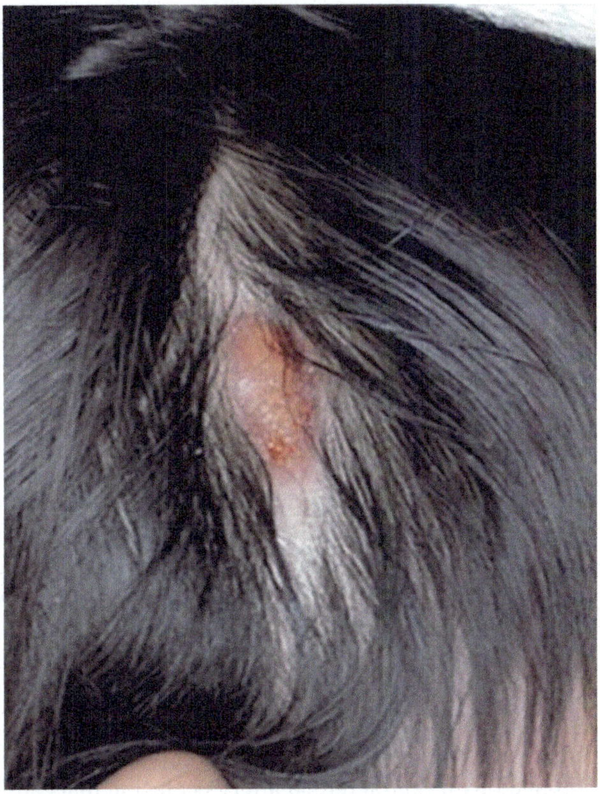

Fig. 19.3 Skin necrosis at the corner of the scalp incision

The cranial bone is protected from tissue layers, including the skin, subcutaneous tissue, galea, temporal muscle, and pericranium. Since revascularization surgery uses part of the scalp tissue and muscle, the skin layer becomes prone to being atrophic. The edge of the titanium fixation plate can penetrate the skin, which requires it to be removed.

(d) Acute bypass spasm/occlusion

During the direct bypass of the STA-middle cerebral artery (MCA) anastomosis, thrombosis at the anastomosis site is more frequent than that in bypass performed for main cerebral artery occlusion due to arteriosclerosis [25]. The occlusion could be associated with increased flow velocity and endothelial damage. Katsuta et al. reported the phenomenon of the reversible occlusion of the STA-MCA bypass during mouth opening in 5 out of 15 procedures and termed it as a *big bite ischemic phenomenon* [26]. During mouth opening, the stretched temporalis muscle may compress the STA against the bone window edge.

(e) Acute brain swelling

Acute brain swelling has been reported after dural opening. Acute brain swelling is associated with hypercapnia; child surgery; small craniotomy; and prone position, including revascularization in the posterior cerebral artery territory. Upon the occurrence of acute brain swelling, measures for reducing intracranial pressure, including normalizing PaCO2, dripping mannitol, and elevating head position should be promptly taken.

(f) Aneurysm at the anastomosis site

Hemodynamic stress may cause postoperative aneurysmal formation after several decades [27, 28]. The reported bleeding timing from an anastomotic aneurysm was 6, 8, 14, 20, and 27 postoperative years [27–30].

(g) Other rare complications

Previous studies have reported other rare complications. De novo formation of arteriovenous malformation has been reported after moyamoya disease diagnosis [31, 32]. Arteriovenous fistula (AVF) has been reported at the STA-MCA anastomosis site [33]. Dural and pial AVF within the prior operative field has been reported in routine 8-month postoperative angiography. Here, AVF spontaneously disappeared without treatment upon a 2-year surveillance cerebral angiogram [34]. Moreover, severe cerebral vasospasm and delayed cerebral infarction have been reported in a 7-year-old girl after intraventricular hemorrhage [35]. A patient with moyamoya disease at 30 years old, after successful pial synangiosis when she was 6 years old, presented with central retinal artery occlusion that caused unilateral blindness [36].

19.6 Perioperative Management to Prevent Complications

Hemodynamic assessment is performed to evaluate the perioperative risk through nuclear medicine examinations and noninvasive MR. [^{123}I]- p-iodoamphetamine/single-photon emission computed tomography (SPECT) or ^{15}O-gas positron emission tomography (PET) are often preferred. Cerebrovascular insufficiency can be evaluated by administering 10 mg/kg acetazolamide on SPECT or by measuring the oxygen-extracting fraction/cerebral blood volume on PET. For critical hemodynamic insufficiency, 500–1000 ml/day intravenous drip for hydration is preoperatively administered (1 to 3 preoperative days). After general anesthesia induction, $PaCO_2$ was strictly maintained above 35–40 mmHg throughout the surgery. Subsequently, both colloids and crystalloids (25% albumin and/or 6% hydroxyethyl starch) were administered for 3 postoperative days. In addition to volume supplementation, fluid administration (1000 ml/day in pediatric patients and 1500 mL/day in adult patients) is continued for 7 postoperative days. Postoperative CBF measurements are performed to detect hyperperfusion on SPECT. Colloid and crystalloid administration is discontinued in the case of abnormal focal increases in the CBF [19]. Systolic blood pressure is maintained within 120–130 mmHg. To avoid temporal muscle bleeding, antiplatelet agents are discontinued between 7 preoperative days and 3 postoperative days. It remains unclear whether preoperative antiplatelet therapy reduces the postoperative stroke rate [16, 37].

19.7 Discussion

Revascularization surgery has an approximate complication rate of 5% [7, 9]. Poor cerebrovascular reserve and ischemic attack episodes are hallmark signs and symptoms for surgical indication. However, recent and frequent ischemic attacks increase the risk of postoperative ischemic complications [9, 38]. In children, surgery should be delayed for approximately 6 weeks after the last ischemic infarction [8].

Postoperative hemorrhage mainly occurs in patients with a previous history of intracranial hemorrhage [15]. Age is positively correlated with the postoperative hemorrhage risk [15]. Although an RCT reported the benefit of direct revascularization for preventing recurrent hemorrhage, the surgical revascularization effect can be diminished by postoperative hemorrhagic complications. This demonstrates the need for detecting the early signs of critical hyperperfusion in surgical and remote areas.

The preference for surgical procedures is based on the technical feasibility and complication rate. The procedure involving direct anastomosis allows an immediate increase in the regional CBF and is associated with good neovascularization. However, compared with indirect anastomosis, the direct procedure is considered to have a greater risk of postoperative complications. Nevertheless, the direct/combined procedure has a lower stroke rate than the indirect procedure in pediatric patients [7]. This is counterintuitive since direct anastomosis is a difficult and time-consuming procedure. It could be attributed to the immediate increase in CBF when hemodynamic conditions are unstable. The immediate increase in the blood flow from direct bypass could compensate for the detrimental effects of anemia, crying-induced hypocapnia, hypotension, and circulation volume loss. Contrastingly, the indirect procedure alone may critically decrease the CBF in the acute period.

Additionally, an excessive increase in intracranial pressure can cause critical ischemia in patients with moyamoya disease. The standard encephaloduroarteriosynangiosis procedure is performed with relatively small craniotomy, which can cause brain protrusion from the craniotomy site. Temporal muscle swelling may also aggravate the increased intracranial pressure [22]. Therefore, patients with severe hemodynamic compromise can postoperatively develop global ischemia [39].

Previous studies have mainly focused on hemodynamic stroke originating from hypocapnia, circulating volume loss, anemia, and hypotension [8, 40, 41] as the main causes of perioperative stroke. The importance of acute occlusive changes remote to the superficial area has been emphasized [5, 11]. This complication may be associated with immediate blood flow alterations. Propofol has been recently shown to increase cerebral perfusion pressure during general anesthesia, [42] which suggests that improved anesthetic management may have decreased the incidence of postoperative stroke.

Skin trouble causes distress to both patients and surgeons. Harvesting of double branches is a routine procedure in conventional combined direct/indirect bypass. STA harvesting is often performed as extensively as possible, particularly in direct STA-ACA anastomosis. After 30 years of experience, the improvement of the harvesting technique has reduced the rate of skin trouble. However, direct STA-ACA anastomosis is not indiscriminately performed because of high frequency of skin trouble.

Temporal muscle swelling complicates combined direct/indirect bypass procedure, in which the muscle bulk is inserted under the bone flap. To reduce this complication, we have attempted splitting the muscle in half and using an indirect procedure. However, this muscle splitting technique was also associated with remarkable swelling of the muscle. A sufficient craniotomy size with an arterialized pedicle and preserved venous drainage is necessary for safe indirect procedures.

Detecting bleeding-prone arterial lesions is essential for prognosis. Revascularization surgery is not always effective for eliminating aneurysms in the perforating artery. Angiographical examination is necessary for patients with a history of intracranial hemorrhage. De novo arteriovenous shunt is occasionally observed as a consequence of acute stroke or revascularization surgery. In clinical settings, excision as primary treatment is difficult, given the stroke-prone brain. Furthermore, subsequent surgery is considered more difficult due to neovascularization.

References

1. Kodama N, Suzuki J. Moyamoya disease associated with aneurysm. J Neurosurg. 1978;48(4):565–9.
2. Suzuki J, Kodama N. Moyamoya disease--a review. Stroke. 1983;14(1):104–9.
3. Sakamoto T, et al. Postoperative neurological deterioration following the revascularization surgery in children with moyamoya disease. J Neurosurg Anesthesiol. 1998;10(1):37–41.
4. Nomura S, et al. Perioperative management protocols for children with moyamoya disease. Childs Nerv Syst. 2001;17(4–5):270–4.
5. Kuroda S, et al. Frontal lobe infarction due to hemodynamic change after surgical revascularization in moyamoya disease--two case reports. Neurol Med Chir (Tokyo). 2000;40(6):315–20.
6. Sato K, Shirane R, Yoshimoto T. Perioperative factors related to the development of ischemic complications in patients with moyamoya disease. Childs Nerv Syst. 1997;13(2):68–72.
7. Kazumata K, et al. The frequency of postoperative stroke in moyamoya disease following combined revascularization: a single-university series and systematic review. J Neurosurg. 2014;121(2):432–40.
8. Kim SH, et al. Risk factors for postoperative ischemic complications in patients with moyamoya disease. J Neurosurg. 2005;103(5 Suppl):433–8.
9. Guzman R, et al. Clinical outcome after 450 revascularization procedures for moyamoya disease. Clinical article. J Neurosurg. 2009;111(5):927–35.
10. Sussman ES, et al. Contralateral acute vascular occlusion following revascularization surgery for moyamoya disease. J Neurosurg. 2018;131(6):1702–8.
11. Huang AP, Tu YK. Progressive PCA steno-occlusive changes after revascularization for moyamoya disease: a neglected' phenomenon. Neurosurgery. 2010;67(6):E1865–6. author reply E1866
12. Hosoda Y, Ikeda E, Hirose S. Histopathological studies on spontaneous occlusion of the circle of Willis (cerebrovascular moyamoya disease). Clin Neurol Neurosurg. 1997;99(Suppl 2):S203–8.

13. Wei W, et al. Risk factors for postoperative stroke in adults patients with moyamoya disease: a systematic review with meta-analysis. BMC Neurol. 2019;19(1):98.
14. Iwama T, Hashimoto N, Yonekawa Y. The relevance of hemodynamic factors to perioperative ischemic complications in childhood moyamoya disease. Neurosurgery. 1996;38(6):1120–5. discussion 1125-6
15. Tokairin K, et al. Postoperative Intracerebral hemorrhage after combined revascularization surgery in Moyamoya disease: profiles and clinical associations. World Neurosurg. 2018;120:e593–600.
16. Schubert, G.A., et al., Perfusion characteristics of Moyamoya disease: an anatomically and clinically oriented analysis and comparison. (1524–4628 (Electronic)).
17. Mesiwala AH, et al. Long-term outcome of superficial temporal artery-middle cerebral artery bypass for patients with moyamoya disease in the US. Neurosurg Focus. 2008;24(2):E15.
18. Kazumata K, et al. Topographic changes in cerebral blood flow and reduced white matter integrity in the first 2 weeks following revascularization surgery in adult moyamoya disease. J Neurosurg. 2017;127(2):260–9.
19. Uchino H, et al. Predictors and clinical features of postoperative hyperperfusion after surgical revascularization for moyamoya disease: a serial single photon emission CT/positron emission tomography study. Stroke. 2012;43(10):2610–6.
20. Fujimura M, et al. Significance of focal cerebral hyperperfusion as a cause of transient neurologic deterioration after extracranial-intracranial bypass for moyamoya disease: comparative study with non-moyamoya patients using N-isopropyl-p-[(123)I]iodoamphetamine single-photon emission computed tomography. Neurosurgery. 2011;68(4):957–64. discussion 964-5
21. Andoh T, et al. Chronic subdural hematoma following bypass surgery--report of three cases. Neurol Med Chir (Tokyo). 1992;32(9):684–9.
22. Fujimura M, et al. Cerebral ischemia owing to compression of the brain by swollen temporal muscle used for encephalo-myo-synangiosis in moyamoya disease. Neurosurg Rev. 2009;32(2):245–9. discussion 249
23. Touho H. Cerebral ischemia due to compression of the brain by ossified and hypertrophied muscle used for encephalomyosynangiosis in childhood moyamoya disease. Surg Neurol. 2009;72(6):725–7.
24. Takanari K, et al. Operative wound-related complications after cranial revascularization surgeries. J Neurosurg. 2015;123(5):1145–50.
25. Mikami T, et al. Predictive factors for acute thrombogenesis occurring immediately after bypass procedure for moyamoya disease. Neurosurg Rev. 2020;43(2):609–17.
26. Katsuta T, et al. Reversible occlusion of donor vessel caused by mouth opening after superficial temporal artery-middle cerebral artery anastomosis in adult moyamoya patients. J Neurosurg. 2015;123(3):670–5.
27. Nishimoto T, et al. A ruptured middle cerebral artery aneurysm originating from the site of anastomosis 20 years after extracranial-intracranial bypass for moyamoya disease: case report. Surg Neurol. 2005;64(3):261–5. discussion 265
28. Hokari M, et al. Intracerebral hemorrhage from a ruptured aneurysm at the site of anastomosis 27 years after superficial temporal artery-middle cerebral artery bypass. Neurol Med Chir (Tokyo). 2010;50(11):1012–4.
29. Yokota H, Yokoyama K, Noguchi H. De novo aneurysm associated with superficial temporal artery to middle cerebral artery bypass: report of two cases and review of literature. World Neurosurg. 2016;92:583.e7–583.e12.
30. Aoki T, et al. Ruptured de novo aneurysm arising at a site remote from the anastomosis 14 years after superficial temporal artery-middle cerebral artery bypass: a case report. Neurosurgery. 2012;71(4):E905–9.
31. Fujimura M, et al. Development of a de novo arteriovenous malformation after bilateral revascularization surgery in a child with moyamoya disease. J Neurosurg Pediatr. 2014;13(6):647–9.
32. Schmit BP, et al. Acquired cerebral arteriovenous malformation in a child with moyamoya disease. Case report. J Neurosurg. 1996;84(4):677–80.
33. Feroze AH, et al. Development of arteriovenous fistula after revascularization bypass for Moyamoya disease: case report. Neurosurgery. 2015;11(Suppl 2):E202–6.

34. Peeters SM, et al. Spontaneous resolution of Dural and Pial Arteriovenous fistulae arising after superficial temporal artery to middle cerebral artery bypass for Moyamoya disease. World Neurosurg. 2020;142:404–7.
35. Inoue K, et al. A case of pediatric moyamoya disease with severe cerebral vasospasm and delayed cerebral infarction following an intraventricular hemorrhage. In: Childs Nerv Syst; 2020.
36. Karsten MB, et al. Central retinal artery occlusion occurring 30 years after successful revascularization surgery for moyamoya disease: case report. In: Acta Neurochir (Wien); 2020.
37. Yamada S, et al. Effects of surgery and antiplatelet therapy in ten-year follow-up from the registry study of research committee on Moyamoya disease in Japan. J Stroke Cerebrovasc Dis. 2016;25(2):340–9.
38. Antonucci MU, et al. Acute preoperative infarcts and poor cerebrovascular reserve are independent risk factors for severe ischemic complications following direct Extracranial-intracranial bypass for Moyamoya disease. AJNR Am J Neuroradiol. 2016;37(2):228–35.
39. Sim YW, et al. Unpredictable postoperative global cerebral infarction in the patient of Williams syndrome accompanying moyamoya disease. J Korean Neurosurg Soc. 2011;50(3):256–9.
40. Iwama T, et al. Peri-operative complications in adult moyamoya disease. Acta Neurochir. 1995;132(1–3):26–31.
41. Parray T, Martin TW, Siddiqui S. Moyamoya disease: a review of the disease and anesthetic management. J Neurosurg Anesthesiol. 2011;23(2):100–9.
42. Kikuta K, et al. Effects of intravenous anesthesia with propofol on regional cortical blood flow and intracranial pressure in surgery for moyamoya disease. Surg Neurol. 2007;68(4):421–4.

Long-Term Outcome in Europe

20

Friedrich Mrosk, Güliz Acker, Kristin Lucia, and Peter Vajkoczy

Abstract

Despite being one of the leading causes for stroke in pediatric patients, Moyamoya Vasculopathy (MMV) is a rare cerebrovascular disease, especially in non-Asian countries. While the epidemiological and clinical aspects of MMV in Europe were comparable to the North American series, major differences are known when compared to East-Asian countries. The surgical treatment strategies worldwide to prevent ischemia or intracranial hemorrhage include direct, indirect and combined revascularization procedures. The aim of this following chapter was to present long-term outcome results of MMV patients treated in Europe. We analyzed the so far published MMV series with a follow-up period with up to 17 years. Overall, 12 studies reporting surgical results of $n = 451$ MMV patients in Europe could be included in this chapter. The majority of the patients presented with ischemic symptoms (mean 77.9%, +/− 14.8%), while intracranial hemorrhage occurred only in few cases (mean 10.9%, +/− 15.7%). Overall, 84.0% of the patients were treated surgically (32.8% direct, 20.1% combined, 47.1% indirect revascularization procedures). These patients reached an estimated good outcome in 87.9% of cases with a bypass patency of 96.5% in mean indicating the long-term benefit of the surgical revascularization also in European

F. Mrosk · K. Lucia · P. Vajkoczy (✉)
Department of Neurosurgery and Center for Stroke Research Berlin (CSB), Charité–Universitätsmedizin Berlin, Berlin, Germany
e-mail: friedrich.mrosk@charite.de; kristin-elizabeth.lucia@charite.de; peter.vajkoczy@charite.de

G. Acker
Department of Neurosurgery and Center for Stroke Research Berlin (CSB), Charité–Universitätsmedizin Berlin, Berlin, Germany

Berlin Institute of Health, Berlin, Germany
e-mail: gueliz.acker@charite.de

S. Kuroda (ed.), *Moyamoya Disease: Current Knowledge and Future Perspectives*, https://doi.org/10.1007/978-981-33-6404-2_20

MMV patients. However, further clinical trials with long-term outcome results of European MMV patients are warranted.

Keywords

Moyamoya disease · Moyamoya syndrome · Long-term outcome · Europe Bypass Revascularization

20.1 Moyamoya Disease in Europe: Overview

Despite being one of the leading causes for stroke in pediatric patients, Moyamoya Vasculopathy (MMV) in Europe is a rare occurring cerebrovascular disease. While Moyamoya disease (MMD) refers to idiopathic MMV, Moyamoya syndrome (MMS) is defined as MMD with an associated underlying disease such as trisomy 21. Studies have shown that when compared to East-Asian countries, not only the incidence but also clinical characteristics significantly vary among the affected patients throughout the countries (Table 20.1) [1–13]. In Japan, for example, epidemiological studies have shown incidences ranging between 0.35 and 0.94 / 100,000 for MMD with an increasing trend over the years [7, 14]. In Europe, however, the incidence was estimated to be ten-times lower [15]. One recent nationwide register study from Denmark supported this estimation with an incidence of 0.047 / 100,000, identifying n = 56 patients during a course of 21 years [2]. Similar incidences were reported in North America [5]. Unfortunately, literature lacks further investigations from other European countries in relation to epidemiological data.

MMV usually becomes apparent due to either ischemic symptoms or intracranial hemorrhage [1]. Seizures or headache also play a role as an onset symptom, especially in children. However, several studies have shown that the onset symptom varies depending on the ethnicity and age. For adult MMD patients, hemorrhagic manifestation was reported only up to 14.6% in the largest North American series, while in Asian countries the so far reported hemorrhage rate ranged between 24.3% and 62.4% [3, 6, 9, 13, 14, 16–18]. An analysis of $n = 153$ MMD patients from our Department of the Charité Berlin in Germany also confirmed that the European MMD population was overall similar to North American series with considerable differences to the East-Asian population [3]. Importantly, only 7.8% of the adult patients overall presented with hemorrhage in our series [3]. Furthermore, it could be shown that hemorrhage was significantly more frequent (12%) in European pediatric MMD patients as compared to other countries [3]. Recent studies also supported the theory that choroidal anastomosis of the anterior and posterior choroidal artery as well as involvement of the posterior cerebral artery predict hemorrhage in MMV [19, 20]. These angiographic findings were particularly seen in Asian patients while European patients were unaffected of these findings [20]. One other difference of European MMD patients characteristics was the age distribution. In Berlin population, patients were distributed with one peak at 11–18 years and one later peak at 40–49 years [3]. In contrast, patients from Japan showed an earlier

Table 20.1 Regional differences in Moyamoya vasculopathy

Country, Reference	Incidence (100.000/year)	Age distribution (years)		Gender (F:M)		Clinical presentation			
						Ischemic events		Hemorrhage	
		MMD	MMS	MMD	MMS	MMD	MMS	MMD	MMS
Europe [2–4]	0.047	P mean: 11.4 A mean: 40.5	P mean: 7.5 A mean: 41.5	P–1.8:1 A–3.3:1	P–3:1 A–2.7:1	P: 72.0% A: 82.8%	P: 85% A: 82.7%	P: 12% A: 7.8%	P: 0% A: 12.2%
North America [5, 6]	0.086	P mean: 10.1 A mean: 39.5	n.a.	P–1:1 A–3:1	n.a.	P: 20–80% A: 35–36%	A + P: 52.4–78.2%	P: 2.1% A: 14.6%	A + P: 4.8%
Japan [7, 8]	0.94	P peak: 5–9 A peak: 45–49	P peak: 0–9 A peak: 40–59	A + P – 2.2:1	A + P – 1.6:1	P: 78.4% A: 53.5%	A + P: 63.4%	P: 2.7% A: 24.3%	A + P: 6.9%
China [9, 10]	0.71–1.19	P peak: 5–9 A peak: 35–39	A peak: 30–40 (unimodal)	A+P– 1.15:1	A + P – 1.1:1	P: 86.0% A: 34.0%	A + P: 70.3%	P: 14.0% A: 62.0%	A + P: 21.9%
Taiwan [11]	0.048	P peak: 0–10 A peak: 31–40	n.a.	A + P – 1.3:1	n.a.	P: 83.0% A: 25.0%	n.a.	P: 17.0% A: 65.0%	n.a.
Korea [12, 13]	1.7–2.3	P mean: 8.2 A mean: 37.1	n.a.	P–2.4:1 A–2.5:1	n.a.	P: 61.2% A: 25.4%	n.a.	P: 9.1% A: 62.4%	n.a.

A adult; *P* pediatric; *F* female; *M* male

manifestation in both groups [21]. Furthermore, European patients tend to show a higher predominance towards the female gender. These findings were also supported by several other European studies which are going to be discussed below.

While MMS occurs more infrequently than MMD, it comes with several important differences [8]. For example, European MMS patients showed less unilateral cases, higher female predominance, and less hemorrhagic clinical presentation in pediatric patients [4]. Furthermore, European MMS patients tend to show a reverse biphasic age distribution as compared to East-Asian and European MMD patients towards younger age [4].

20.2 Surgical Treatment of Moyamoya Patients in our Institute

To prevent ischemia to the brain and intracranial hemorrhage in MMD patients, surgical treatment options include direct or indirect revascularization or both combined procedures [22]. While indirect vascularization relies on delayed neovascularization through pedicled vascularized flaps which were placed onto the brain surface, direct revascularization, i.e. bypass surgery, provides immediate blood flow augmentation [22]. Treatment strategies vary not only throughout the countries, but also throughout the different departments since there is still lack of prospective randomized trials for ischemic MMV patients. However, recent meta analyses confirmed the superiority of direct revascularization also in these patients [23, 24]. Thus, our treatment algorithm always aims for a direct revascularization with or without an indirect technique. In the following section, the treatment algorithm of our Neurosurgical Department of the Charité is going to be further explained as an example.

If MMV is suspected, a standardized diagnostic workup needs to be performed. Since MMV is mostly diagnosed in patients with stroke or ischemic events, often being recurrent, MRI scans of the brain with TOF-vessel imaging are usually the first diagnostic modalities that come to light. In our department, we then perform an angiography to assess not only the brain vessel configuration but also the superficial temporal artery on both sides which will serve as bypass graft. Furthermore, SPECT or PET-scans need to be performed to determine the cerebrovascular reserve capacity (CVRC). In cases of asymptomatic MMV patients, reduced CVRC indicates a higher likelihood of developing ischemic events in the future, most of all due to the progressive natural course of this disease [25].

In cases of bilateral MMV, we prefer a two-staged strategy where the symptomatic brain hemisphere should be treated first. In adult patients, we prefer a direct (superficial temporal artery (STA) to the M3-segment of the middle cerebral artery (MCA)) or a combined revascularization procedure. As the additional indirect revascularization, we use an encephalodurosynangiosis (EDS) and/or an encephalomyosynangiosis (EMS) [26]. Since the craniotomy is performed temporally at the end of the Sylvian fissure, the skin incision depends on the targeted branch of the STA [26].

Czabanka et al. showed that for adult patients, combined revascularization procedures are superior compared to indirect procedures only [27]. Furthermore, the authors stated that in pediatric patients, bypass surgery has a higher failure rate while indirect revascularization procedures seem to have higher success rates [27]. We therefore prefer in these cases the combination of STA-MCA bypass with indirect revascularization procedures, primarily encephalomyosynangiosis (EMS). Some authors suggest to perform encephaloduroarteriosynangiosis (EDAS) or encephaloduroarteriomyosynangiosis (EDAMS) for children [28, 29]. This indirect revascularization procedure involves the placement of the STA onto the pial surface. The goal in these cases is the additional augmentation through the STA. However, this also implicates the sacrifice of this vessel for further bypass operations. In our opinion, even if the direct revascularization fails, indirect procedures such as EMS should provide sufficient delayed flow augmentation in the later course. Therefore, for juvenile patients combined revascularization should always be attempted [30].

One important aspect in perioperative management is the use of antiplatelet therapy before and after bypass surgery. One study supports the evidence that aspirin improves the outcome in patients with MMD after surgery while perioperative strokes and bypass patency was not afflicted [31]. In our daily practice, we favor the use of aspirin and qualify it with specific platelet function lab tests to evaluate the metabolic response of the patient.

Postoperatively, we perform first a CT-angiography to evaluate bypass patency and rule out periprocedural complications. After 3 months and second bypass surgery of the contralateral hemisphere (if needed), a conventional angiography should be done to determine bypass patency and anastomosis pattern. Afterwards, scheduled follow-ups should be performed with conventional angiographies and MRI on a regular base.

20.3 Long-Term Outcome of Moyamoya Patients in Europe

Since MMV is a rare cerebrovascular disease in Europe, patients are usually referred to few neurosurgical departments which have specialized in treating these patients. Table 20.1 shows the so far published long-term results of European Moyamoya patients. Due to small numbers of reports, we also included two short-term outcome studies with mean follow-up times from 3 to 6 months and focused on MMV also including MMS instead of MMD only.

Overall, 12 studies reporting surgical results for MMV patients in Europe while our study only included MMS patients (Table 20.2) [4, 27, 32–41]. In total, $n = 451$ patients were included in this analysis to summarize the long-term outcome of MMV patients in Europe based on so far published series. The mean follow-up time ranged between 3 months and 17.3 years. Most of the patients were children with an age between 0 and 18 years (ratio 1.47:1) and with a female predominance. Patients mostly presented with ischemic symptoms (mean 77.9%, +/− 14.8%), while the presence of hemorrhage was between 1–48% (mean 10.9%, +/− 15.7%).

Table 20.2 Long-term outcomes of MMV patients in Europe

Author	Study Design	Country	Cases (n=)	Pathology	Pediatric: Adults	Gender (F:M)	Onset Symptom	Treatment modality	Mean Follow-Up	Bypass patency	Outcome	Recurrent Hemorrhage	Recurrent Ischemic Events
Khan (2003)	R	Switzerland	23	MMV	4.8:1	1.6:1	Ischemic–96% Seizure–13%	Combined–70% Direct–30%	6 Mo	100%	Improved / stable–96% Death–4%	–	4.3%
Hänggi (2008)	R	Germany	9	MMV	0:1	3.5:1	Ischemic–89% Hemorrhagic–11%	Direct - 77% Combined–11% Indirect–11%	3–6 Mo	100%	Improved–67% Stable–22% Worsen–11%	0%	11.0%
Czabanka (2011)	R	Germany	30	MMV	1:3.3	1.5:1	TIA–83% Stroke–16% Psychological–23%	Combined–100%	12 Mo	94%	Improved–80% Stable–16% Worsen–3%	–	0%
Ulrich (2011)	R	Germany	19	MMV	1:0	1.7:1	Epilepsy–89% TIA–79% Mental retardation–58%	Indirect–63% Combined–21% Direct–16%	17.3 Yrs	91%	Improved / stable–94%	–	0%
Acker (2016)	R	Germany	61	MMS only	1:2	2.8:1	Ischemic–83% Hemorrhage–8% Seizure–3% Headache–2% Cognition–2%	Combined–68/61% Direct–23/25% Indirect–9/14% Conservative–8%	51 Mo	97%	Improved / stable–88%	n.a.	18.0%* *analyzed only in operated patients
Jecko (2016)	R	France	9	MMV	2:1	n.a.	Ischemic–67% Hemorrhage–33%	Indirect–100%	4.7 Yrs	–	mRS 0–2–44.4% mRS 2–6–55.6%	0%	0%
Lanterna (2016)	P	Italy	23	MMV	n.a	3:1	Hemorrhage–48% Stroke–30% TIA–22%	Combined–61% Direct–39%	2.2 Yrs	100%	Improved / stable–96% Recurrent hemorrhage–9%	9.0%	0%
Kraemer (2018)	R + P	Germany	54	MMV	n.a.	2.6:1	n.a.	Direct–100%	38.2 Mo	100%	Improved / stable–100% Patients satisfaction 9.2/10 mean	0%	0%
Tho-Calvi (2018)	R	United kingdom	88	MMV	1:0	1.8:1	Stroke–41% TIA–33% Hemorrhage–1% Seizure–5% Headache–11%	Indirect–63% Conservative–37%	43 Mo	–	Indirect: mRS 0–2–63.5% mRS 3–6–36.5% Conservative: mRS 0–2–60.6% mRS 3–6–39.4%	n.a.	Overall –75.6% Indirect –60.0%

Savolainen (2019)	R	Finnland	61	MMV	1:5.1	4.5:1	Ischemic–57% Hemorrhage–13% Seizure–5% Headache–11% Asymptom–13%	Direct–26% Indirect- 18% Conservative–56%	9.5 Yrs	n.a.	NIHSS (mean)–1 mRS (mean)–1 BI (mean)–97% WHOQOL-BREF–53-79 / 100	37.5%	20.0%
Blauwbomme (2019)	R	France	64	MMV	1:0	1:1.1	Stroke–47% TIA–34% Hemorrhage–6% Headache–5% Asymptom–8%	Indirect–100%	4.2 Yrs	–	Stable / improved–98%	0%	2.0%
Aboukais (2019)	P	France	10	MMV	0:1	n.a.	Stroke–80% Headache–20%	Direct–100%	24 Mo	90%	mRS 0–2–90%	–	12.5%

Study Design: *R* retrospective, *P* prospective; MMV includes MMD and MMS; Pediatrics: 0–18 yrs.; BI: Barthel-Index; Divided numbers in study number 4 at treatment modality is referred to first and second treated hemisphere. Bypass patency, recurrent hemorrhage and ischemic events refer to the time of latest follow-up

Eight studies reported the results from either direct or combined revascularization procedures while three authors performed indirect revascularization procedures only. In detail, these indirect revascularization surgeries consisted of mainly EDAS, followed by EMS and multiple burr hole surgery (MBH). For the direct revascularization, the most common type of bypass used was STA-MCA as described above. Overall, most of the patients (84.0%) were treated surgically (32.8% direct, 20.1% combined, 47.1% indirect procedures), while only 16.0% were treated conservatively.

The outcome assessments were also different among the studies while the modified ranking score was the most common score. "Good outcome" was considered if the report stated improved or stable neurological outcome or the modified ranking score (mRS) ranged between 0 and 2. The overall reported rate of good patient outcome was 87.9% (CI 95–78.8%; 97.0%). Importantly, the rate for good outcome reached only 68.6% (CI 95–43.5%; 93.7%) in three studies with only indirect revascularization procedures as surgical treatment.

Two studies compared surgical intervention with conservative care for MMV patients. Antiplatelet therapy was the conservative treatment of choice. While one study showed no differences in patients treated either surgically or conservatively [39], Tho-Calvi et al. demonstrated slightly improved outcomes in the interventional group (63.5% mRS 0–2 versus 60.6% mRS 0–2) [38]. Bypass patency was confirmed at follow-up in 96.5% of cases in mean (ranging between 90 and 100% of the cases) demonstrating the duration of this surgical treatment.

Reccurrent ischemic events occurred in 11.9% of the ischemic MMV patients on average with a wide range of 0 to 75.6%. Besides the study with the highest reported recurrent event rate, these incidences were referred to the latest follow-up, since many initially reported recurrent ischemic events tended to resolve during the first weeks to months after surgery without any intervention [27, 34, 41]. Interestingly, if the study with 75% was excluded, then the highest reported recurrent ischemic event rate was 20% [39]. If we look closer to this study with 75.6% recurrent ischemic events that only included pediatric patients and performed only indirect revascularization as surgical treatment, this high rate may furthermore be explained by the involvement of other symptoms as "recurrent events" unlike ischemic events only. Although perioperative events were also included in the recurrent event rate in this cohort, these were still lower with 60% for the operated children ($n = 33$) in comparison to the whole cohort including also conservatively treated children ($n = 88$). In addition, despite the high rate of recurrent events, the severity and frequency of ischemic events could be reduced in 67.2% of the surgically treated patients. Furthermore, if we only concentrate on the studies with surgically treated patients, then the recurrent ischemic events were between 0 and 18% [4, 27, 32–37, 40, 41]. This observation again reflects the need for surgical revascularization in MMV patients also in Europe.

In cases of hemorrhagic MMV, rebleeding is the major issue. The JAM trial showed a mean risk between 30 and 37% without any intervention, which could be reduced to 11.9% at 5 years after bypass surgery [39]. Overall, hemorrhage is a rare onset symptom in Europe as indicated above with only 10.9% in mean summarized in this analysis. However, rebleeding is still relevant. In the European studies referred in Table 20.1, rebleeding rates varied from 0 to 37.5% (mean 7.8%, +/– 15.0%). In the study with the highest rebleeding rates of 37.5%, 3 patients suffered from recurrent hemorrhage where one patient was treated conservatively, and the remaining 2 patients were treated by either direct and combined revascularization surgery [39].

These studies does not enable a differentiated analysis of long-term outcome between MMD and MMS patients in Europe, but our study specifically about the MMS patients confirmed the comparable success of the revascularization surgery with stable and improved neurological symptoms in 88% of cases [4].

20.4 Conclusion

Overall, patients treated for MMV in Europe reached an estimated good outcome in 94.9% of the patients with a bypass patency of 96.5% in mean. While direct and combined revascularization procedures yielded slightly better outcomes than indirect revascularization procedures, one study also showed the superiority of treating these patients surgically as compared to conservative approaches. Overall, the comparison of recurrent ischemic events also highlighted the benefit of revascularization surgery in long term for European MMV patients. However, the present data regarding the long-term outcome in Europe is sparse with mainly small patient series. Thus, further clinical studies with long-term outcomes of European patients are warranted. In this regard, we currently analyze the 10-years results of all surgically treated Moyamoya patients at our Berlin neurosurgical department.

References

1. Research Committee on the Pathology and Treatment of Spontaneous Occlusion of the Circle of Willis. Guidelines for diagnosis and treatment of Moyamoya disease (spontaneous occlusion of the circle of Willis). Neurol Med Chir (Tokyo). 2012;52(5):245–66.
2. Birkeland P, Lauritsen J. Incidence of moyamoya disease in Denmark: a population-based register study. Acta Neurochir Suppl. 2018;129:91–3.
3. Acker G, Goerdes S, Schneider UC, Schmiedek P, Czabanka M, Vajkoczy P. Distinct clinical and radiographic characteristics of moyamoya disease amongst European Caucasians. Eur J Neurol. 2015;22(6):1012–7.
4. Acker G, Goerdes S, Schmiedek P, Czabanka M, Vajkoczy P. Characterization of clinical and radiological features of quasi-Moyamoya disease among European Caucasians including surgical treatment and outcome. Cerebrovasc Dis. 2016;42(5–6):464–75.
5. Uchino K, Johnston SC, Becker KJ, Tirschwell DL. Moyamoya disease in Washington state. Neurology. 2005;65:956–8.
6. Guzman R, Lee M, Achrol A, Bell-Stephens T, Kelly M, Do HM, et al. Clinical outcome after 450 revascularization procedures for moyamoya disease: clinical article. J Neurosurg. 2009;111(5):927–35.
7. Ikezaki K, Inamura T, Kawano T, Fukui M. Clinical features of probable Moyamoya disease in Japan. Clinical Neurology and Neurosurgery. 1997;99(SUPPL. 2)

8. Hayashi K, Horie N, Izumo T, Nagata I. Nationwide survey on quasi-moyamoya disease in Japan. Acta Neurochir. 2014;156(5):935–40.
9. Miao W, Zhao PL, Zhang YS, Liu HY, Chang Y, Ma J, et al. Epidemiological and clinical features of Moyamoya disease in Nanjing, China. Clin Neurol Neurosurg. 2010;112(3):199–203.
10. Zhao M, Lin Z, Deng X, Zhang Q, Zhang D, Zhang Y, et al. Clinical characteristics and natural history of quasi-Moyamoya disease. J Stroke Cerebrovasc Dis. 2017;26(5):1088–97.
11. Hung CC, Tu YK, Su CF, Lin LS, Shih CJ. Epidemiological study of Moyamoya disease in Taiwan. Clin Neurol Neurosurg. 1997;99(SUPPL. 2):97–9.
12. Ahn IM, Park DH, Hann HJ, Kim KH, Kim HJ, Ahn HS. Incidence, prevalence, and survival of moyamoya disease in Korea: a nationwide, population-based study. Stroke. 2014;45(4):1090–5.
13. Han DH, Kwon OK, Byun BJ, Choi BY, Choi CW, Choi JU, et al. A co-operative study: clinical characteristics of 334 Korean patients with moyamoya disease treated at neurosurgical institutes (1976-1994). Acta Neurochir. 2000;142(11):1263–74.
14. Baba T, Houkin K, Kuroda S. Novel epidemiological features of moyamoya disease. J Neurol Neurosurg Psychiatry. 2008;79(8):900–4.
15. Yonekawa Y, Ogata N, Kaku Y, Taub E, Imhof H-G. Moyamoya disease in Europe, past and present status. Clin Neurol Neurosurg. 1997 Oct;99:S58–60.
16. Hallemeier CL, Rich KM, Grubb RL, Chicoine MR, Moran CJ, Cross DWT, et al. Clinical features and outcome in north American adults with moyamoya phenomenon. Stroke. 2006;37(6):1490–6.
17. Chen PC, Yang SH, Chien KL, Tsai IJ, Kuo MF. Epidemiology of moyamoya disease in Taiwan: a nationwide population-based study. Stroke. 2014;45(5):1258–63.
18. Gross BA, Du R. The natural history of Moyamoya in a north American adult cohort. J Clin Neurosci. 2013;20(1):44–8.
19. Funaki T, Takahashi JC, Houkin K, Kuroda S, Takeuchi S, Fujimura M, et al. Angiographic features of hemorrhagic moyamoya disease with high recurrence risk: a supplementary analysis of the Japan adult Moyamoya trial. J Neurosurg. 2018;128(3):777–84.
20. Hori S, Kashiwazaki D, Yamamoto S, Acker G, Czabanka M, Akioka N, et al. Impact of interethnic difference of collateral Angioarchitectures on prevalence of hemorrhagic stroke in Moyamoya disease. Clin Neurosurg. 2019;85(1):134–45.
21. Hoshino H, Izawa Y, Suzuki N. Epidemiological features of Moyamoya disease in Japan. Neurol Med Chir. 2012;52(5):295–8.
22. Acker G, Fekonja L, Vajkoczy P. Surgical management of moyamoya disease. Stroke. 2018;49(2):476–82.
23. Qian C, Yu X, Li J, Chen J, Wang L, Chen G. The efficacy of surgical treatment for the secondary prevention of stroke in symptomatic moyamoya disease a meta-analysis. Medicine (United States). 2015;94(49):1–6.
24. Jeon JP, Kim JE, Cho WS, Bang JS, Son YJ, Oh CW. Meta-analysis of the surgical outcomes of symptomatic moyamoya disease in adults. J Neurosurg. 2018;128(3):793–9.
25. Kuroda S, Hashimoto N, Yoshimoto T, Iwasaki Y. Radiological findings, clinical course, and outcome in asymptomatic moyamoya disease: results of multicenter survey in Japan. Stroke. 2007;38(5):1430–5.
26. Acker G, Schlinkmann N, Fekonja L, Grünwald L, Hardt J, Czabanka M, et al. Wound healing complications after revascularization for moyamoya vasculopathy with reference to different skin incisions. Neurosurgical Focus. 2019;46(2).
27. Czabanka M, Peña-Tapia P, Scharf J, Schubert GA, Münch E, Horn P, et al. Characterization of direct and indirect cerebral revascularization for the treatment of european patients with moyamoya disease. Cerebrovasc Dis. 2011;32(4):361–9.
28. Liu JJ, Steinberg GK. Direct versus indirect bypass for Moyamoya disease. Neurosurg Clin N Am. 2017 Jul;28(3):361–74.
29. Ravindran K, Wellons JC, Dewan MC. Surgical outcomes for pediatric moyamoya: a systematic review and meta-analysis. J Neurosurg Pediatr. 2019;24(6):663–72.

30. Czabanka M, Vajkoczy P, Schmiedek P, Horn P. Age-dependent revascularization patterns in the treatment of moyamoya disease in a European patient population. Neurosurg Focus. 2009;26(4):1–6.
31. Zhao Y, Zhang Q, Zhang D, Zhao Y. Effect of aspirin in postoperative Management of Adult Ischemic Moyamoya Disease. World Neurosurg. 2017;105:728–31.
32. Khan N, Schuknecht B, Boltshauser E, Capone A, Buck A, Imhof HG, et al. Moyamoya disease and Moyamoya syndrome: experience in Europe; choice of revascularisation procedures. Acta Neurochir. 2003;145(12):1061–71.
33. Hänggi D, Mehrkens JH, Schmid-Elsaesser R, Steiger H-J. Results of direct and indirect revascularisation for adult European patients with Moyamoya angiopathy. In: Changing aspects in stroke surgery: aneurysms, dissections, Moyamoya Angiopathy and EC-IC bypass. Vienna: Springer Vienna. p. 119–22.
34. Ulrich PT, Januschek E. Revascularisation Surgery and Long-Term Follow-up in Juvenile Moyamoya Syndrome: A Retrospective Analysis. In: Tsukahara T, Regli L, Hänggi D, Turowski B, Steiger H-J, editors. Vienna: Springer Vienna; 2011. p. 39–43. (Acta Neurochirurgica Supplementum; vol. 112).
35. Jecko V, Penchet G, Champeaux C. Traitement de la maladie de Moya-Moya par synangiose piale. L'expérience bordelaise. Neurochirurgie. 2016;62(4):190–6.
36. Lanterna LA. Brembilla C, Gritti P, Bernucci C. universal bypass for treatment of symptomatic Moyamoya disease or Moyamoya syndrome. Analysis of a personal case series on behalf of the Italian Moyamoya association. In: trends in cerebrovascular surgery. Acta Neurochirurgica Supplement 123. 2016:129–32.
37. Kraemer M, Karakaya R, Matsushige T, Graf J, Albrecht P, Hartung HP, et al. Efficacy of STA–MCA bypass surgery in moyamoya angiopathy: long-term follow-up of the Caucasian Krupp hospital cohort with 81 procedures. J Neurol.
38. Tho-Calvi SC, Thompson D, Saunders D, Agrawal S, Basu A, Chitre M, et al. Clinical features, course, and outcomes of a UK cohort of pediatric moyamoya. Neurology. 2018;90(9):E763–70.
39. Savolainen M, Mustanoja S, Pekkola J, Tyni T, Uusitalo AM, Ruotsalainen S, et al. Moyamoya angiopathy: long-term follow-up study in a Finnish population. J Neurol. 2019;266(3):574–81.
40. Aboukais R, Verbraeken B, Leclerc X, Gautier C, Henon H, Vermandel M, et al. Superficial temporal artery-middle cerebral artery anastomosis patency correlates with cerebrovascular reserve in adult moyamoya syndrome patients. Neurochirurgie.
41. Blauwblomme T, Mathon B, Naggara O, Kossorotoff M, Bourgeois M, Puget S, et al. Long-term outcome after multiple burr hole surgery in children with moyamoya angiopathy: a single-center experience in 108 hemispheres. Neurosurgery. 2017;80(6):950–6.

Long-Term Outcomes in the USA

21

Syed Uzair Ahmed and Gary K. Steinberg

Abstract

Moyamoya disease (MMD) was first described in the Japanese population, and remains significantly more common in Asia. The etiology of the disease remains unknown, but it is a chronic cerebrovascular disorder that manifests as progressive stenosis and occlusion of the large intracranial arteries, and formation of abnormal collateral vascular supply as a compensatory mechanism. The disease has since been recognized as a clinical entity in non-Asian populations, but its true incidence in these populations remains unclear. MMD in the USA is of growing interest in recent years, and multiple authors have contributed series of long-term outcomes after treatment for MMD, which are now available.

Keywords

Moyamoya disease · Cerebral bypass · Revascularization surgery

Abbreviations

CBF	cerebral blood flow
CT	computed tomography
DSA	digital subtraction angiography
DWI	diffusion weighted imaging
ECIC	extracranial-intracranial

S. U. Ahmed · G. K. Steinberg (✉)
Department of Neurosurgery and Stanford Stroke Center, Stanford University School of Medicine, Stanford, CA, USA
e-mail: uahmed@stanford.edu; gsteinberg@stanford.edu

S. Kuroda (ed.), *Moyamoya Disease: Current Knowledge and Future Perspectives*, https://doi.org/10.1007/978-981-33-6404-2_21

EDAS	Encephaloduroarteriosynangiosis
ICA	internal carotid artery
ICH	intracerebral hemorrhage
IPH	intraparenchymal hemorrhage
IVH	intraventricular hemorrhage
MAP	mean arterial pressure
MMD	moyamoya disease
MRI	magnetic resonance imaging
mRS	modified Rankin Score
OR	odds ratio
PET	positron emission tomography
SAH	subarachnoid hemorrhage
SPECT	single photon emission computed tomography
STA	superficial temporal artery
TIA	transient ischemic attack

21.1 Introduction

Moyamoya disease (MMD) is an idiopathic steno-occlusive disease of the large intracranial arteries. The disease was first described in Japan [1], and has a significantly higher prevalence in East Asian populations. The disease is named after the angiographic "puff of smoke" appearance of the dilated intracranial collateral vessels that arise in the setting of the disease, purportedly as a result of severe chronic ischemia secondary to the stenosis. The etiology of MMD remains unknown; however, a primary pathological feature of the affected arteries from MMD patients is fibro-cellular thickening of the intima related to proliferation of vascular smooth muscle cells and/or endothelial cells, as well as accumulation of matrix components [2–5]. The incidence and prevalence of the disease in non-Asian populations are lower than in Asia, but there has been an increase in the number of diagnosed cases over time. This chapter reviews the epidemiology, presentation, natural history, treatment, and outcomes of MMD in the USA, and compares these factors to those found in the Asian population.

21.2 Epidemiology of Moyamoya Disease in the USA

The incidence of MMD in non-Asian populations has been the subject of much interest, with limited data available. Greater awareness of the disease has meant that the diagnosis of MMD has been made with increasing frequency in the USA in recent years. A 2005 study in the western US states of California and Washington found the incidence to be 0.086/100,000 persons/year [6], while a subgroup analysis found the incidence in Asian-Americans to be 0.28/100,000 persons/year. A more recent study in 2012 reported a US incidence of 0.57/100,000 persons/year [7]. The adjusted incidence ratios compared to Caucasians in this study were 4.6-times higher incidence for Asian-Americans, 2.2 for African Americans, and 0.5 for Hispanics [6]. The incidence of MMD in Asian-Americans in this study was lower than that found in Japanese epidemiological studies, which report the incidence of MMD to range between 0.54 and 0.94/100,000 persons/year, with a prevalence of 6–10.5/100,000 [8, 9].

A study in Hawaii found the incidence of MMD in Japanese-Hawaiians to be comparable to that in Japan, and the overall incidence of MMD to be significantly higher compared to the rest of the USA, which was an expected finding, with Asians and Pacific Islanders making up 56% of the Hawaiian population, compared to 3% of the population in the USA overall [10].

Local population trends within the USA may make it difficult to extrapolate the data to the entire country, as most of the current studies reflect local population and referral patterns. California and Hawaii have some of the highest percentages of Asian ethnicity within the USA. Our published series of 329 MMD Stanford patients consisted of 59% Caucasian, 32% Asian, 5% African-American, and 4% Hispanic patients [11], and our current total series of 1230 moyamoya patients comprise 51% Caucasians, 32% Asians, 5% African-Americans, and 8% Hispanics, which was similar to the epidemiological data from California and Washington [6]. By comparison, a recent single-center cohort in Maryland consisted of 43% Caucasian, 23% African American, 23% Asian, and 12% patients of other ethnicities [12]. Other US studies have also contained predominantly Caucasian and African American patients [13, 14]. National trends in extracranial-to-intracranial bypass surgeries confirm that the Western United States consistently accounted for the highest proportion of bypasses, with MMD accounting for the highest proportion of these, at 60% [15].

MMD affects females more commonly than males; however, the ratio of female/male patients is higher in the USA than what has been reported in the Asian literature. Our current series of 1230 patients had a female/male ratio of 2.5:1 (F882:M348). Other American series have found comparable ratios [13, 14, 16], while some American series have had female/male ratios between 3.6 and 6:1 [12, 16]. The female/male ratio in the Asian literature is between 1.6 and 1.8:1 [8, 9].

MMD has a bimodal distribution, with patients presenting in childhood with peak incidence at 5–10 years, and in adulthood with peak incidence in their 40s [8]. In our current series, we observed two peaks of age at presentation, at 10 for the pediatric cohort, and 39 years for adults. A nation-wide survey of pediatric admissions for revascularization in MMD found the mean age of presentation in patients who underwent revascularization to be 9.6 years [17].

Approximately 6–15% of MMD cases are familial in the Asian population [8, 18]. The familial disease indicates an autosomal dominant mode of inheritance, with incomplete penetrance [19]. In a US study of 537 pediatric patients, Gaillard and colleagues found 3.4% of the patients to have familial MMD, while a sub-analysis of Asian-American patients in this cohort revealed a 5.5% rate of familial

MMD [20]. In our patients, we identified a positive family history of MMD in 13.9% of pediatric and 20.8% of adult patients, which is higher than what has been identified in the Asian literature. True rates of familial MMD in the American population remain unknown [2].

21.3 Presentation

Presenting symptoms in MMD have been grouped broadly into ischemic and hemorrhagic types. In our series, we have observed a larger percentage of patients presenting with ischemic symptoms (ischemic stroke or TIA) than with hemorrhagic symptoms, which is different from the Asian literature. In our series, 13%(127/963) of adult patients presented with intracerebral hemorrhage, while 68%(654/963) presented with ischemic stroke, and 49%(471/963) with TIAs. This is similar to the presentation characteristics in other American series showing 70% [14] and 74% [13] of patients presenting with ischemic symptoms, and 15% [14] and 17% [13] presenting with hemorrhagic symptoms. Multiple large Asian series of MMD have shown higher rates of adult patients with hemorrhagic presentations, particularly in the Korean population. A study comparing Korean and Japanese MMD patients found the incidence of hemorrhage in Korean patients to be 42.2%, compared with 19.1% in Japanese patients, while the incidence of ischemic stroke was lower in both Korean (27.3%) and Japanese (14.9%) patients [21].

In a subgroup analysis, we compared our adult Asian (69) and Caucasian (137) patients and found no statistically significant difference in the incidence of ischemic stroke (67 versus 65%) and TIA (61 versus 67%). The rate of hemorrhagic presentation was higher in Asian-American as compared to Caucasian (24 versus 16%), but did not reach statistical significance ($p = 0.08$). There was a statistically non-significant higher incidence of stroke and lower incidence of hemorrhage in African-American patients [22].

Another study comparing 31 Asian-American and 109 Non-Asian patients (including adult and pediatric patients) found 47% incidence of hemorrhage in Asian patients, compared to 16% in Non-Asians ($p = 0.02$), while 53% of Asians and 84% of non-Asians presented with ischemic stroke [12].

Pediatric patients with MMD present less commonly with hemorrhage. In our cohort, 7%(18/267) of pediatric patients presented with hemorrhage, compared to 13% of adults. Other US studies, including our previously published series, have found even lower rates of hemorrhagic presentation, of 2.1% [11] and 2.8% [23].

Headaches have been described as an independent presenting symptom of MMD in both adult [24] and pediatric populations [25]. Several theories have been posited to explain headaches in these patients, including hypoperfusion [26, 27], and dural nociceptor stimulation via dilatation of meningeal collaterals [25]. A significant number of our patients presented with a history of moderate-severe headaches, with 50% of adult and 44% of pediatric patients reporting headaches as a symptoms on presentation [11]. This is similar to the rates of headache as a presenting symptom reported in the Asian literature [25, 28].

21.4 Natural History in the USA

Few studies exist on the natural history of MMD in the USA. However, it is widely accepted to be a progressive disease with significant risk of recurrent stroke. From a clinical perspective, Asian and American data agree that when left untreated MMD is a devastating disease even in initially asymptomatic patients.

The 5-year cumulative risk for any recurrent ipsilateral stroke among medically treated hemispheres with impaired hemodynamic reserve, as defined by increased oxygen extraction fraction on PET, is approximately 65% and, in patients with bilateral disease, the stroke risk increases to 82% over 5 years [14]. Another American study showed a cumulative 5-year stroke risk of 40%, with 18% stroke risk in the first year following presentation [13]. In the Japanese population, the stroke risk has been studied to be similar to that in the American population. Furthermore, a study of asymptomatic MMD patients in Japan found a stroke risk of 3.2%/year in conservatively treated hemispheres [28].

Unilateral MMD is present in up to 18% of patients. Japanese studies have reported rates of angiographic progression to bilateral disease of up to 36.4% [29]. In our experience with 217 patients presenting with unilateral MMD, angiographic progression to bilateral disease was seen in 8.3% of patients, with an average time-to-progression of 5.8 years [30]. Asian patients included in this series (31% of patients) had a higher rate of progression (HR 2.26), but this was not statistically significant [30].

21.5 Treatment Trends

There is significant debate concerning the best method for revascularization in MMD with regard to safety and efficacy of the technique. Many indirect methods have been tried and compared to the direct revascularization technique. No randomized trial exists to compare direct and indirect revascularization techniques, and reviews of the literature have not shown improved efficacy or lower surgical morbidity of one technique over another [31]. In general, the treatment strategy is to provide direct revascularization in adults, and indirect revascularization in pediatric patients. However, several large American series have utilized mainly indirect bypass in all adult and pediatric patients [32–34]. Some authors prefer indirect revascularization as it theoretically reduces the risk of hyperperfusion in the perioperative period, which has been blamed for increased risk of perioperative stroke [35].

We recently published the results of our single-center study that utilized an individualized patient strategy to assign patients to direct versus indirect bypass procedures. Patients with at least 1 of these 4 criteria underwent indirect bypass: (1) mild to moderate ICA or M1 segment stenosis, (2) preserved cerebrovascular reserve, (3) intra-operative M4 segment anterograde flow (indicating flow away from the sylvian fissure) ≥8 ml/min, and (4) the absence of frequent and severe TIAs, clinical strokes, or MRI evidence of chronic watershed infarction. By contrast, the criteria for direct bypass were severe ICA or M1 segment stenosis or occlusion, impaired cerebrovascular reserve or steal phenomenon, intra-operative M4 segment retrograde flow or anterograde flow <8 ml/min, and the presence of frequent and severe TIAs or clinical strokes. Using these criteria, 133 direct and 62 indirect bypasses were performed. We observed major post-operative strokes in 4.7% of direct and 6.8% of indirect bypasses, but this result was not statistically significant. The degree of collateralization on follow-up angiography at 6 months was greater in the direct bypass group [36].

Our current treatment philosophy is to attempt direct revascularization in all patients. The main advantage of this approach is that it provides immediate augmentation of blood flow after surgery, provides higher and more consistent extent of angiographic collateralization, and is superior to indirect revascularization at restoring post-bypass cerebrovascular reserve capacity [37]. If possible, direct revascularization is our preferred strategy in cases of repeat revascularization as well, and we consider repeat revascularization in patients who have ongoing or new neurological symptoms [38].

American series have shown neurological complication rates of 3.5–13% per surgical hemisphere [11, 32, 34, 39–41], which is comparable to results reported in the Japanese literature utilizing mainly direct revascularization procedures [42, 43]. In our experience of over 1200 (predominantly direct) procedures, the 30-day major stroke risk was found to be 6.5%; this varied according to age with patients <18 years showing a 1.9%, 19–39 years a 4.8%, 40–59 years a 11.3%, and ≥ 60 a 15.0% major stroke rate.

A study of the US National Inpatient Sample examining all ECIC bypass procedures (4753) performed for MMD between 2002 and 2014 found perioperative rates of 3.8% ischemic or hemorrhagic stroke, 4.3% all neurological morbidity, and 0.3% mortality. The overall complication rate in this sample was 13.2% after cerebral bypass for MMD. This study did not stratify patients based on direct versus indirect bypass for MMD [15].

Mitigation of these risk factors can be achieved through several factors. High-volume surgical centers [17], specialized surgical teams, rigorous intra-operative and post-operative blood pressure control, intra-operative neuromonitoring [44], and possibly mild intra-operative hypothermia [45] are factors contributing to successful outcomes after revascularization surgery.

Studies have attempted to identify risk factors for predicting perioperative morbidity in cerebral revascularization for MMD. Sakamoto and colleagues found that a high frequency of preoperative TIA (>1–4/months; OR 4.8, $p = 0.01$) and indirect revascularization (OR 5.8, $p = 0.01$) were predictors of perioperative stroke risk, in a study of 368 revascularization procedures [42]. Frequent TIAs are a sign of cerebral hemodynamic instability and put the patient at higher risk of perioperative stroke in the setting of intra-operative hypercapnia or hypotension [46]. In our institutional experience, older age, angiographic severity of the disease, presence and acuity of previous infarcts on MRI, and status of the hemodynamic reserve were found to be associated with higher risk of perioperative stroke [47].

Additional syndromes associated with MMD have also been found to confer higher risk of perioperative morbidity. A study of patients with Down's syndrome-associated MMD reported a stroke risk of 12.5% perioperatively [48].

21.6 Outcomes

Cerebral revascularization for MMD has the goal of prevention of future ischemic or hemorrhagic events. American studies have generally shown reduced risk of stroke and TIA in surgically treated hemispheres. Several American studies of the long-term outcomes following cerebral revascularization are now available and are summarized in Table 21.1.

Our long-term MMD outcome data estimates the stroke risk to be 0.59%/patient year after bypass, over a mean follow-up duration of 7.3 years. The estimated mean stroke-free survival was 23.8 years. Favorable neurological outcomes were observed with regard to the mRS score after revascularization. While 25.6% of our patients had mRS 0–1 and 53.7% of patients mRS 2 preoperatively, at last follow-up (mean 7.3 years) 75% of patients had mRS 0–1, i.e. normal or with mild symptoms, but able to carry out all activities without limitations.

Most American studies report similarly successful long-term outcomes with revascularization in MMD.

In MMD patients presenting with intracranial hemorrhage, our results have been similarly successful. In a study of 104 MMD patients with 172 hemispheres revascularized (91.3% direct bypasses) and a mean follow-up of 5.1 years, 72.1% of patients had mRS 0–1 at last follow-up, compared to 66.3% of patients preoperatively. Eight patients had recurrent hemorrhages (7.7%), and there were 4 cases of mortality [51]. Our observed rates of recurrent hemorrhage are lower than the up-to 18% re-hemorrhage rates previously reported in the Japanese literature [52].

1.4% of patients in our institutional long-term series required repeat revascularization, predominantly for continuing ischemic symptoms. Repeat revascularization rates were 4% for indirect bypasses compared to 1% for direct bypasses, when stratified by initial revascularization procedure ($p = 0.03$). The mean time to repeat revascularization surgery was similar between indirect and direct bypass groups (48.8 and 47.4 months, respectively), and at a mean follow-up of 4.8 years, 81% of these patients had no further neurological events [38].

Neurocognitive outcomes following revascularization for MMD are scarcely reported in the literature. We studied neurocognitive performance using a structured battery of 13 tests in 84 MMD adult patients, at presentation and 6 months post-revascularization. In this cohort, 14% of patients showed statistically significant decline in cognition, while 11% improved, and 75% had unchanged cognitive status. These results did not vary in unilateral versus bilateral revascularization. This data shows stability of neurocognition post-bypass, but long-term studies are needed [53].

Table 21.1 Demographics, clinical presentation, procedures, and outcomes in American studies of moyamoya disease

Author	Year	Patients	Ethnicity	Sex (F)	Age (mean)	Presentation	Treatment	Mean Follow-up (yr)	Outcomes
Yilmaz et al. [49]	2001	19 (13 pediatric; 6 adults)	90% Caucasian; 10% African American	60%	Ped.: 8 Adult: 35	Ischemic: 100% ped. 86% adult;	STA-MCA bypass; EDAS; medical (38% ped.)	3	1 stroke in medical group; none in surgical groups; Mean mRS 2 (surgical) versus 1.8 (medical)
Scott et al. [23]	2004	143 (pediatric)	89% Caucasian; 11% Asian	62%	7.1	Ischemic: 67.8% Hemorrhagic: 2.8%	EDAS	5.1	11 post-op stroke (7.7%) 7 delayed neuro. events (5.6%) 71% mRS 0–1
Mesiwala et al. [39]	2008	39 (adult)	69% Caucasian; 31% Asian	77%	34	Ischemic: 85% Hemorrhagic: 13%	STA-MCA bypass: 91%; EDAS	3.6	3 post-op deaths (7.7%) 92% stable or improved functional status
Starke et al. [40]	2009	43 (adult)	65% Caucasian; 21% Asian	65%	40	Stroke: 60% TIA: 58% Hemorrhage: 2%	EDAS; + Burr holes in 35%	3.4	2 deaths (5%) 6 stroke (9%) 88% improved/ stable independence

Guzman et al. [11]	2009	329 (272 adult; 96 pediatric)	59% Caucasian; 32% Asian	70%	Ped: 10.1 Adult: 39.5	Ischemic: 57% adult; 51% ped. Hemorrhagic: 14.6% adult; 2.1% ped.	STA-MCA bypass: 97% adult; 68% ped.; EDAS	4.9	3% post-op stroke; 2.6% post-op hem 5.5% 5-year stroke risk 68% had improvement of 1–2 points on mRS; 71% improved QoL
Abla et al. [16]	2013	92 (68 adult; 24 pediatric)	N/A	71%	Ped: 10.6 Adult: 43.6(D)/40.3(I)	Ischemic: 33% ped.; 48%(D)/33%(I) adult	STA-MCA bypass: 29 adults, 4 peds; EDAS (39 adults; 20 peds)	2.1–3.9	2% ped.; 7.3% adult (D); 5.1% adult (I) post-op stroke 12.2% ped; 12.5% adult (D); 6.8% adult (I) delayed stroke Mean mRS: 1.29 ped.; 1.09 adult (D); 1.94 adult (I)
Lin et al. [50]	2014	36 (adult)	17% Asian	83%	27.5	Stroke: 67% TIA: 78% Hemorrhage: 8.3%	Pial synangiosis	5.8	1 death (3%) 3 stroke (8%) 91% mRS 0–2
Agarwalla et al. [32]	2014	37 (adult)	78% Caucasian; 3% Asian	81%	38	Stroke: 49% TIA: 35% Hemorrhage: 13.5%	EDAS	2.7	3 post-op strokes (6%) 3 delayed strokes (6%) 78% mRS 0–1

(continued)

Table 21.1 (continued)

Author	Year	Patients	Ethnicity	Sex (F)	Age (mean)	Presentation	Treatment	Mean Follow-up (yr)	Outcomes
Riordan et al. [34]	2019	59 (pediatric)	10% Asian	64%	6.2	Stoke: 73% TIA: 37% Hemorrhage: 3.4%	Pial synangiosis	20.6	6 deaths (10.%) 1 stroke (2%) 82% independent
Feghali et al. [41]	2019	85 (59 adults; 26 pediatric)	43% Caucasian; 27% Asian	71%	Ped.: 9 Adult: 40	Ischemic: 86% Hemorrhagic: 16.5%	14% direct; 63% indirect; 23% combined bypass	4.6	8% perioperative stroke 3% delayed stroke 88% mRS 0–2
Abhinav et al. [51]	2020	104	42% Caucasian; 45% Asian	66%	38	Hemorrhagic: 100%	STA-MCA bypass: 91% EDAS	5.1	1 perioperative ICH/death 3 perioperative stroke (2.9%) 7.7% re-hemorrhage rate 85% mRS 0–2
Stanford	2020	769 (564 adult; 205 pediatric)	53% Caucasian; 32% Asian	71%	Ped.: 11 Adult: 41	Ischemic: 83.2% adult; 79.5% peds Hemorrhagic: 15.2% adult; 7.3% ped.	STA-MCA bypass: 96% adult, 76% ped.; EDAS	7.3	75% mRS 0–1 6.5% 30-day risk of perioperative stroke 4% rate of long-term stroke

D direct bypass, *I* indirect bypass

21.7 Conclusions

MMD is rare in the American population; however, the diagnosis has been made more frequently in recent years, with increasing awareness of the disease. The Asian-American population has similar characteristics to those reported in the Asian literature in terms of disease presentation. Fewer US patients present with hemorrhagic MMD, but Asian-American populations show comparable rates to the Asian population. Cerebral revascularization remains the mainstay of treatment in the USA, and long-term outcomes of revascularization are quite favorable compared to the devastating natural clinical course of MMD.

References

1. Suzuki J, Takaku A. Cerebrovascular "moyamoya" disease. Disease showing abnormal net-like vessels in base of brain. Arch Neurol. 1969;20(3):288–99.
2. Achrol AS, Guzman R, Lee M, Steinberg GK. Pathophysiology and genetic factors in moyamoya disease. Neurosurg Focus. 2009;26(4):E4.
3. Kuroda S, Houkin K. Moyamoya disease: current concepts and future perspectives. Lancet Neurol. 2008;7(11):1056–66.
4. Takekawa Y, Umezawa T, Ueno Y, Sawada T, Kobayashi M. Pathological and immunohistochemical findings of an autopsy case of adult moyamoya disease. Neuropathology. 2004;24(3):236–42.
5. Weinberg DG, Arnaout OM, Rahme RJ, Aoun SG, Batjer HH, Bendok BR. Moyamoya disease: a review of histopathology, biochemistry, and genetics. Neurosurg Focus. 2011;30(6):E20.
6. Uchino K, Johnston SC, Becker KJ, Tirschwell DL. Moyamoya disease in Washington state and California. Neurology. 2005;65(6):956–8.
7. Starke RM, Crowley RW, Maltenfort M, Jabbour PM, Gonzalez LF, Tjoumakaris SI, et al. Moyamoya disorder in the United States. Neurosurgery. 2012;71(1):93–9.
8. Baba T, Houkin K, Kuroda S. Novel epidemiological features of moyamoya disease. J Neurol Neurosurg Psychiatry. 2008;79(8):900–4.
9. Kuriyama S, Kusaka Y, Fujimura M, Wakai K, Tamakoshi A, Hashimoto S, et al. Prevalence and clinicoepidemiological features of moyamoya disease in Japan: findings from a nationwide epidemiological survey. Stroke. 2008;39(1):42–7.
10. Graham JF. Matoba a. a survey of moyamoya disease in Hawaii. Clin Neurol Neurosurg. 1997;99(Suppl 2):S31–5.
11. Guzman R, Lee M, Achrol A, Bell-Stephens T, Kelly M, Do HM, et al. Clinical outcome after 450 revascularization procedures for moyamoya disease. Clinical article. J Neurosurg. 2009;111(5):927–35.
12. Feghali J, Xu R, Yang W, Liew J, Tamargo RJ, Marsh EB, et al. Racial phenotypes in moyamoya disease: a comparative analysis of clinical presentation and natural history in a single multiethnic cohort of 250 hemispheres. J Neurosurg. 2019:1–7.
13. Chiu D, Shedden P, Bratina P, Grotta JC. Clinical features of moyamoya disease in the United States. Stroke. 1998;29(7):1347–51.
14. Hallemeier CL, Rich KM, Grubb RL Jr, Chicoine MR, Moran CJ, Cross DT 3rd, et al. Clinical features and outcome in north American adults with moyamoya phenomenon. Stroke. 2006;37(6):1490–6.
15. Winkler EA, Yue JK, Deng H, Raygor KP, Phelps RRL, Rutledge C, et al. National trends in cerebral bypass surgery in the United States, 2002–2014. Neurosurg Focus. 2019;46(2):E4.
16. Abla AA, Gandhoke G, Clark JC, Oppenlander ME, Velat GJ, Zabramski JM, et al. Surgical outcomes for moyamoya angiopathy at barrow neurological institute with comparison of adult

indirect encephaloduroarteriosynangiosis bypass, adult direct superficial temporal artery-to-middle cerebral artery bypass, and pediatric bypass: 154 revascularization surgeries in 140 affected hemispheres. Neurosurgery. 2013;73(3):430–9.
17. Titsworth WL, Scott RM, Smith ER. National Analysis of 2454 pediatric Moyamoya admissions and the effect of hospital volume on outcomes. Stroke. 2016;47(5):1303–11.
18. Bao XY, Duan L, Yang WZ, Li DS, Sun WJ, Zhang ZS, et al. Clinical features, surgical treatment, and long-term outcome in pediatric patients with moyamoya disease in China. Cerebrovasc Dis. 2015;39(2):75–81.
19. Mineharu Y, Takenaka K, Yamakawa H, Inoue K, Ikeda H, Kikuta KI, et al. Inheritance pattern of familial moyamoya disease: autosomal dominant mode and genomic imprinting. J Neurol Neurosurg Psychiatry. 2006;77(9):1025–9.
20. Gaillard J, Klein J, Duran D, Storey A, Scott RM, Kahle K, et al. Incidence, clinical features, and treatment of familial moyamoya in pediatric patients: a single-institution series. J Neurosurg Pediatr. 2017;19(5):553–9.
21. Ikezaki K, Han DH, Kawano T, Inamura T, Fukui M. Epidemiological survey of moyamoya disease in Korea. Clin Neurol Neurosurg. 1997;99(Suppl 2):S6–10.
22. Guzman R, Khan N, Steinberg GK. Moyamoya disease in North America. In: Moyamoya disease update [Internet]. Tokyo: Springer; 2010.
23. Scott RM, Smith JL, Robertson RL, Madsen JR, Soriano SG, Rockoff MA. Long-term outcome in children with moyamoya syndrome after cranial revascularization by pial synangiosis. J Neurosurg. 2004;100(2 Suppl Pediatrics):142–9.
24. Iwama T, Yoshimura S. Present status of Moyamoya disease in Japan. Acta Neurochir Suppl. 2008;103:115–8.
25. Seol HJ, Wang KC, Kim SK, Hwang YS, Kim KJ, Cho BK. Headache in pediatric moyamoya disease: review of 204 consecutive cases. J Neurosurg. 2005;103(5 Suppl):439–42.
26. Olesen J, Friberg L, Olsen TS, Andersen AR, Lassen NA, Hansen PE, et al. Ischaemia-induced (symptomatic) migraine attacks may be more frequent than migraine-induced ischaemic insults. Brain. 1993;116(Pt 1):187–202.
27. Park-Matsumoto YC, Tazawa T, Shimizu J. Migraine with aura-like headache associated with moyamoya disease. Acta Neurol Scand. 1999;100(2):119–21.
28. Kuroda S, Hashimoto N, Yoshimoto T, Iwasaki Y. Research committee on Moyamoya disease in J. radiological findings, clinical course, and outcome in asymptomatic moyamoya disease: results of multicenter survey in Japan. Stroke. 2007;38(5):1430–5.
29. Kuroda S, Ishikawa T, Houkin K, Nanba R, Hokari M, Iwasaki Y. Incidence and clinical features of disease progression in adult moyamoya disease. Stroke. 2005;36(10):2148–53.
30. Church EW, Bell-Stephens TE, Bigder MG, Gummidipundi S, Han SS, Steinberg GK. Clinical course of unilateral Moyamoya disease. Neurosurgery. 2020; https://doi.org/10.1093/neuros/nyaa293.
31. Veeravagu A, Guzman R, Patil CG, Hou LC, Lee M, Steinberg GK. Moyamoya disease in pediatric patients: outcomes of neurosurgical interventions. Neurosurg Focus. 2008;24(2):E16.
32. Agarwalla PK, Stapleton CJ, Phillips MT, Walcott BP, Venteicher AS, Ogilvy CS. Surgical outcomes following encephaloduroarteriosynangiosis in north American adults with moyamoya. J Neurosurg. 2014;121(6):1394–400.
33. Gonzalez NR, Dusick JR, Connolly M, Bounni F, Martin NA, Van de Wiele B, et al. Encephaloduroarteriosynangiosis for adult intracranial arterial steno-occlusive disease: long-term single-center experience with 107 operations. J Neurosurg. 2015;123(3):654–61.
34. Riordan CP, Storey A, Cote DJ, Smith ER, Scott RM. Results of more than 20 years of follow-up in pediatric patients with moyamoya disease undergoing pial synangiosis. J Neurosurg Pediatr. 2019:1–7.
35. Yu J, Shi L, Guo Y, Xu B, Xu K. Progress on complications of direct bypass for Moyamoya disease. Int J Med Sci. 2016;13(8):578–87.
36. Nielsen TH, Abhinav K, Sussman ES, Han SS, Weng Y, Bell-Stephens T, et al. Direct versus indirect bypass procedure for the treatment of ischemic moyamoya disease: results of an individualized selection strategy. J Neurosurg. 2020:1–12.

37. Teo MK, Madhugiri VS, Steinberg GK. Editorial: direct versus indirect bypass for moyamoya disease: ongoing controversy. J Neurosurg. 2017;126(5):1520–2.
38. Teo M, Johnson J, Steinberg GK. Strategies for and outcome of repeat revascularization surgery for Moyamoya disease: an American institutional series. Neurosurgery. 2017;81(5):852–9.
39. Mesiwala AH, Sviri G, Fatemi N, Britz GW, Newell DW. Long-term outcome of superficial temporal artery-middle cerebral artery bypass for patients with moyamoya disease in the US. Neurosurg Focus. 2008;24(2):E15.
40. Starke RM, Komotar RJ, Hickman ZL, Paz YE, Pugliese AG, Otten ML, et al. Clinical features, surgical treatment, and long-term outcome in adult patients with moyamoya disease. Clinical article. J Neurosurg. 2009;111(5):936–42.
41. Feghali J, Xu R, Yang W, Liew J, Tamargo RJ, Marsh EB, et al. Differing surgical outcomes in a multiethnic cohort suggest racial phenotypes in Moyamoya disease. World Neurosurg. 2019;128:e865–e72.
42. Sakamoto H, Kitano S, Yasui T, Komiyama M, Nishikawa M, Iwai Y, et al. Direct extracranial-intracranial bypass for children with moyamoya disease. Clin Neurol Neurosurg. 1997;99(Suppl 2):S128–33.
43. Fujimura M, Kaneta T, Tominaga T. Efficacy of superficial temporal artery-middle cerebral artery anastomosis with routine postoperative cerebral blood flow measurement during the acute stage in childhood moyamoya disease. Childs Nerv Syst. 2008;24(7):827–32.
44. Lopez JR. Neurophysiologic intraoperative monitoring of pediatric cerebrovascular surgery. J Clin Neurophysiol. 2009;26(2):85–94.
45. Choi R, Andres RH, Steinberg GK, Guzman R. Intraoperative hypothermia during vascular neurosurgical procedures. Neurosurg Focus. 2009;26(5):E24.
46. Iwama T, Hashimoto N, Yonekawa Y. The relevance of hemodynamic factors to perioperative ischemic complications in childhood moyamoya disease. Neurosurgery. 1996;38(6):1120–5. discussion 5–6
47. Teo M, Furtado S, Kaneko OF, Azad TD, Madhugiri V, Do HM, et al. Validation and application for the Berlin grading system of Moyamoya disease in adult patients. Neurosurgery. 2020;86(2):203–12.
48. Jea A, Smith ER, Robertson R, Scott RM. Moyamoya syndrome associated with down syndrome: outcome after surgical revascularization. Pediatrics. 2005;116(5):e694–701.
49. Yilmaz EY, Pritz MB, Bruno A, Lopez-Yunez A, Moyamoya BJ. Indiana university medical center experience. Arch Neurol. 2001;58(8):1274–8.
50. Lin N, Aronson JP, Manjila S, Smith ER, Scott RM. Treatment of Moyamoya disease in the adult population with pial synangiosis. J Neurosurg. 2014;120(3):612–7.
51. Abhinav K, Furtado SV, Nielsen TH, Iyer A, Gooderham PA, Teo M, et al. Functional outcomes after revascularization procedures in patients with hemorrhagic Moyamoya disease. Neurosurgery. 2020;86(2):257–65.
52. Ikezaki K, Inamura T, Kawano T, Fukui M. Clinical features of probable moyamoya disease in Japan. Clin Neurol Neurosurg. 1997;99(Suppl 2):S173–7.
53. Zeifert PD, Karzmark P, Bell-Stephens TE, Steinberg GK, Dorfman LJ. Neurocognitive performance after cerebral revascularization in adult Moyamoya disease. Stroke. 2017;48(6):1514–7.

Long-Term Outcome in China

22

Ni Wei, Yu Lei, Han-Qiang Jiang, Yu-Xiang Gu, and Ying Mao

Abstract

Moyamoya disease (MMD) is not rarely detected in China. Currently, more than 50 neurosurgical institutions and 200 neurosurgeons are engaging in treating this complicated vascular disorder. In this chapter, we retrospectively reviewed the demographic data, clinical features, surgical strategies, and long-term outcomes of patients based on the literatures published by Chinese neurosurgical centers. In China, large national epidemiologic studies are still required. The largest series showed that the median age for the onset of symptoms was 30.36 years with the highest peak detection rate at 35–45 years of age and a smaller peak at 5–9 years of age. The disease occurred mainly in the Han people and was rarely seen in minority ethnicity. Treating modalities include direct bypass, indirect bypass, and combined bypass. Multimodal neuroimaging guided bypass surgery is also developing in some qualified centers. Based on Chinese reports, revascularization can help prevent further ischemic and hemorrhagic attacks. It can also improve the cognitive function in patients with cognitive impairment. Indirect bypass showed encouraging effect in pediatric patients. Although MMD is not rare in China, the management has not reached a consensus. More randomized controlled trials are needed to update the concepts and future perspectives in MMD.

Keywords

Moyamoya disease · China · Combined revascularization · Modified revascularization · Long-term outcome · Cognitive status

N. Wei · Y. Lei · H.-Q. Jiang · Y.-X. Gu · Y. Mao (✉)
Department of Neurosurgery, Huashan Hospital, Fudan University, Shanghai, China
e-mail: hsniwei@fudan.edu.cn; maoying@fudan.edu.cn

S. Kuroda (ed.), *Moyamoya Disease: Current Knowledge and Future Perspectives*, https://doi.org/10.1007/978-981-33-6404-2_22

22.1 Introduction

Moyamoya disease (MMD) is an uncommon chronic cerebrovascular disease characterized by an unusual vascular network at the base of the brain caused by progressive stenosis or occlusion of the supraclinoid internal carotid artery (ICA) and its main branches around the circle of Willis [1]. To the author's knowledge, MMD appears to be relatively rare in Western countries. In Asia, however, it is a common cause of stroke in patients younger than 50 years. With the development of non-invasive imaging modalities, more and more cases of MMD have been detected in China [2]. Accordingly, more than 50 neurosurgical institutions and 200 neurosurgeons are engaging in treating this complicated vascular disorder. In the past 20 years, Chinese neurosurgeons have gained rich experience on the clinical characteristics, natural history, and long-term outcome. Based on our experience, we published *Expert Consensus on Moyamoya in China* in 2015 to guide the diagnosis and treatment. In the recent years, great progress has been made on both basic studies and clinical practices for MMD. In this chapter, we retrospectively reviewed the demographic data, clinical features, surgical strategies, and long-term outcomes of patients based on the literatures published by Chinese neurosurgical centers.

22.2 Epidemiology

22.2.1 General Epidemiology

The epidemiological characteristics of MMD show obvious regional differences. The incidence of MMD is high in East Asia and low in other regions [3]. In China, large national epidemiologic studies are still required. A single-center study summarized the epidemiological characteristics of MMD in Nanjing, China [2]. In this study, an increasing incidence rate of MMD was observed during the period of 2000–2007, with an average detection rate of 0.43 cases per 100,000 persons/year (prevalence 3.92/100,000 persons). The incidence of ischemia associated with the disease was 0.16 cases/100,000 people-years and the incidence of hemorrhage was 0.22 cases/100,000 people-years. A population-based study in Taiwan province showed that during the 12-year period, 422 patients were identified in Taiwan, representing an annual incidence of 0.15/100,000 person-years [4].

Recently, a single-center report of a cohort including 4128 patients in China with MMD [5] showed that the median age for the onset of symptoms was 30.36 years. The age distribution of patients with MMD was bimodal, with the highest peak detection rate at 35–45 years of age and a smaller peak at 5–9 years of age. The ratio of female-to-male patients was 1:1. The disease occurred mainly in the Han people and was rarely seen in minority ethnicity. In our cohort, transient ischemic attack was the most common initial clinical manifestation (48.13%). The other initial manifestations included infarction (22.62%), hemorrhage (16.45%), and headache 230/4128 (5.57%). In north and northeast China, the ischemic type was more predominated while the hemorrhagic type was relatively rare. However, the percentage of hemorrhagic type in East China was higher than anywhere else in China.

22.2.2 Genetic Epidemiology

A high incidence of MMD has been reported in some ethnic groups and pedigrees, suggesting that genetic factors may be involved. In recent years, there have been more and more studies on genetic epidemiology of MMD. RNF213 gene located on chromosome 17q25.3 is a susceptibility gene for MMD in East Asian population, and c.14429G > A (p.R4810K or rs112735431) is particularly relevant to the occurrence and development of MMD [6–9].

Domestic genetic research on MMD is also being carried out. In one study by Li et al., polymorphisms of the MATRIX metalloproteinase 3 gene at 1171 loci were found to be closely associated with MMD. Another study carried out by Wu Z et al [10] concluded that RNF213 mutations are associated with MMD susceptibility in Han Chinese. The ischemic type MMD is particularly related to the R4810K mutation. A4399T is also a susceptible variant for MMD, primarily associated with hemorrhage. A recent study from Wang Y et al. involving 1385 Chinese patients with MMD and 2903 normal control showed an trend that the carrying rate of p.R4810K gradually decreased when moving from coastal cities in northeast, north, and east China to southern cities or inland areas; higher frequencies of p.R4810K were observed in patients with MMD compared with control participants (odds ratio, 48.1; 95% confidence interval, 29.1–79.6; = 1.6 × 10) [11].

A recent Meta-Analysis demonstrated that the fixed-effect odds ratios (95% CI) in allelic model of MMP-2 rs243865 were 0.60 (0.41–0.88) ($P = 0.008$) [12]. In the country-based subgroup analysis, the fixed-effect odds ratios (95% CI) of RNF213 rs112735431 in allelic model were China, 39.74 (26.63–59.31), Japan, 74.65 (42.79–130.24), and Korea, 50.04 (28.83–86.88; all $P < 0.00001$). In the sensitivity analysis, the fixed-effect odds ratios (95% CI) of allelic and dominant models were the rs148731719 variant, 2.17 (1.36–3.48; =0.001), 2.20 (1.35–3.61; =0.002), the rs8179090 variant, 0.33 (0.25–0.43; <0.00001), 0.88 (0.65–1.21; =0.440), and the rs3025058 variant, 0.61 (0.47–0.79; =0.0002), 0.55 (0.41–0.75; =0.0001), respectively.

In general, although China has a high incidence of MMD, the epidemiological researches on MMD in China are still regional based. There is still a lack of national epidemiological studies of MMD in China.

22.3 Treating Modality

22.3.1 Revascularization

Surgical treatment is the most effective method to restore the blood supply and increase cerebral perfusion in order to prevent secondary stroke for ischemic MMD and stabilize hemodynamics to prevent bleeding [13, 14]. In surgical practice, revascularization including direct, indirect, and combined bypass surgery is often applied. Bypass surgery is more effective than conservative treatment to prevent future strokes [15].

22.3.2 Varied Kinds of Revascularization

Direct revascularization via an anastomosis of the superficial temporal artery to middle cerebral artery (STA-MCA bypass) has been the most common procedure that mainly addresses the MCA territory and supports the anterior cerebral artery (ACA) territory via leptomeningeal anastomoses. Particularly, Tong et al. from Tianjin Huanhu Hospital reported the application of occipital artery to vertebral artery bypass for the treatment of posterior circulation ischemia [5]. Furthermore, large caliber grafts might provide a fallback strategy in some cases. A saphenous vein graft for high-flow bypass or radial artery graft for intermediate-flow bypass has also been reported. However, potential risk of hyperperfusion needs to be concerned in such techniques. According to the previous study, the anastomosis patency rate of direct bypass was more than 88% in long-term angiographic follow-up. Multiple literatures have confirmed that direct revascularization is more effective in preventing recurrent ischemic strokes for adult ischemic-type MMD [16, 17]. While direct bypass is challenging in children where bypass patency rates have been reported to be lower. Meanwhile, the presence of hemorrhage and dilated anterior choroidal artery for some MMD may result in poor postoperative collateral formation [15].

Indirect revascularization relies on neovascularization of the cortical surface via angiogenic mechanisms from pedicle-based grafts like pial and temporal muscle, which is generally easier to perform but hemodynamic effects may take months to develop and less predictable. After indirect bypass surgery, arterial neoangiogenesis development can be observed within 6 months. And interestingly, the growth of veins might continue after 6 months [17]. Previous study confirmed that indirect bypass surgery could provide encouraging long-term improvement in clinical outcome and prevention of recurrent stroke in children with MMD. Duan et al. from 307th Hospital of PLA have also proved that encephalo-duro-arterio-synangiosis (EDAS) was beneficial for patients with hemorrhagic MMD during long-term follow-up [5]. Multiple burr hole technique was also underlined in pediatric MMD, resulting in good collateral revascularization, which can improve cerebral perfusion with low perioperative risk. In addition, many literatures analyzed patients with MMD treated with omental transposition or transplantation with 98% improvement in cerebral revascularization. Due to the variety of indirect techniques, it still remains unknown which of these techniques is superior [15, 16]. Although indirect bypass is easier to perform, the hemodynamic alteration may take months to develop and is less predictable in terms of clinical outcome. Notably, the cerebrovascular plasticity in patients with MMD seems to be age dependent, from which indirect revascularization may show a lower stroke protective effect in adult MMD patients.

Combined revascularization includes the direct bypass and the indirect bypass, which aims at immediate and further hemodynamic improvement [16]. Multiple literatures have confirmed that combined revascularization would be the best choice to prevent not only ischemic events but hemorrhagic stroke by improving anterior choroidal artery-posterior communicating artery dilation and extension [18]. Besides, combined revascularization may improve cognitive function for MMD patients with the evidence of postsurgical brain functional imaging. Different neurosurgical centers may choose various kinds of incisions according to the distribution of STA and cortical branches of MCA. For example, procedures in Beijing Xuanwu hospital and Wuhan Zhongnan hospital are generally performed with straight cut. Meanwhile, pterional approach is preferred in Huashan hospital and Henan Provincial hospital. Similarly, different combination of direct and indirect bypass is applied in different hospital like STA-MCA bypass and EDMS, STA-MCA bypass and EDMAPS, STA-MCA bypass and EDAS, etc. However, postoperative hyperperfusion syndrome (HPS) such as aphasia, epileptic seizures and even new cerebral hemorrhage or ischemia are experienced frequently in the acute phase after such combined revascularization [5]. Thus, the selection of recipient vessels is still controversial and hemodynamic changes after revascularization have not been revealed. Some studies revealed that direct anastomoses to parasylvian cortical arteries with antegrade from the MCA had a high risk of postoperative HPS.

22.3.3 Modified Revascularization

Although surgical revascularization is the most successful treatment to improve cerebral perfusion and decrease the incidence of recurrent stroke events, postoperative complications such as hyperperfusion syndrome, cerebral infarction, and epilepsy are still common due to hemodynamic abnormalities [19]. Previous studies confirmed that the redistribution of cerebral perfusion and hemodynamic remodeling effect (i.e., water shift phenomenon) are highly suspected factors to explain such situation. Furthermore, the choice of recipient vessel is always based on the experience from operators with lacking objective evidence [20]. As the development and application of advanced neuroimaging evaluation, modified method of operation can be achieved based on multimodal neuro-information to help choose appropriate recipient artery for the purpose of reducing the risk of postoperative complications [21]. According to the pathogenesis of MMD, factors including angioarchitecture, global and regional perfusion status, and electrical activity of neurons need to be involved for precise bypass. It is generally accepted that digital subtraction angiography (DSA) could reflect the distribution and structural characteristics of cerebral arteries with high spatial resolution. Both arterial spin labeling (ASL) and positron emission tomography (PET) could evaluate the cerebral perfusion and metabolism level. Electroencephalogram (EEG) and electrocorticogram (ECoG) can imply the functional connections and regional neuronal activities of brain. All these factors could be taken into consideration to clarify hypoperfusion cortical area and localize optional recipient arteries in such modified bypass surgery [22]. Varies kinds of neuro-information can be integrated in neuro-navigating system and projected into the surgical area under microscope via augmented reality (AR) technique intraoperatively. After fully exposion of surgical area, regional hemodynamic status based on indocyanine green angiography (ICG-FLOW800) and neuron electronic activities from ECoG could be achieved and compared among optional arteries. All the information can be evaluated for surgical decision making to choose the appropriate

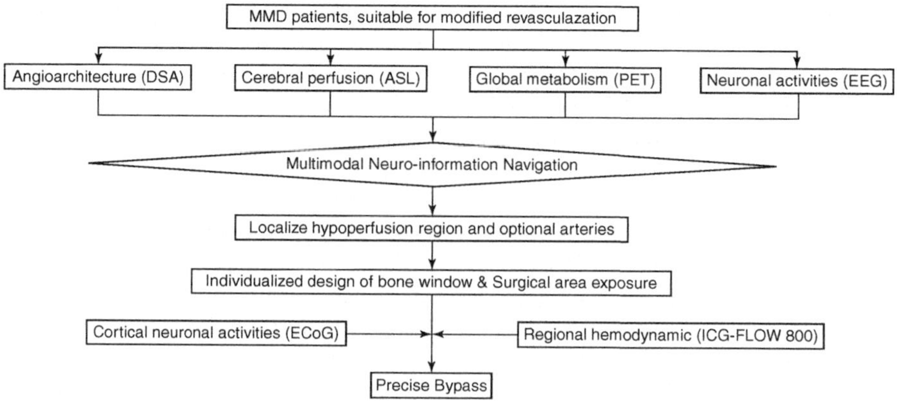

Fig. 22.1 The flowchart of precise revascularization for MMD in Huashan Hospital, Fudan University

artery. After anastomosis, regional blood flow and neuron electronic level can be compared with before to confirm the effectiveness of bypass and monitor abnormal wave of cerebral cortex, which may be helpful to distinct patients with high risk of HPS and adapt postoperative medication. Such kind of multimodal neuroimaging guided bypass surgery was first reported in Huashan hospital and the clinical outcome was improved (Fig. 22.1).

22.4 Ischemic Moyamoya Disease in China and Its Long-Term Outcomes

22.4.1 Cognitive Status of MMD in China

Cognitive impairment of MMD can be traced back to 1990, when Sato et al. reported 13 pediatric MMD with cognitive impairment in Japan [23]. In China, the first published MMD with cognitive impairment was reported in a Master's thesis in 2008. Interestingly, the 8 patients with cognitive impairment were also children less than 5 years old.

Cognitive impairment of Chinese adult MMD has been assessed by neuropsychological testing. He et al. reported that as compared with healthy subjects, asymptomatic patients with MMD exhibited varying degrees of deficits in the intelligence, spatial imagination, working memory, and computational ability [19]. Furthermore, patients with history of stroke had more severe impairment in word short-term memory and complex arithmetic. Referring to pediatric MMD, Li et al. recruited 21 patients, and found that 15 (71.4%) patients showed various degrees of cognitive impairment [15]. Considering as a kind of vascular cognitive impairment (VCI), cognitive impairment of MMD is also studied in accordance with the AHA/ASA statement of VCI, in which the four cognitive domains of attention/executive function, memory, language, and visual-spatial function should be studied [24]. Lei et al. revealed that the attention/executive function was severely impaired by using the neuropsychological testing of both the Trail Making Test Part B and the executive subtests of Memory and Executive Screening [17]. In addition, Fang et al. adopted 5 typical executive function tests, and the ischemic MMD exhibited worse working memory and poorer sustained attention than the hemorrhagic MMD [25].

In a single-center review of Huashan hospital, 45% (28–58% in different provinces) of the 466 adult patients with MMD who received neuropsychological testing were with VCI. Besides, the mild VCI accounted for more than half of the whole cohort. In addition, based on this single-center data, the numbers of patients with deficits of memory was similar with that of patients with attention/executive function impairment. This conclusion is different from the features of VCI summarized by the AHA/ASA [24], which is characterized as primary attention/executive function deficits. We hypothesize that the features of VCI in MMD are due to its unique and complicated hemodynamic disturbances, in which, frontal, parietal, and temporal hypoperfusion have no fixed patterns.

The electroencephalogram (EEG) is also a sensitive measurement to evaluate cognitive status of healthy and diseased brain [26]. The EEG characteristics of adult MMD have been investigated by authors of this chapter. We found that although ischemic and hemorrhagic MMD share some similarities in EEG metrics, they are totally different in electrophysiological processes. This information is very helpful not only in understanding the MMD, but also in developing a sensitive tool to investigate the VCI of ischemic cerebrovascular diseases.

22.4.2 Long-Term Outcomes of Ischemic MMD in China

22.4.2.1 Overall Outcomes

There are still rare data of long-term outcomes in Chinese patients with ischemic MMD. In one cohort reported by Duan et al., the follow-up period was 26.3 months, and the stroke risk was 10.1% at 2 years and 12.7% at 5 years after surgery [22]. In another cohort, Bao et al. reported the long-term outcomes of ischemic MMD after the indirect bypass surgery, and results showed that after 141.4 months, the permanent morbidity rate were 1.2%/operation and 2.0%/person [5]. The annual rates of stroke were 0.73%/person/year. And the actuarial stroke of 1/5/10 years was 2.1%, 6.8%, and 8.9%, respectively. Besides, Yu et al. involved 346 patients with ischemic MMD and followed up for 4 years. They reported that the annual subsequent stroke rate beyond 30 days after surgery was 1.2% [27].

Referring to pediatric ischemic MMD, Zhao et al. reported a cohort of 223 pediatric patients with MMD, among which, 34 patients received direct bypass and 104 patients received indirect bypass [17]. After a mean follow-up period of 71.9 months for the direct bypass group and 60.2 months for the indirect bypass group, the direct bypass group showed a longer stroke-free time. Besides, good neurological outcome was noted in 32 (94.1%) of the direct bypass group, and 34 (100%) of the indirect bypass group. Furthermore, both groups exhibited a significant decreased MRS score at last follow-up than at admission.

22.4.2.2 Neurocognitive and Neuroimaging Outcomes

In a fMRI study of Huashan hospital, Lei et al. followed the cognitive function and fMRI changes 6 months after direct bypass surgery [17]. Results showed that only the left PCu, bilateral PCC, and right DLPFC presented with significant postoperative ALFF changes (Fig. 22.2). Furthermore, the follow-up changes (△) of the hemodynamics, ALFF, and executive function (MES-EX scores) were calculated and compared based on brain lobes. Results showed that only the right frontal lobe exhibited significant positive correlations between postoperative radiological changes and cognitive improvement. Thus, the right DLPFC was noted to be the only node which met all the above standards. Therefore, we concluded that the nodal changes of the right DLPFC might be the primary marker for predicting postoperative cognitive improvement, while the nodal changes of the left PCu and bilateral PCC may act as autoregulation to topological changes.

Lu et al. involved 683 surgically treated patients with ischemic MMD and investigated their possibility of hemorrhagic transformation (HT) during the follow-up [19]. Results showed that the HT only accounted for 4.3% of all patients, and the normal cerebral perfusion (CT perfusion) was recognized as a factor associated with HT through multivariate analysis. They concluded that recognition of HT might contribute to an improved outcome in adult ischemic MMD.

Interestingly, Ge et al. included 188 bypass procedures and followed for an averaged 18 months. They noted that postoperative collateral formation was

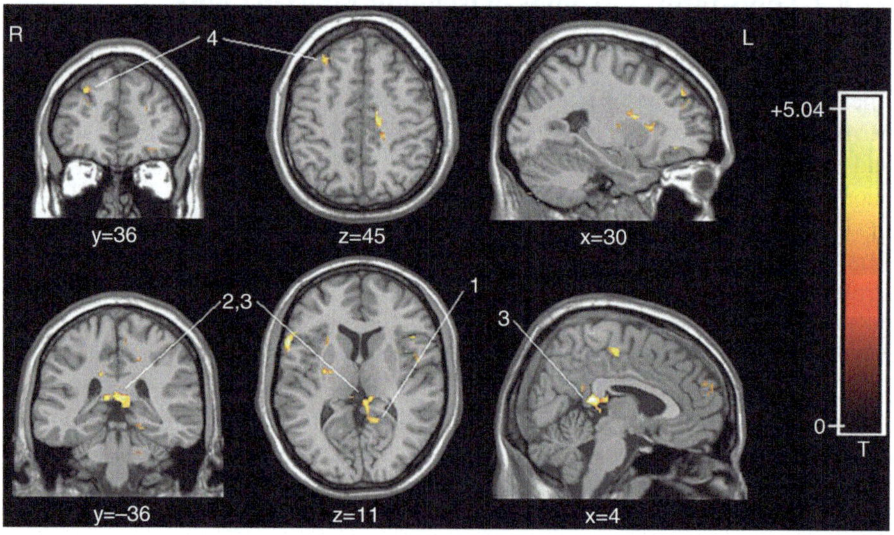

Fig. 22.2 The paired-sample t-test shows the regions with significant ALFF changes after cerebral revascularization. The left precuneus (1), bilateral posterior cingulate cortex (2), and right dorso-lateral prefrontal cortex (3) were generated

associated with the patency of the anastomosis [15]. Besides, the older age and presence of hemorrhage were both associated with poor postoperative collateral formation.

In conclusion, the long-term outcomes of ischemic stroke in MMD are still unclear, especially in China. More studies and clinics are needed to get involved in the study of ischemic MMD and its long-term outcomes.

22.5 Long-Term Outcomes in Hemorrhagic MMD

22.5.1 Natural History of Hemorrhagic MMD in China

Recently, Kang et al. reported the natural history of hemorrhagic MMD, and the risk factors for rebleeding [28]. A total of 128 conservatively treated patients with hemorrhagic MMD and complete follow-up data were included. After a median follow-up time of 10.1 years, 47 (36.7%) patients experienced 59 rebleeding episodes, rendering an average annual incidence of 4.5%. Among them, 9 patients (19.1%) died and 12 patients had severe disability. The cumulative rebleeding rate was 7.8% at 5 years, 22.6% at 10 years, and 35.9% at 15 years. Multivariate analysis showed that smoking was an independent risk factor for rebleeding. The results revealed that rebleeding was common and the main cause of deaths or severe disability in patients with hemorrhagic MMD. Furthermore, the risk of rebleeding increased and neurological function deteriorated during long-term follow-up. Much earlier, Liu et al. reported the long-term results of 43 conservatively managed patients [29]. After a median follow-up of 7.1 years, 17 of 43 (37.1%) patients experienced rebleeding. In summary, the natural history of hemorrhagic MMD was similar with that in other countries, showing a high rebleeding rate and a poor outcome during long-term follow-up.

22.5.2 Long-Term Outcome of Surgically Treated Hemorrhagic MMD in China

22.5.2.1 Direct Revascularization

Direct revascularization often referred to superficial temporal artery to middle cerebral artery (STA-MCA) bypass. The anterior or posterior branch of STA was dissected and sutured to the cortical branch of MCA by end-to-side anastomosis. In China, the long-term outcomes of direct revascularization for hemorrhagic MMD almostly demonstrated the safety and efficacy of preventing rebleeding. Recently, Kang et al. recruited 312 patients (319 hemispheres) with hemorrhagic MMD, including 186 hemispheres (58.3%) with direct revascularization and 133 hemispheres (41.7%) with indirect revascularization [30]. The result showed that direct revascularization was superior to indirect revascularization for prevention of rebleeding. The regression of original collaterals and establishment of revascularization collaterals after revascularization were more significant in hemispheres with direct revascularization than those with indirect revascularization. Earlier, Liu et al. described the long-term outcomes of patients with hemorrhagic MMD treated with direct revascularization [29]. 44 patients were included in this study; only 3 patients (6.8%) experienced rebleeding during a median follow-up time of 39 months. The results revealed that direct revascularization could improve cerebral perfusion and had a positive impact in preventing rebleeding in patients with hemorrhagic MMD.

22.5.2.2 Indirect Revascularization

Encephalodurosynangiosis (EDAS) was a common indirect revascularization modality for hemorrhagic MMD in China. However, the long-term outcomes of EDAS for hemorrhagic MMD were uncertain. Recently, Zhang et al. reported the long-term outcomes of 44 patients with hemorrhagic MMD receiving EDAS, revealing that EDAS could reduce the risk of rebleeding [22]. Ge et al. also used EDAS for hemorrhagic MMD and investigated the postoperative collateral formation after indirect bypass for hemorrhagic MMD [19]. The results revealed that anterior hemorrhage was significantly related to good postoperative collateral formation after indirect bypass. Wang et al. recently reviewed 95 patients with hemorrhagic MMD who were treated with EDAS [5]. After a median follow-up duration of 8.5 years, 16 of 95 patients (16.8%) suffered from rebleeding. The annual rebleeding rate was 2.2% per person per year. The results revealed that EDAS proved beneficial for patients with hemorrhagic MMD. However, there were also negative results. Recently, Kang et al. retrospectively collected patients with hemorrhagic MMD, including 133 hemispheres with indirect revascularization [30]. The result of indirect revascularization was inferior to direct revascularization. Furthermore, the risk of postoperative rebleeding was higher in those with indirect revascularization.

22.5.2.3 Combined Revascularization

In general, the long-term outcomes of combined revascularization for hemorrhagic MMD in China showed the efficacy in terms of preventing rebleeding. Recently, Zhao et al. compared the 5-year prognosis of combined STA-MCA bypass and EDAS and EDAS alone in hemorrhagic MMD [22]. 123 patients were included in this study, with 79 patients receiving combined STA-MCA bypass and EDAS, 44 patients receiving EDAS alone. The results revealed that both combined revascularization and EDAS alone could reduce the risk of rebleeding in hemorrhagic MMD. However, combined revascularization was found to be superior to EDAS alone in terms of preventing rebleeding. Jiang et al. prospectively recruited 113 patients with hemorrhagic MMD, who received combined STA-MCA bypass and EDMS [31]. The medium follow-up results demonstrated that annual rebleeding rate was 1.87%/person/year, combined revascularization provided a benefit over conservative therapy for hemorrhagic MMD. The 5-year long-term follow-up results also revealed that combined revascularization surgery might help prevent ipsilateral rebleeding [18].

22.6 Long-Term Outcomes in Pediatric MMD

MMD is the most important cause of stroke or transient ischemic attack (TIA) in pediatric patients, especially in East Asian countries. However, the epidemiological features of pediatric MMD in china are still unknown. Prof. Duan retrospectively analyzed 802 patients with MMD in china and found the percentage of patients younger than 10 years was lower than patients older than age 18 years(26.9% vs 61.6%) [22]. An epidemiological study in Taiwan showed the incidence of pediatric MMD was 0.2 /100,000, which was higher than in adult population (0.14/100,000) [4]. Therefore, the epidemiological data on children with MMD in China was still lacked and a national epidemiological study of pediatric MMD in China was urgent needed. It is well known that there are two age peaks of incidence in MMD (at about 10 years and 30–40 years old) [3]. An epidemiological study on the area of Nanjing demonstrated that the age peak of MMD incidence rate in patients age less than 18 in child was at 5–9 years of age [2], which was almost the same as in Taiwan, Japan, and South Korea. In addition, the sex ratio of pediatric MMD patients was 1:1 in China, which was varied from Japan and South Korea.

Most pediatric patients with MMD present with ischemic symptoms, such as TIA and cerebral infarction, while adults present with both hemorrhagic and ischemic manifestations at almost equal proportion. About 61.4% pediatric MMD patients present with TIA initially [32] and recurrent TIAs can result in subsequent stroke. The incidence of pediatric hemorrhagic MMD was reported to be 4.2–10.5% in China [32, 33], which was low compared with adults (14%) [22]. Previous studies also demonstrated that the symptoms of headaches and seizures are more common in pediatric patients with MMD than in adults. A Chinese cohort study included 288 pediatric patients with MMD showed the incidence of initial symptom of headache and seizure was 12.8% and 2%, respectively [32]. In addition, cognitive dysfunction is a specific symptom of pediatric patients with MMD and many children presented with mental decline due to the lack of cerebral perfusion. Therefore, MMD has tremendous effects on the intelligence of children.

22.6.1 Treatments

At present, there is no definitive medical therapy to delay or even reverse the progression of MMD. The current medical therapy for MMD patients just only targets its clinical symptoms, such as ischemia and hemorrhage. In addition, conservative treatment can be used as an auxiliary approach to surgical treatment in children patients with MMD. Previous study demonstrated that calcium channel blocker nicardipine could exhibit a positive effect in improving the hemodynamics of children with MMD.

Surgical treatment is the most effective therapy for children with MMD and the main surgical treatment in MMD is revascularization, including direct revascularization, indirect revascularization, and combined revascularization. The direct bypass is performed to anastomose the STA and MCA directly. However, the surgical success rate in children with MMD is not ideal because the branch vessels of cortical artery and superficial temporal artery are too slender and fragile in children. In addition, various complications are often observed in many pediatric MMD patients after direct bypass. Indirect surgery is considered to be safer and easier to perform than direct surgery, especially for pediatric patients. Indirect surgery could also have a good effect for children patients with MMD and the efficacy of indirect bypass in children with MMD is better than that in adults. Therefore, the majority of pediatric MMD patients are performed indirect bypass in China. Now, the indirect bypass includes encephalomyosynangiosis (EMS), encephalo-duro-arteriosynangiosis (EDAS), encephalo-duro-myosynangiosis (EDMS), encephalo-duro-arterio-myosynangiosis (EDAMS), multiple burr hole surgery (MBHS), and transplantation of the greater omentum. As we all known, MMD is a progressive cerebrovascular disease; therefore, it is recommended that pediatric MMD patients should achieve surgical revascularization as soon as possible. Early intervention before irreversible brain damage can obtain favorable clinical outcome in children.

22.6.2 Long-Term Clinical Outcome

Compared to adult patients, children with MMD can have a good prognosis if early diagnosis and early active surgical treatment are achieved. Surgical revascularization can prevent recurrent ischemic and hemorrhagic stroke in pediatric patients with MMD. Furthermore, previous study also reported that the symptom of headache and seizure may disappear after revascularization by improving cerebral vascular perfusion. Currently, the majority of studies about clinical outcome in pediatric MMD patients are almost single-center retrospective researches, there are still lacking Randomized Controlled Trial to demonstrate the long-term clinical outcome in pediatric patients with MMD in China.

There are many prognostic factors for pediatric MMD outcome after cerebral revascularization, such as preoperative multiple cerebral infarctions, younger age of symptom onset, high Suzuki stages, decreased vascular reserve, the surgical procedure itself, and perioperative ischemic events [34–36]. As we all known, successful direct bypass could improve blood flow immediately after surgery. Therefore, direct or combined bypass is recognized as the optimal choice for MMD patients. However, direct bypass for pediatric patients with MMD is technically challenging. So, children with MMD are commonly performed with indirect bypass. Direct and combined surgeries are only performed in some adolescent patients with MMD, whose donor and recipient vessels are approximately adult-sized. There are a number of studies on the effects of indirect bypass in pediatric patients with MMD. Bao et al. reported a long-term clinical outcome in 288 Chinese pediatric patients with MMD achieved EDAS operation and estimated stroke risk in the first 2 years and 5 years were 5% and 9%, respectively [32]. In a cohort consisting of 100 patients, the 5-and 10-year cumulative risks of any stroke were 2.6% and 3.5% after indirect revascularization, the risk of stroke was 0.33%/person-year, and about 92% of pediatric patients achieved independent life with no significant disability at the last follow-up [37]. Another retrospective study of 67 pediatric patients with MMD in China demonstrated the stroke rate for pediatric patients who underwent EDAS procedure was 7.1% per patients-years and 97% of pediatric patients achieve favorable outcomes at last follow-up [38]. Therefore, indirect bypass is a safe and effective treatment for pediatric MMD and can reduce the risk of stroke events and improve the quality of life. However, the long-term outcome of direct bypass in pediatric patients with MMD is lacking. Zhao et al. [33] reported a long-term outcome consisting of 95 adolescent patients with MMD. A total of 42 patients (44.2%) underwent direct/combined bypass surgery, who had significantly lower risk of future stroke events compared to those who underwent indirect bypass. In addition, revascularization could also decrease the rate of recurrent hemorrhage in children with hemorrhagic MMD [39, 40]. Therefore, the surgical choice for each pediatric patient should be specific and direct/combined bypass may be a preferred choice for some adolescent patients.

22.7 Conclusion

Although MMD is not rare in China, the management has not reached a consensus. A number of prospective studies have reported the encouraging outcome; however, the complication rate could not be ignored in patients with significant risk factors. Further investigations are needed to figure out the patients who might get benefits from the surgical procedures. Nationwide randomized controlled trials might help to clarify the efficacy of different treating style for the prevention of the recurrent stroke. Further epidemiological and follow-up studies may help us get more detailed understanding of the natural course of MMD in China. We hope to refine the guidelines for medical and surgical treatments for MMD based on our data in the near future.

References

1. Suzuki J, Takaku A. Cerebrovascular "moyamoya": disease. Disease showing abnormal net-like vessels in base of brain. Arch Neurol. 1969 Mar;20(3):288–99.
2. Miao W, Zhao PL, Zhang YS, et al. Epidemiological and clinical features of Moyamoya disease in Nanjing. China Clin Neurol Neurosurg. 2010 Apr;112(3):199–203.
3. Kim JS. Moyamoya disease: epidemiology, clinical features, and diagnosis. J Stroke. 2016 Jan;18(1):2–11.
4. Chen PC, Yang SH, Chien KL, Tsai IJ, Kuo MF. Epidemiology of moyamoya disease in Taiwan: a nationwide population-based study. Stroke. 2014 May;45(5):1258–63.
5. Bao XY, Wang QN, Zhang Y, et al. Epidemiology of Moyamoya disease in China: single-center, population-based study. World Neurosurg. 2019 Feb;122:e917–e23.
6. Ge P, Ye X, Liu X, et al. Association between p.R4810K variant and postoperative collateral formation in patients with Moyamoya disease. Cerebrovasc Dis. 2019;48(1–2):77–84.
7. Sun X, Luo M, Li J, et al. Prevalence of RNF213 variants in symptomatic intracranial arterial stenosis/occlusion in China. Mol Genet Genomics. 2020 May;295(3):635–43.

8. Wang Y, Zhang Z, Wei L, et al. Predictive role of heterozygous p.R4810K of RNF213 in the phenotype of Chinese moyamoya disease. Neurology. 2020 Feb 18;94(7):e678–e86.
9. Zhang Q, Liu Y, Yu L, et al. The Association of the RNF213 p.R4810K Polymorphism with Quasi-Moyamoya disease and a review of the pertinent literature. World Neurosurg. 2017 Mar;99:701-8e1.
10. Wu, Z., Jiang, H., Zhang, L., Xu, X., Zhang, X., Kang, Z., Song, D., Zhang, J., Guan, M., Gu, Y., 2012. Molecular Analysis of RNF213 Gene for Moyamoya Disease in the Chinese Han Population. PLOS ONE 7, e48179. https://doi.org/10.1371/journal.pone.0048179.
11. Wang Y, Zhang Z, Wei L, et al. RNF213Predictive role of heterozygous p.R4810K of in the phenotype of Chinese moyamoya disease. Neurology. 2020;94(7):e678–e86.
12. Wang X, Wang Y, Nie F, et al. Association of Genetic Variants with Moyamoya Disease in 13000 individuals: a meta-analysis. Stroke. 2020;51(6):1647–55.
13. Acker G, Fekonja L, Vajkoczy P. Surgical management of moyamoya disease. Stroke. 2018 Feb;49(2):476–82.
14. Alexandrov AV. Current and future recanalization strategies for acute ischemic stroke. J Intern Med. 2010 Feb;267(2):209–19.
15. Correction to: 2018 Guidelines for the early Management of Patients with Acute Ischemic Stroke: a guideline for healthcare professionals from the American Heart Association/ American Stroke Association. Stroke. 2018 Jun;49(6):e233–e4.
16. Deng X, Gao F, Zhang D, et al. Direct versus indirect bypasses for adult ischemic-type moyamoya disease: a propensity score-matched analysis. J Neurosurg. 2018 Jun;128(6):1785–91.
17. Campbell BCV, Mitchell PJ, Churilov L, et al. Effect of intravenous Tenecteplase dose on cerebral reperfusion before Thrombectomy in patients with large vessel occlusion ischemic stroke: the EXTEND-IA TNK part 2 randomized clinical trial. JAMA. 2020 Feb 20;323(13):1257–65.
18. Cao J, Zhuang Y, Zhang J, et al. Leucine-rich repeat kinase 2 aggravates secondary brain injury induced by intracerebral hemorrhage in rats by regulating the P38 MAPK/Drosha pathway. Neurobiol Dis. 2018 Nov;119:53–64.
19. Alexander LD, Black SE, Gao F, Szilagyi G, Danells CJ, McIlroy WE. Correlating lesion size and location to deficits after ischemic stroke: the influence of accounting for altered perinecrotic tissue and incidental silent infarcts. Behav Brain Funct. 2010;6:6.
20. Cao S, Zhu P, Yu X, et al. Hydrogen sulfide attenuates brain edema in early brain injury after subarachnoid hemorrhage in rats: possible involvement of MMP-9 induced blood-brain barrier disruption and AQP4 expression. Neurosci Lett. 2016 May 16;621:88–97.
21. Watchmaker JM, Frederick BD, Fusco MR, et al. Clinical use of cerebrovascular compliance imaging to evaluate revascularization in patients with Moyamoya. Neurosurgery. 2019 Jan 1;84(1):261–71.
22. Duan L, Bao XY, Yang WZ, et al. Moyamoya disease in China: its clinical features and outcomes. Stroke. 2012 Jan;43(1):56–60.
23. Sato H, Sato N, Tamaki N, Matsumoto S. Chronic low-perfusion state in children with moyamoya disease following revascularization. Child's Nervous System: ChNS: Official Journal of the International Society for Pediatric Neurosurgery. 1990 May;6(3):166–71.
24. Gorelick PB, Scuteri A, Black SE, et al. Vascular contributions to cognitive impairment and dementia: a statement for healthcare professionals from the American heart association/ American stroke association. Stroke. 2011 Sep;42(9):2672–713.
25. Andrade-Barazarte H, Jagersberg M, Belkhair S, et al. The extended lateral supraorbital approach and extradural anterior Clinoidectomy through a Frontopterio-orbital window: technical note and pilot surgical series. World Neurosurg. 2017 Apr;100:159–66.
26. Niedermeyer E. The clinical relevance of EEG interpretation. Clin Electroencephalogr. 2003 Jul;34(3):93–8.
27. Hill MD, Goyal M, Menon BK, et al. Efficacy and safety of nerinetide for the treatment of acute ischaemic stroke (ESCAPE-NA1): a multicentre, double-blind, randomised controlled trial. Lancet. 2020 Mar 14;395(10227):878–87.

28. Wang X, Sun G, Feng T, et al. Sodium oligomannate therapeutically remodels gut microbiota and suppresses gut bacterial amino acids-shaped neuroinflammation to inhibit Alzheimer's disease progression. Cell Res. 2019 Oct;29(10):787–803.
29. Chen Y, Dai D, Fang Y, et al. Endovascular treatment of ruptured large or wide-neck basilar tip aneurysms associated with Moyamoya disease using the stent-assisted coil technique. J Stroke Cerebrovasc Dis. 2015 Oct;24(10):2229–35.
30. Kang K, Lu J, Ju Y, et al. Clinical and radiological outcomes after revascularization of hemorrhagic Moyamoya disease. Front Neurol. 2020;11:382.
31. Gu Q, Huang P, Xuan M, et al. Greater loss of white matter integrity in postural instability and gait difficulty subtype of Parkinson's disease. The Canadian journal of neurological sciences. J Can Sci Neurol. 2014 Nov 7:1–6.
32. Bao XY, Duan L, Yang WZ, et al. Clinical features, surgical treatment, and long-term outcome in pediatric patients with moyamoya disease in China. Cerebrovasc Dis. 2015;39(2):75–81.
33. Zhao M, Zhang D, Wang S, et al. Adolescents with moyamoya disease: clinical features, surgical treatment and long-term outcomes. Acta Neurochir. 2017 Nov;159(11):2071–80.
34. Matsushima Y, Aoyagi M, Suzuki R, Tabata H, Ohno K. Perioperative complications of encephalo-duro-arterio-synangiosis: prevention and treatment. Surg Neurol. 1991 Nov;36(5):343–53.
35. Kim SK, Cho BK, Phi JH, et al. Pediatric moyamoya disease: an analysis of 410 consecutive cases. Ann Neurol. 2010 Jul;68(1):92–101.
36. Scott RM, Smith JL, Robertson RL, Madsen JR, Soriano SG, Rockoff MA. Long-term outcome in children with moyamoya syndrome after cranial revascularization by pial synangiosis. J Neurosurg. 2004 Feb;100(2 Suppl Pediatrics):142–9.
37. Zhang Y, Bao XY, Duan L, et al. Encephaloduroarteriosynangiosis for pediatric moyamoya disease: long-term follow-up of 100 cases at a single center. J Neurosurg Pediatr. 2018 Aug;22(2):173–80.
38. Wang C, Zhao M, Wang J, et al. Encephaloduroarteriosynangiosis for pediatric Moyamoya disease: a single-center experience with 67 cases in China. J Child Neurol. 2018 Dec;33(14):901–8.
39. Ge P, Zhang Q, Ye X, Wang S, Zhang D, Zhao J. Clinical features, surgical treatment, and long-term outcome in children with hemorrhagic Moyamoya disease. J Stroke Cerebrovasc Dis. 2018 Jun;27(6):1517–23.
40. Liu P, Han C, Li DS, Lv XL, Li YX, Duan L. Hemorrhagic Moyamoya disease in children: clinical, angiographic features, and long-term surgical outcome. Stroke. 2016 Jan;47(1):240–3.

Long-Term Outcome of Revascularization Surgery for Moyamoya Disease in Korea

23

Jeong Eun Kim and Chang Wan Oh

Abstract

Moyamoya disease (MMD) is a rare chronic cerebral ischemic disease with unknown etiology that shows characteristic angiographic features of intracranial collateral vessels. Revascularization surgery (RVS) is a well-known method for the augmentation of cerebral perfusion in MMD. Based on the surgical procedures, RVS for MMD is classified as direct, indirect, and combined. For RVS, there are many aspects to consider, such as age (pediatric vs. adult), surgical indication, and selection of surgical procedures (indirect vs. direct vs. combined). Along with these aspects, we analyzed and described the outcome of RVS in both pediatric and adult MMD in Korea with a review of pertinent literature.

Keywords

Moyamoya disease · Surgical outcome · Revascularization · Pediatric · Adult · Korea

J. E. Kim
Department of Neurosurgery, Seoul National University College of Medicine, Seoul, South Korea

Seoul National University Hospital, Seoul, South Korea
e-mail: eunkim@snu.ac.kr

C. W. Oh (✉)
Department of Neurosurgery, Seoul National University College of Medicine, Seoul, South Korea

Seoul National University Bundang Hospital, Seongnam-si, South Korea
e-mail: wanoh@snu.ac.kr

S. Kuroda (ed.), *Moyamoya Disease: Current Knowledge and Future Perspectives*, https://doi.org/10.1007/978-981-33-6404-2_23

23.1 Introduction

Revascularization surgery (RVS) involves establishing a vascular connection between the brain and extracranial vessels or vascularized tissues for blood flow augmentation to the ischemic brain. RVS techniques for moyamoya disease (MMD) are classified into direct, indirect, and combined RVS procedures.

According to data from the National Health Insurance Service in South Korea, from 2008 to 2019, 18,056 patients were newly diagnosed with MMD [1, 2]. The number of newly diagnosed adult patients with MMD increased by 67.0% over the 11-year period, with 1,590 adult patients diagnosed with MMD in 2019. For adult MMD, the crude incidence in 2019 was calculated as 3.75 per 100,000 person-years, which increased by 76.9% over the 11-year period (Fig. 23.1) [1, 2]. The number of newly diagnosed pediatric patients with MMD decreased by 16.2% from 296 in 2008 to 248 in 2019. This is thought to be caused by a significant decrease in the birth rate; however, the crude incidence did not decrease as the detection rate increased. For pediatric MMD, the crude incidence in 2019 was calculated as 2.76 per 100,000 person-years, which increased by 11.1% over the 11-year period [1, 2].

Regarding the treatment for MMD in Korea, the total number of RVS for adult MMD increased to 389 by 2012, and then slightly decreased to 364 in 2016. The number of direct RVS cases, including combined RVS cases, peaked at 266 in 2014 and then showed plateaus status to 2016. The proportion of cases in which indirect RVS was performed alone decreased from 62.5% in 2008 to 31.3% in 2016. (Fig. 23.2a) Meanwhile, RVS for pediatric MMD declined significantly over the

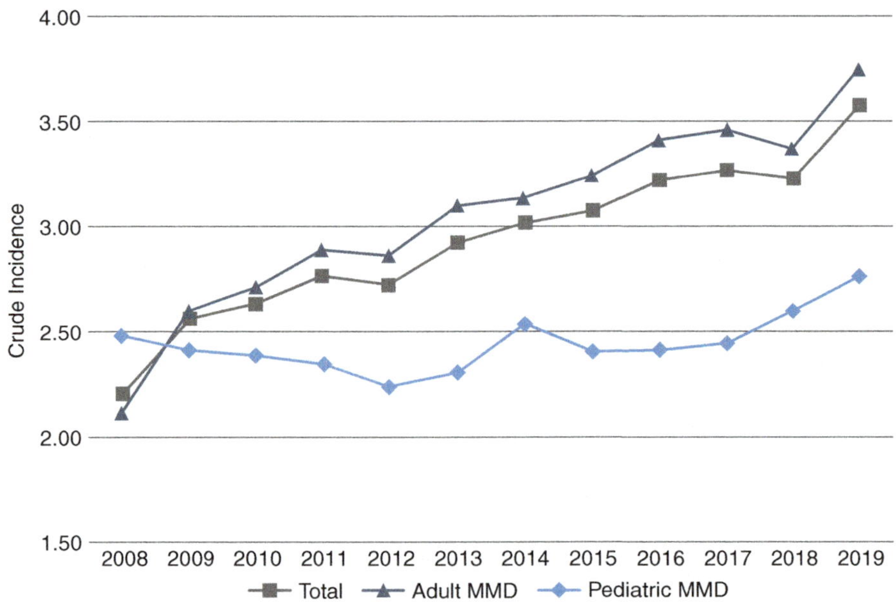

Fig. 23.1 The crude incidence of moyamoya disease (MMD) in Korea. The crude incidence of adult MMD in 2019 was calculated as 3.75 per 100,000 person-years, which increased by 76.9% throughout 2008–2019. For pediatric MMD, the crude incidence was 2.76 per 100,000 person-years in 2019, which increased by 11.1% from 2008

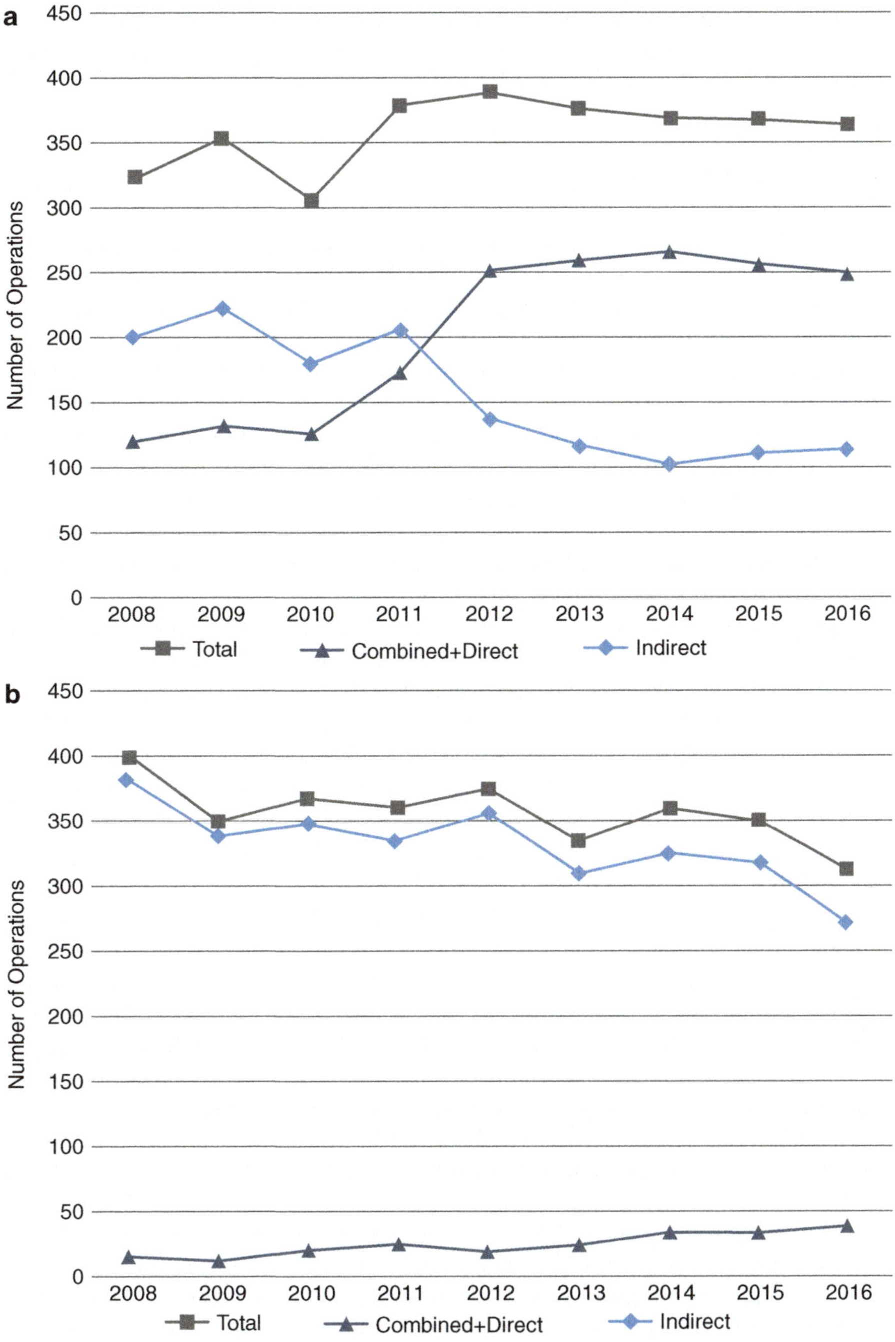

Fig. 23.2 The treatment for moyamoya disease (MMD) in Korea. (**a**) The total number of revascularization surgeries (RVS) for adult MMD increased to 389 by 2012 and then decreased to 364 in 2016. The number of direct RVS cases, including combined RVS cases, peaked in 2014 and then showed plateau status. The proportion of indirect RVS alone decreased from 62.5% in 2008 to 31.3% in 2016. (**b**) Operations for pediatric MMD declined significantly over the 9-year period, with 399 and 313 operations performed in 2008 and 2016, respectively

9-year period, with 399 and 313 operations performed in 2008 and 2016, respectively, although the number of direct RVS cases, including cases of combined RVS, increased steadily over the 9-year period (Fig. 23.2b) [1, 2].

23.2 Procedure of RVS

Indirect RVS is the procedure of shifting the external carotid artery branches supplying vascularized tissue from the scalp to the surface of the ischemic brain for provoking spontaneous leptomeningeal anastomoses [3, 4]. There are various types of indirect RVS procedures. The most standard and generally used procedures for indirect RVS are encephalo-duro-arteriosynangiosis (EDAS) [5, 6], encephalo-myo-synangiosis (EMS) [7], and encephalo-duro-arterio-myo-synangiosis (EDAMS) [8]. The choice of donor tissue, such as the superficial temporal artery (STA), dura (middle meningeal artery), temporalis muscle (deep temporal artery), galea, and periosteum vary according to the operator or the institute's preference [9–11]. The advantages of indirect RVS over direct RVS are its relatively easy surgical technique, short operation time, and a relatively low risk of postoperative hyperperfusion syndrome. However, because indirect RVS procedures require the process of angiogenesis, neovascularization takes time to occur in the repositioned tissue adjacent to the ischemic brain, which is not effective for immediate blood flow augmentation [10, 12]. In some cases, sufficient collateral vessels do not grow even after the indirect RVS procedure [9, 13]. Due to concerns about incomplete RVS [14–18], a combination of different indirect RVS procedures is used for a wide extent of revascularizations. These include procedures such as EDAS plus bifrontal encephalo-galeo-periosteal-synangiosis (EGPS) [9], multiple EDAS [19], ribbon EDAMS [20], and multiple burr holes [21].

Direct RVS, usually represented by the STA to middle cerebral artery (MCA) anastomosis, is the most used technique in adult MMD. Other variations include the occipital artery to posterior cerebral artery anastomosis and the STA to anterior cerebral artery anastomosis. Direct extracranial–intracranial artery anastomosis enables prompt flow augmentation because it does not require angiogenesis and only requires remodeling of the arterio-arterial anastomosis site called arteriogenesis [12]. However, immediate changes in hemodynamics can cause perioperative complications such as postoperative hyperperfusion syndrome [22, 23].

Combined RVS with both direct and indirect RVS is the most effective technique currently used. As the revascularization process continues after surgery, both direct bypass and indirect bypass play an important role because they have different formation processes and patterns [24]. Direct bypass plays a major role in early flow augmentation in the early postoperative period; however, the area revascularized by direct revascularization may decrease due to occlusion of the distal cerebral artery over time. In such cases, collateral vessels by the indirect bypass can play a complementary role [10]. In some cases, synergistic increases are seen in the area revascularized by both direct and indirect bypasses without regression of the flow by direct bypass [25].

23.3 Indication of RVS

The common idea of RVS in patients with MMD is the enhancement of intrinsic compensatory mechanisms in the nature of MMD [26]. Revascularization surgery preserves the brain that is vulnerable to stroke from cerebral ischemia by improving cerebral blood flow and preventing cerebral hemorrhage by reducing hemodynamic stress [27].

In pediatric MMD, RVS is an irreplaceable option regardless of disease severity. The young developing brain, which requires high cerebral oxygen metabolism, justifies timely RVS surgery [9, 28–31]. The younger the age at which MMD is diagnosed, the worse the clinical prognosis, which means that the earlier the surgery, the better the clinical outcome [9, 29, 30, 32].

In contrast to pediatric MMD, treatment strategies for adult MMD are selected depending on the disease state. RVS is primarily considered in adult ischemic MMD with the presence of symptoms and hemodynamic compromise [27, 33, 34]. Recently, bilateral direct RVS has been reported as an effective treatment for adult hemorrhagic MMD, reducing hemorrhagic recurrence, and improving patient prognosis since the Japan Adult Moyamoya trial [35].

As the use of magnetic resonance imaging (MRI) for diagnostic purposes increases, patients with asymptomatic MMD are increasing [1, 2]. However, the long-term clinical course and prognosis of asymptomatic MMD are indeterminate, and treatment strategies for asymptomatic MMD are unclear. Kuroda et al. [36] reported 23.8% (15/63 patients) of disease progression, with a mean time to progression from diagnosis of 60 months (1.5–8 years). MMD progression occurs in both bilateral and unilateral MMD, both the anterior and posterior circulation, and symptomatic and asymptomatic cases [36]. Yamada et al. [37] reported that 21.2% (6/33 patients) of the patients with asymptomatic MMD became symptomatic within the mean follow-up duration of 44 months. In a prospective study of patients with asymptomatic MMD [38], silent cerebral infarct and decreased cerebral hemodynamics accounted for 20% and 40%, respectively. During a mean follow-up duration of 43.7 months, seven patients experienced cerebrovascular events (transient ischemic attack, $n = 3$; ischemic stroke, $n = 1$; hemorrhagic stroke, $n = 3$) among 34 non-surgically treated patients (3.2% of estimated annual stroke risk). Unlike previous studies that did not separate the hemodynamic state and the presence of symptoms, Cho et al. [39] investigated the natural course of adult patients with MMD ($n = 241$) who were hemodynamically stable during a mean follow-up duration of 82.5 months. While the overall annual stroke rate was 4.5% per person-year (hemorrhagic presenting group, 4.3%; ischemic presenting group, 3.0%), the annual stroke rate in hemodynamically stable patients with asymptomatic MMD was 3.4% (hemorrhagic stroke, 2.5%; ischemic stroke, 0.8%). As asymptomatic MMD is not a fixed but dynamic disease, regular follow-up is necessary. Through MRI/MR angiography (MRA), disease progression, as well as silent cerebral infarction or microbleeding, can be confirmed. In this regard, it would be helpful to know the long-term clinical course and prognosis through the ongoing asymptomatic moyamoya registry (AMORE) study [40].

After a statement by the Research Committee of MMD of the Japanese Ministry of Health, Labour, and Welfare in 2015, unilateral MMD has also been modified to include diagnostic criteria for definitive MMD. Compared with bilateral MMD, unilateral MMD has a higher proportion of adult patients with a range of progression rates between 14.6% and 50% [41, 42]. The younger the patients' age, the more frequently [43–46] and faster [43, 47, 48] contralateral progression occurs. In patients under 2 years of age, concurrent bilateral surgery is considered due to the high likelihood of contralateral progression and poor prognosis [32]. Except for an extremely young age, the usual treatment strategy for unilateral pediatric and adult MMD is to treat the symptomatic side first and then wait.

The surgical indications for adult MMD at our institution are as follows: (1) symptomatic manifestations including ischemic and hemorrhagic events; (2) asymptomatic patients with disease progression proven on computed tomography angiography (CTA), MRA, or conventional angiography; (3) functionally independent with the Karnofsky Performance Scale over 70; (4) no acute cerebral infarction or hemorrhage within 4 weeks at the time of surgery; and (5) hemodynamically unstable demonstrated by acetazolamide challenge single-photon emission computed tomography and perfusion CT or MRI [49, 50].

23.4 Selection of the RVS Procedure

The selection of the RVS procedure has the following limitations: heterogeneity of MMD according to age proportion, racial and geographical distribution; diversity of surgical methods by the preference of institutions and operators; relatively small number of patients; and lack of randomized controlled trials.

For a good surgical outcome for MMD, preoperative hemodynamic compromise should be considered first before the choice of surgical procedure. Without preoperative hemodynamic compromise, neovascularization would not occur, regardless of the extent of surgery [51]. Satisfactory angiographic revascularization assumes the correct location of the vascularized donor tissues or correct selection of the recipient artery on the surface of the on-demanding ischemic brain [51].

In pediatric MMD, both direct and indirect RVS procedures are comparable in surgical outcomes [52–56]. If there are no issues with the surgeon's technique and facility policy, direct with indirect revascularization can be considered [25, 57]. However, in children, satisfactory revascularization can also be accomplished with only indirect bypass procedures [32, 58, 59]. In younger patients with MMD, direct RVS procedures have technical limitations because of the small size of the STA and the cortical branch of the MCA. Therefore, children under 4 years of age are not candidates for direct RVS [34]. Patients older than 5 years can be appropriate candidates for direct RVS [25, 57]. Direct flow augmentation by direct RVS can diminish the risk of perioperative stroke [25, 56, 60]. However, the possibility of watershed shift or hyperperfusion syndrome should be kept in mind [61, 62], although those chances are less likely than in adults [60, 63–65]. With well-developed moyamoya collateral vessels compared with adults, there is less likelihood of postoperative stroke due to progressive occlusion of the main cerebral artery [60]. In patients who experience frequent transient ischemic attacks (TIA) with severe hemodynamic compromise, it is better to consider direct revascularization for the rapid formation of collaterals [25, 56, 60].

In adult ischemic MMD, a combination of both direct and indirect RVS is the main treatment of choice [24, 25, 66–68]; however, the role of indirect bypass has been reported continuously [69–72]. In cases of adult hemorrhagic MMD, bilateral combined RVS for improving hemodynamic stress is considered an effective treatment [35, 73].

23.5 Long-term Outcome of RVS for Patients with MMD in Korea (Table 23.1)

A majority of the pediatric patients with MMD in Korea present with TIAs or cerebral infarcts (98%), while hemorrhagic manifestations occur in only around 2% of the patients [74]. In a retrospective study of indirect RVS for pediatric patients with MMD (629 patients with 1,283 surgeries) in Korea, who were followed up for more than 5 years, with a mean clinical follow-up duration of 12 years, 95% of the patients showed favorable clinical outcomes. The annual risk of developing symptomatic hemorrhage or cerebral infarction was 0.04% and 0.08%, respectively. The 10-year event-free survival rates without symptomatic infarction and hemorrhage were 99.2% and 98%, respectively [74]. Based on a comparison study between EDAS with bifrontal EGPS and simple EDAS in Korea, which showed larger revascularization with better hemodynamic improvement and more favorable outcomes in combined surgery [9], combined indirect RVS methods with bifrontal EGPS, occipital EDAS, or multiple burr hole surgery are actively utilized during the careful surveillance of disease progression. Although indirect bypass has been attempted in pediatric patients with hemorrhagic MMD, with good outcomes in a few studies, there are few reports to establish strong evidence [74, 79].

Poor social outcomes with cognitive dysfunction are major concerns among pediatric patients with MMD. Despite satisfactory RVS without complications, patients who had preoperative neurological deficits tend to experience adaptation difficulties in their education or occupation due to intellectual impairment [80]. Patients with preoperative neurological impairment and major cerebral infarct showed poor social outcomes [32, 80, 81]. Regardless of the presence of major or borderzone infarctions, RVS can prevent further neurocognitive declination [81]. There are no comparative reports on social outcomes according to the type of revascularization.

Compared with conservative treatment [39], RVS is considered to improve cerebral hemodynamics and prevent subsequent ischemic stroke in adult ischemic MMD [24, 66, 67]. Direct or combined revascularization is a common surgical method for adult ischemic MMD. To achieve optimal surgical outcomes, combined RVS is preferred in most studies [24, 66, 67, 82]. The combined RVS is a technique for obtaining advantages of both direct and indirect RVS. Along with direct RVS for

Table 23.1 Long-term outcomes of revascularization surgery for moyamoya disease patients in Korea

Authors (Year)	Age	No of patients	Clinical presentation	Revascularization procedure	Follow-up duration	Annual stroke rate	5-year event-free survival	Other outcomes
Kim et al. (2002) [9]	Ped	159 (314[a])	Ischemic and hemorrhage	Indirect (EDAS alone or EDAS with biF. EGPS)	45 months	–	–	EDAS with biF. EGPS compared with EDAS; More favorable outcomes (62% vs 36%); Better ACA RV (79% vs 16%); More hemodynamic improvement (70% vs 52%)
Kim et al. (2010) [28]	Ped	410	Ischemic and hemorrhage	Indirect (EDAS alone or EDAS with biF. EGPS)	61 months	–	–	81% favorable clinical outcome (event free)
Ha et al. (2019) [74]	Ped	629	Ischemic and hemorrhage	Indirect (EDAS)	12 years	0.08% for symptomatic infarct; 0.04% for symptomatic hemorrhage	–	Favorable outcome: 95% of the patients; 10-year event-free survival for infarction/hemorrhage: 99.2%/99.8%
Cho et al. (2014) [24]	Adult	60 (77[a])	Ischemic only	Combined (STA-MCA + EDGS)	71 ± 10.1 months	0.2% for symptomatic infarct; 0.4% for symptomatic hemorrhage	98.70%	–

Kim et al. (2016) [66]	Adult	301	Ischemic only	Combined (STA-MCA + EDGS/EDAS/EGS/EMS/EDAMS); Direct (single/double barrel STA-MCA)	44.9 ± 34.4 months	0.8% for symptomatic infarct; 0.8% for symptomatic hemorrhage	–	1–/5–/10-year cumulative incidence rate of ischemic stroke: 2.7/2.7/3.9%; 1–/5–/10-year cumulative incidence rate of hemorrhagic stroke: 2.4/2.7/5.6%
Bang et al. (2012) [67]	Adult	75	Ischemic and hemorrhage	Combined (STA-MCA + EDAS/EDAMS/EMS); Direct (STA-MCA); Indirect (EDAS)	64 months	–	–	Ischemic stroke recurrence: 7.1% in indirect RVS group, 1.7% in combined/direct RVS group; Hemorrhagic stroke recurrence: 7.1% in indirect RVS group, 0% in combined/direct RVS group
Kim et al. (2012) [75]	Adult	96 (134[a])	Ischemic only	Combined (STA-MCA + EDAGS); Indirect (EDAGS)	40.2 months	–	–	Angiographic revascularization: combined RVS > indirect RVS

(continued)

Table 23.1 (continued)

Authors (Year)	Age	No of patients	Clinical presentation	Revascularization procedure	Follow-up duration	Annual stroke rate	5-year event-free survival	Other outcomes
Lee et al. (2012) [76]	Adult	124 (147[a])	Ischemic and hemorrhage	Combined (STA-MCA + EDAGS); Direct (STA-MCA); Indirect (EDAS/EDAMS/EMS)	54.5 months	1.6% in ischemic MMD after combined/direct bypass; 6.0% in ischemic MMD after indirect bypass; 2.5% in hemorrhagic MMD after combined/direct bypass; 4.7% in hemorrhagic MMD after indirect bypass	–	Incidence of recurrent stroke 8/25.5/4.3% (direct/indirect/combined RVS); Stroke free time: $78.5 \pm 8.8/71.5 \pm 6.6/87.1 \pm 11.4$ months (direct/indirect/combined RVS)

Kim et al. (2017) [77]	Adult	70	Hemorrhage only	Combined (STA-MCA + EDGS); Indirect (EDAS)	83 months	0.5% after combined bypass; 1.8% after indirect bypass	–	–
Choi et al. (2013) [78]	Adult	44	Hemorrhage only	Combined (STA-MCA + EDAGS); Direct (STA-MCA); Indirect (EDAS/EDAMS/EMS)	55.4 months	–	–	Incidence of rebleeding 11.1/22.2/12.5% (direct/indirect/combined RVS); Stroke free time: 70.3 ± 7.5/77.4 ± 5.8/81.1 ± 9.6 months (direct/indirect/combined RVS)

EDAS encephaloduroarteriosynangiosis, *EGPS* encephalogaleoperiosteal synangiosis, *STA–MCA* superficial temporal artery-middle cerebral artery anastomosis, *EDGS* encephalodurogaleosynangiosis, *EDAMS* encephaloduroarteriomyosynangiosis, *EMS* encephalomyosynangiosis, *RVS* revascularization surgery, *EGS* encephalogaleosynangiosis, *No* number, *VS* versus, *ACA* anterior cerebral artery territory, *RV* revascularization, *biF* bifrontal, *Ped* pediatric

[a]Number of hemispheres

immediate flow augmentation, indirect RVS mobilizes as many vasogenic potent tissues as possible to create a revascularization channel. The revascularization area is the largest in combined RVS, followed by direct and indirect RVS [67, 83]. According to angiographic follow-up after 6–12 months of surgery, revascularization by both direct and indirect RVS explains the complementary relationships between the two methods [75]. In a prospective study of combined RVS for adult patients with ischemic MMD (77 hemispheres, 60 patients) in Korea, the annual risk of developing symptomatic hemorrhage or a cerebral infarct was 0.4% and 0.2%, respectively. The patients showed improvement in clinical, angiographic, and hemodynamic aspects until 6 months after surgery. The 5-year event-free survival rate without symptomatic hemorrhage and cerebral infarction was 98.7% [24]. According to a comparative study of patients presenting with ischemia, the 1-year and 5-year incidences of symptomatic ischemic stroke were not lower in patients who underwent combined RVS in comparison to those in the conservative treatment group because perioperative stroke offsets the benefit [66]. It was not until 10 years later that the benefit of RVS was confirmed, with the absolute risk reduction for ischemic stroke being 9.4%, and the number required for treatment was 11. Briefly, while the benefit of combined RVS for conservative treatment is generally acceptable, it depends on perioperative stroke control. Perioperative stroke developed with various incidences (2.7–13.0%) [24, 66, 67]. Although patients with an advanced Suzuki stage with a poorer perfusion status seem to be prone to perioperative stroke development, little has been reported about factors related to perioperative stroke [76].

Indirect RVS in adult patients with ischemic MMD results in a lower incidence of recurrent stroke compared with conservative treatment, although it did not show more satisfactory outcomes than a direct bypass [67, 75, 84].

A study of the natural history of hemorrhagic MMD showed that the overall estimated rate of hemorrhagic recurrence was 16.9% per person at 5 years and 26.3% per person at 10 years after the onset of initial hemorrhage [77]. Recurrent hemorrhage is the most significant poor prognostic factor in hemorrhagic MMD [77]. Hemodynamic failure in patients with hemorrhagic MMD is an independent risk factor for subsequent hemorrhage [85]. In a retrospective study of adult patients with hemorrhagic MMD in Korea (44 patients), the incidence of recurrent hemorrhage was 11.1% after direct revascularization, 22.2% after indirect revascularization, and 12.5% after combined revascularization [78].

23.6 Conclusion

RVS for MMD can improve radiological and clinical outcomes. The selection of the RVS procedure is determined by the patient's age, the degree of hemodynamic compromise, the patient's symptoms, the condition of the donor/recipient vessel, and the surgeon's preference.

Acknowledgement The authors appreciate Dr. Jin Woo Bae, Si Un Lee, and Tackeun Kim for helping with the preparation of this manuscript.

References

1. Lee SU, Kim T, Kwon OK, Bang JS, Ban SP, Byoun HS, et al. Trends in the incidence and treatment of cerebrovascular diseases in Korea: part II. Cerebral infarction, cerebral arterial stenosis, and Moyamoya disease. J Korean Neurosurg Soc. 2020;63(1):69–79.
2. Oh CW. The overall trends of neurosurgical diseases in Korea: analysis of the incidence of diseases and treatment modalities using NHIS data from 2010 to 2016. Health Insurance Review & Assessment Service; 2017.
3. Spetzler RF, Roski RA, Kopaniky DR. Alternative superficial temporal artery to middle cerebral artery revascularization procedure. Neurosurgery. 1980;7(5):484–7.
4. Suzuki J, Takaku A. Cerebrovascular "moyamoya" disease. Disease showing abnormal net-like vessels in base of brain. Arch Neurol. 1969;20(3):288–99.
5. Matsushima Y, Fukai N, Tanaka K, Tsuruoka S, Inaba Y, Aoyagi M, et al. A new surgical treatment of moyamoya disease in children: a preliminary report. Surg Neurol. 1981;15(4):313–20.
6. Matsushima Y, Inaba Y. Moyamoya disease in children and its surgical treatment. Introduction of a new surgical procedure and its follow-up angiograms. Childs Brain. 1984;11(3):155–70.
7. Karasawa J, Kikuchi H, Furuse S, Sakaki T. Yoshida Y. a surgical treatment of "moyamoya" disease "encephalo-myo synangiosis". Neurol Med Chir. 1977;17(1 Pt 1):29–37.
8. Kinugasa K, Mandai S, Kamata I, Sugiu K, Ohmoto T. Surgical treatment of moyamoya disease: operative technique for encephalo-duro-arterio-myo-synangiosis, its follow-up, clinical results, and angiograms. Neurosurgery. 1993;32(4):527–31.
9. Kim SK, Wang KC, Kim IO, Lee DS, Cho BK. Combined encephaloduroarteriosynangiosis and bifrontal encephalogaleo(periosteal)synangiosis in pediatric moyamoya disease. Neurosurgery. 2002;50(1):88–96.
10. Houkin K, Kuroda S, Ishikawa T, Abe H. Neovascularization (angiogenesis) after revascularization in moyamoya disease. Which technique is most useful for moyamoya disease? Acta Neurochir. 2000;142(3):269–76.
11. Matsushima T, Inoue T, Katsuta T, Natori Y, Suzuki S, Ikezaki K, et al. An indirect revascularization method in the surgical treatment of moyamoya disease--various kinds of indirect procedures and a multiple combined indirect procedure. Neurol Med Chir. 1998;38(Suppl):297–302.
12. Saito N, Imai H. Insights on the revascularization mechanism for treatment of Moyamoya disease based on the histopathologic concept of angiogenesis and arteriogenesis. World Neurosurg. 2011;75(2):204–5.
13. Nakashima H, Meguro T, Kawada S, Hirotsune N, Ohmoto T. Long-term results of surgically treated moyamoya disease. Clin Neurol Neurosurg. 1997;99(Suppl 2):S156–61.
14. Shim KW, Park EK, Kim JS, Kim DS. Cognitive outcome of pediatric Moyamoya disease. J Korean Neurosurg Soc. 2015;57(6):440–4.
15. Pandey P, Steinberg GK. Outcome of repeat revascularization surgery for moyamoya disease after an unsuccessful indirect revascularization. Clinical article. J Neurosurg. 2011;115(2):328–36.
16. Miyamoto S, Kikuchi H, Karasawa J, Nagata I, Yamazoe N, Akiyama Y. Pitfalls in the surgical treatment of moyamoya disease. Operative techniques for refractory cases. J Neurosurg. 1988;68(4):537–43.
17. Matsushima Y. Failure of encephalo-duro-arterio-synangiosis procedure in moyamoya disease. Pediatr Neurosci. 1985;12(6):326–7.
18. Cahan LD. Failure of encephalo-duro-arterio-synangiosis procedure in moyamoya disease. Pediatr Neurosci. 1985;12(1):58–62.
19. Tenjin H, Ueda S, Multiple EDAS. (Encephalo-duro-arterio-synangiosis). Additional EDAS using the frontal branch of the superficial temporal artery (STA) and the occipital artery for

pediatric moyamoya patients in whom EDAS using the parietal branch of STA was insufficient. Child's Nervous System: ChNS: Official Journal of the International Society for Pediatric Neurosurgery. 1997;13(4):220–4.
20. Kinugasa K, Mandai S, Tokunaga K, Kamata I, Sugiu K, Handa A, et al. Ribbon enchephalo-duro-arterio-myo-synangiosis for moyamoya disease. Surg Neurol. 1994;41(6):455–61.
21. Sainte-Rose C, Oliveira R, Puget S, Beni-Adani L, Boddaert N, Thorne J, et al. Multiple bur hole surgery for the treatment of moyamoya disease in children. J Neurosurg. 2006;105(6 Suppl):437–43.
22. Kim JE, Oh CW, Kwon OK, Park SQ, Kim SE, Kim YK. Transient hyperperfusion after superficial temporal artery/middle cerebral artery bypass surgery as a possible cause of postoperative transient neurological deterioration. Cerebrovasc Dis (Basel, Switzerland). 2008;25(6):580–6.
23. Fujimura M, Kaneta T, Mugikura S, Shimizu H, Tominaga T. Temporary neurologic deterioration due to cerebral hyperperfusion after superficial temporal artery-middle cerebral artery anastomosis in patients with adult-onset moyamoya disease. Surg Neurol. 2007;67(3):273–82.
24. Cho WS, Kim JE, Kim CH, Ban SP, Kang HS, Son YJ, et al. Long-term outcomes after combined revascularization surgery in adult moyamoya disease. Stroke. 2014;45(10):3025–31.
25. Uchino H, Kim JH, Fujima N, Kazumata K, Ito M, Nakayama N, et al. Synergistic interactions between direct and indirect bypasses in combined procedures: the significance of indirect bypasses in Moyamoya disease. Neurosurgery. 2017;80(2):201–9.
26. Fujimura M, Tominaga T. Lessons learned from moyamoya disease: outcome of direct/indirect revascularization surgery for 150 affected hemispheres. Neurol Med Chir. 2012;52(5):327–32.
27. Kim JE, Jeon JS. An update on the diagnosis and treatment of adult Moyamoya disease taking into consideration controversial issues. Neurol Res. 2014;36(5):407–16.
28. Kim SK, Cho BK, Phi JH, Lee JY, Chae JH, Kim KJ, et al. Pediatric moyamoya disease: an analysis of 410 consecutive cases. Ann Neurol. 2010;68(1):92–101.
29. Suzuki Y, Negoro M, Shibuya M, Yoshida J, Negoro T, Watanabe K. Surgical treatment for pediatric moyamoya disease: use of the superficial temporal artery for both areas supplied by the anterior and middle cerebral arteries. Neurosurgery. 1997;40(2):324–9. discussion 9–30
30. Matsushima Y, Aoyagi M, Masaoka H, Suzuki R, Ohno K. Mental outcome following encephaloduroarteriosynangiosis in children with moyamoya disease with the onset earlier than 5 years of age. Child's Nervous System: ChNS: Official Journal of the International Society for Pediatric Neurosurgery. 1990;6(8):440–3.
31. Scott RM, Smith JL, Robertson RL, Madsen JR, Soriano SG, Rockoff MA. Long-term outcome in children with moyamoya syndrome after cranial revascularization by pial synangiosis. J Neurosurg. 2004;100(2 Suppl Pediatrics):142–9.
32. Kim SK, Seol HJ, Cho BK, Hwang YS, Lee DS, Wang KC. Moyamoya disease among young patients: its aggressive clinical course and the role of active surgical treatment. Neurosurgery. 2004;54(4):840–4. discussion 4–6
33. Narisawa A, Fujimura M, Tominaga T. Efficacy of the revascularization surgery for adult-onset moyamoya disease with the progression of cerebrovascular lesions. Clin Neurol Neurosurg. 2009;111(2):123–6.
34. Guzman R, Lee M, Achrol A, Bell-Stephens T, Kelly M, Do HM, et al. Clinical outcome after 450 revascularization procedures for moyamoya disease. Clinical article. J Neurosurg. 2009;111(5):927–35.
35. Miyamoto S, Yoshimoto T, Hashimoto N, Okada Y, Tsuji I, Tominaga T, et al. Effects of extracranial-intracranial bypass for patients with hemorrhagic moyamoya disease: results of the Japan adult Moyamoya trial. Stroke. 2014;45(5):1415–21.
36. Kuroda S, Ishikawa T, Houkin K, Nanba R, Hokari M, Iwasaki Y. Incidence and clinical features of disease progression in adult moyamoya disease. Stroke. 2005;36(10):2148–53.
37. Yamada M, Fujii K, Fukui M. [clinical features and outcomes in patients with asymptomatic moyamoya disease--from the results of nation-wide questionnaire survey]. No shinkei geka. Neurol Surg. 2005;33(4):337–42.

38. Kuroda S, Hashimoto N, Yoshimoto T, Iwasaki Y. Radiological findings, clinical course, and outcome in asymptomatic moyamoya disease: results of multicenter survey in Japan. Stroke. 2007;38(5):1430–5.
39. Cho WS, Chung YS, Kim JE, Jeon JP, Son YJ, Bang JS, et al. The natural clinical course of hemodynamically stable adult moyamoya disease. J Neurosurg. 2015;122(1):82–9.
40. Kuroda S. Asymptomatic moyamoya disease: literature review and ongoing AMORE study. Neurol Med Chir. 2015;55(3):194–8.
41. Lee SC, Jeon JS, Kim JE, Chung YS, Ahn JH, Cho WS, et al. Contralateral progression and its risk factor in surgically treated unilateral adult moyamoya disease with a review of pertinent literature. Acta Neurochir. 2014;156(1):103–11.
42. Hayashi K, Horie N, Izumo T, Nagata I. A nationwide survey on unilateral moyamoya disease in Japan. Clin Neurol Neurosurg. 2014;124:1–5.
43. Smith ER, Scott RM. Progression of disease in unilateral moyamoya syndrome. Neurosurg Focus. 2008;24(2):E17.
44. Houkin K, Abe H, Yoshimoto T, Takahashi A. Is "unilateral" moyamoya disease different from moyamoya disease? J Neurosurg. 1996;85(5):772–6.
45. Hayashi K, Suyama K, Nagata I. Clinical features of unilateral moyamoya disease. Neurol Med Chir. 2010;50(5):378–85.
46. Kawano T, Fukui M, Hashimoto N, Yonekawa Y. Follow-up study of patients with "unilateral" moyamoya disease. Neurol Med Chir. 1994;34(11):744–7.
47. Park EK, Lee YH, Shim KW, Choi JU, Kim DS. Natural history and progression factors of unilateral moyamoya disease in pediatric patients. Child's Nervous System: ChNS: Official Journal of the International Society for Pediatric Neurosurgery. 2011;27(8):1281–7.
48. Yeon JY, Shin HJ, Kong DS, Seol HJ, Kim JS, Hong SC, et al. The prediction of contralateral progression in children and adolescents with unilateral moyamoya disease. Stroke. 2011;42(10):2973–6.
49. Kim JE, Pang CH. Diagnosis and treatment of adult Moyamoya disease. Journal of the Korean Medical Association/Taehan Uisa Hyophoe Chi. 2019;62(11):577–85.
50. Kim JE, Kim KM, Kim JG, Kang HS, Bang JS, Son YJ, et al. Clinical features of adult moyamoya disease with special reference to the diagnosis. Neurol Med Chir. 2012;52(5):311–7.
51. Nariai T, Suzuki R, Matsushima Y, Ichimura K, Hirakawa K, Ishii K, et al. Surgically induced angiogenesis to compensate for hemodynamic cerebral ischemia. Stroke. 1994;25(5):1014–21.
52. Fung LW, Thompson D, Ganesan V. Revascularisation surgery for paediatric moyamoya: a review of the literature. Child's Nervous System: ChNS: Official Journal of the International Society for Pediatric Neurosurgery. 2005;21(5):358–64.
53. Veeravagu A, Guzman R, Patil CG, Hou LC, Lee M, Steinberg GK. Moyamoya disease in pediatric patients: outcomes of neurosurgical interventions. Neurosurg Focus. 2008;24(2):E16.
54. Zheng J, Yu LB, Dai KF, Zhang Y, Wang R, Zhang D. Clinical features, surgical treatment, and long-term outcome of a multicenter cohort of pediatric Moyamoya. Front Neurol. 2019;10:14.
55. Matsushima T, Inoue T, Suzuki SO, Fujii K, Fukui M, Hasuo K. Surgical treatment of moyamoya disease in pediatric patients--comparison between the results of indirect and direct revascularization procedures. Neurosurgery. 1992;31(3):401–5.
56. Zhao Y, Lu J, Yu S, Li J, Deng X, Zhang Y, et al. Comparison of long-term effect between direct and indirect bypass for pediatric ischemic-type Moyamoya disease: a propensity score-matched study. Front Neurol. 2019;10:795.
57. Ikezaki K. Rational approach to treatment of moyamoya disease in childhood. J Child Neurol. 2000;15(5):350–6.
58. Adelson PD, Scott RM. Pial synangiosis for moyamoya syndrome in children. Pediatr Neurosurg. 1995;23(1):26–33.
59. Bao XY, Duan L, Yang WZ, Li DS, Sun WJ, Zhang ZS, et al. Clinical features, surgical treatment, and long-term outcome in pediatric patients with moyamoya disease in China. Cerebrovasc Dis (Basel, Switzerland). 2015;39(2):75–81.

60. Kazumata K, Ito M, Tokairin K, Ito Y, Houkin K, Nakayama N, et al. The frequency of postoperative stroke in moyamoya disease following combined revascularization: a single-university series and systematic review. J Neurosurg. 2014;121(2):432–40.
61. Heros RC, Scott RM, Kistler JP, Ackerman RH, Conner ES. Temporary neurological deterioration after extracranial-intracranial bypass. Neurosurgery. 1984;15(2):178–85.
62. Hayashi T, Shirane R, Fujimura M, Tominaga T. Postoperative neurological deterioration in pediatric moyamoya disease: watershed shift and hyperperfusion. J Neurosurg Pediatr. 2010;6(1):73–81.
63. Uchino H, Kuroda S, Hirata K, Shiga T, Houkin K, Tamaki N. Predictors and clinical features of postoperative hyperperfusion after surgical revascularization for moyamoya disease: a serial single photon emission CT/positron emission tomography study. Stroke. 2012;43(10):2610–6.
64. Fujimura M, Kaneta T, Tominaga T. Efficacy of superficial temporal artery-middle cerebral artery anastomosis with routine postoperative cerebral blood flow measurement during the acute stage in childhood moyamoya disease. Child's Nervous System: ChNS: Official Journal of the International Society for Pediatric Neurosurgery. 2008;24(7):827–32.
65. Rashad S, Fujimura M, Niizuma K, Endo H, Tominaga T. Long-term follow-up of pediatric moyamoya disease treated by combined direct-indirect revascularization surgery: single institute experience with surgical and perioperative management. Neurosurg Rev. 2016;39(4):615–23.
66. Kim T, Oh CW, Kwon OK, Hwang G, Kim JE, Kang HS, et al. Stroke prevention by direct revascularization for patients with adult-onset moyamoya disease presenting with ischemia. J Neurosurg. 2016;124(6):1788–93.
67. Bang JS, Kwon OK, Kim JE, Kang HS, Park H, Cho SY, et al. Quantitative angiographic comparison with the OSIRIS program between the direct and indirect revascularization modalities in adult moyamoya disease. Neurosurgery. 2012;70(3):625–32. discussion 32–3
68. Kuroda S, Houkin K, Ishikawa T, Nakayama N, Iwasaki Y. Novel bypass surgery for moyamoya disease using pericranial flap: its impacts on cerebral hemodynamics and long-term outcome. Neurosurgery. 2010;66(6):1093–101. discussion 101
69. Bao XY, Zhang Y, Wang QN, Zhang Q, Wang H, Zhang ZS, et al. Long-term outcomes after Encephaloduroarteriosynangiosis in adult patients with Moyamoya disease presenting with ischemia. World Neurosurg. 2018;115:e482–e9.
70. Dusick JR, Gonzalez NR, Martin NA. Clinical and angiographic outcomes from indirect revascularization surgery for Moyamoya disease in adults and children: a review of 63 procedures. Neurosurgery. 2011;68(1):34–43. discussion
71. Gross BA, Du R. The natural history of moyamoya in a north American adult cohort. Journal of Clinical Neuroscience: Official Journal of the Neurosurgical Society of Australasia. 2013;20(1):44–8.
72. Hallemeier CL, Rich KM, Grubb RL Jr, Chicoine MR, Moran CJ, Cross DT 3rd, et al. Clinical features and outcome in north American adults with moyamoya phenomenon. Stroke. 2006;37(6):1490–6.
73. Takahashi JC, Funaki T, Houkin K, Kuroda S, Fujimura M, Tomata Y, et al. Impact of cortical hemodynamic failure on both subsequent hemorrhagic stroke and effect of bypass surgery in hemorrhagic moyamoya disease: a supplementary analysis of the Japan adult Moyamoya trial. J Neurosurg. 2020:1–6.
74. Ha EJ, Kim KH, Wang KC, Phi JH, Lee JY, Choi JW, et al. Long-term outcomes of indirect bypass for 629 children with Moyamoya disease: longitudinal and Cross-sectional analysis. Stroke. 2019;50(11):3177–83.
75. Kim DS, Huh PW, Kim HS, Kim IS, Choi S, Mok JH, et al. Surgical treatment of moyamoya disease in adults: combined direct and indirect vs. indirect bypass surgery. Neurol Med Chir. 2012;52(5):333–8.
76. Kim T, Bang JS, Kwon OK, Hwang G, Kim JE, Kang HS, et al. Hemodynamic changes after unilateral revascularization for Moyamoya disease: serial assessment by quantitative magnetic resonance angiography. Neurosurgery. 2017;81(1):111–9.

77. Kim KM, Kim JE, Cho WS, Kang HS, Son YJ, Han MH, et al. Natural history and risk factor of recurrent hemorrhage in hemorrhagic adult Moyamoya disease. Neurosurgery. 2017;81(2):289–96.
78. Choi WS, Lee SB, Kim DS, Huh PW, Yoo DS, Lee TG, et al. Thirteen-year experience of 44 patients with adult hemorrhagic Moyamoya disease from a single institution: clinical analysis by management modality. Journal of cerebrovascular and endovascular neurosurgery. 2013;15(3):191–9.
79. Ahn JH, Wang KC, Phi JH, Lee JY, Cho BK, Kim IO, et al. Hemorrhagic moyamoya disease in children: clinical features and surgical outcome. Child's Nervous System: ChNS: Official Journal of the International Society for Pediatric Neurosurgery. 2012;28(2):237–45.
80. Phi JH, Wang KC, Cho BK, Lee MS, Lee JH, Yu KS, et al. Long-term social outcome in children with moyamoya disease who have reached adulthood. J Neurosurg Pediatr. 2011;8(3):303–9.
81. Lee JY, Phi JH, Wang KC, Cho BK, Shin MS, Kim SK. Neurocognitive profiles of children with moyamoya disease before and after surgical intervention. Cerebrovasc Dis (Basel, Switzerland). 2011;31(3):230–7.
82. Jeon JP, Kim JE, Cho WS, Bang JS, Son YJ, Oh CW. Meta-analysis of the surgical outcomes of symptomatic moyamoya disease in adults. J Neurosurg. 2018;128(3):793–9.
83. Choi IJ, Cho SJ, Chang JC, Park SQ, Park HK. Angiographic results of indirect and combined bypass surgery for adult moyamoya disease. J Cerebrovasc Endovasc Neurosurg. 2012;14(3):216–22.
84. Lee SB, Kim DS, Huh PW, Yoo DS, Lee TG, Cho KS. Long-term follow-up results in 142 adult patients with moyamoya disease according to management modality. Acta Neurochir. 2012;154(7):1179–87.
85. Jo KI, Kim MS, Yeon JY, Kim JS, Hong SC. Recurrent bleeding in hemorrhagic Moyamoya disease : prognostic implications of the perfusion status. J Korean Neurosurg Soc. 2016;59(2):117–21.

Indirect Bypass Surgery for Moyamoya Disease

24

Tadashi Nariai

Abstract

Recent animal experimental and human autopsy studies have revealed that the mechanism of indirect bypass surgery is the induction of "arteriogenesis," the main trigger of which is the inter-tissue gradient of perfusion pressure. Knowing this helps us to understand why indirect bypass surgery is effective for the chronic ischemic condition of moyamoya disease, how better to apply this technique, and what this technique's limitations are.

In this chapter, we review various aspects of the use of indirect bypass surgery for moyamoya disease. As part of our discussion, the characteristic hemodynamic condition of moyamoya disease is summarized. Special emphasis is placed on the importance of using clinical imaging for precise measurement of regional cerebral perfusion pressures, so that indirect bypass surgery can be most effectively used for the treatment of moyamoya disease.

Keywords

Moyamoya disease · Arteriogenesis · Angiogenesis · Bypass surgery · Cerebral perfusion pressure · Acetazolamide · PET · MRI

T. Nariai (✉)
Department of Neurosurgery, Tokyo Medical and Dental University, Tokyo, Japan
e-mail: nariai.nsrg@tmd.ac.jp

S. Kuroda (ed.), *Moyamoya Disease: Current Knowledge and Future Perspectives*, https://doi.org/10.1007/978-981-33-6404-2_24

24.1 Introduction

Use of indirect bypass surgery was originally conceived as an alternative to direct bypass surgery when performing the latter was technically difficult. The present author's department originated the encephalo-duro-arterio-synangiosis (EDAS) procedure [1], one of the major techniques of indirect bypass surgery, and has been actively using it for the treatment of moyamoya disease (MMD) for approximately 40 years. During this period, around 450 patients have received around 550 operations and have been closely followed to obtain long-term outcome data [2].

A review of the surgical results suggests that indirect bypass surgery might not only be a second-line alternative to direct bypass surgery, but might in fact be a first-line method to ameliorate chronic cerebral ischemia using the biological compensatory mechanism that is inherent to human beings.

In this chapter, the history, physiological mechanism, method of practical clinical use, and advantages and limitations of indirect bypass surgery for MMD will be reviewed.

24.2 History and Mechanism of Indirect Bypass Surgery

Attempts to surgically treat chronic cerebral ischemia without direct vessel-to-vessel suturing were first undertaken in Europe. The first case report of encephalo-myo-synangiosis (EMS) was published by German physicians in 1950 [3]. In the 1970s, animal experiments to examine the effectiveness of omentum transplantation were conducted in both Europe and the USA [4, 5]. While this technique did not take root as a general tool for ameliorating chronic cerebral ischemia, it did gain sway as a procedure for treating MMD. Thereafter, most of the subsequent developments in the indirect bypass technique were reported from Japan [1, 6–8], where active surgical treatment for this disease started earlier than in other countries. The question arises: Why was indirect bypass effective for MMD but not for atherosclerotic internal carotid occlusion? The answer lies in both the biological mechanism of indirect bypass surgery and the characteristic hemodynamic condition of MMD.

There are two ways new blood vessels are formed: "angiogenesis" and "arteriogenesis" [9]. "Angiogenesis" produces a capillary bed induced by ischemia or a wound-healing process. "Arteriogenesis" is the formation of new arteries in this capillary bed, as triggered by large differences in inter-tissue perfusion pressure. A recent experimental study using a pig model of chronic cerebral ischemia [10] and a human autopsy study [11] revealed that newly appeared vessels connecting the external and internal carotid systems after indirect bypass were "arteries" with thick, three-layer vessel walls (Fig. 24.1): in other words, the indirect bypass surgery was shown to induce newly formed vessels by arteriogenesis. More specifically, the formation of vessels by indirect bypass surgery can be considered to have two steps: (1) the formation of a capillary bed in the operative field, and (2) the formation of arteries within this capillary bed, which occurs only when there is a large difference in perfusion pressure between the external carotid system and internal carotid system.

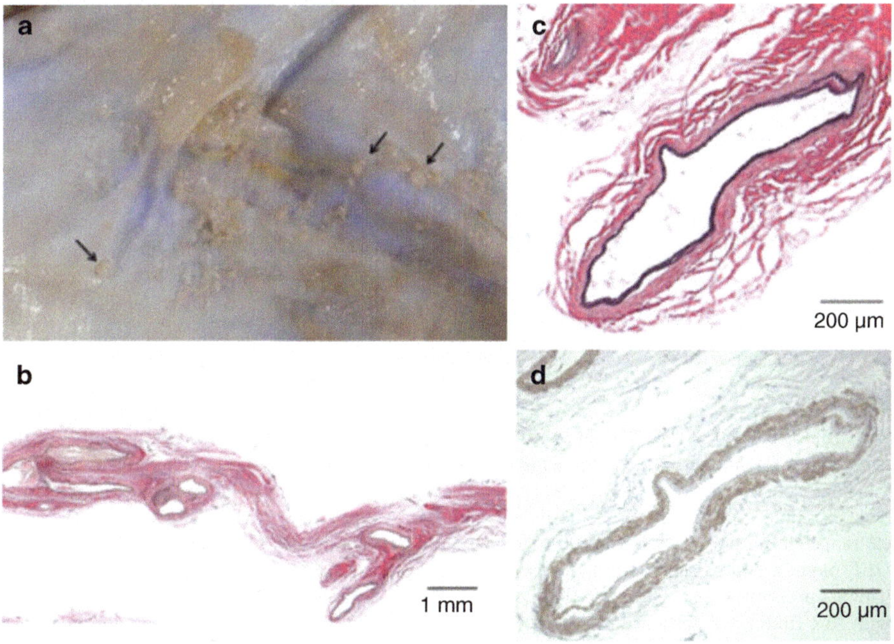

Fig. 24.1 Autopsy analysis of an arterial network that was induced by indirect bypass surgery. This histology was obtained from the dura mater of a 39-year-old woman with MMD who underwent bilateral indirect bypass surgery 22 years earlier. The ends of many protruding cords can be seen (*arrows*) on the internal side of the dura mater (**a**). Numerous arteries run through the internal side of the dura mater (**b**). Some of these arteries sprout to the brain (**c**). The 3-layer structure of the vascular walls is maintained in the new arteries generated (**d**). The media is thin, sparse, and composed mainly of smooth muscle actins. It clearly differs in structure from the media of preexisting vessels. Elastic van Gieson stain (**b** and **c**) and smooth muscle actin stain (**d**). The figure was used with permission from an article by Mukawa et al. [11]

24.3 The Hemodynamic Characteristics of Moyamoya Disease

One might ask, why is indirect bypass surgery effective for MMD but not for atherosclerotic internal carotid occlusion? The answer relates to the characteristics of moyamoya disease. Nariai et al. examined hemodynamic condition of MMD with positron emission tomography (PET) and reported that the hemodynamics of this disease is not uniform but varies according to disease subtype [12]. When patients presented with transient ischemic attack (TIA), the cerebral blood volume (CBV) reached twice that of the normal condition with only mild reduction of cerebral blood flow (CBF) (Fig. 24.2). Depending on the theoretical consideration of compensatory mechanism described by Powers [13], the cerebral perfusion pressure (CPP) correlates with CBF/CBV. In MMD, many patients with TIA may have 50% reduction of CPP without severe reduction of CBF. By contrast, atherosclerotic internal carotid occlusion generally does not cause large increases in CBV [14], so

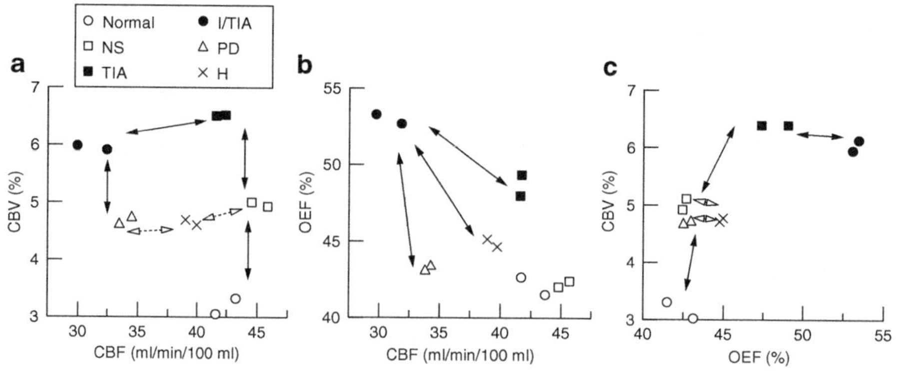

Fig. 24.2 Correlation among PET-measured hemodynamic factors (**a**) CBF vs VBV, (**b**) CBF vs OEF, (**c**) OEF vs CBV) of patients with moyamoya diseases is plotted. The average value of the frontal cortex is plotted according to the clinical presentation. Note that patients presenting with transient ischemic attack (TIA and I/TIA) had twice the average CBV values of normal controls. Note also that, even when OEF is highly elevated (I/TIA type), reduction of CBF is not in the critical range (more than 30 ml/min/100 ml). *CBF* cerebral blood flow, *CBV* cerebral blood volume, *OEF* oxygen extraction fraction, *Normal* normal volunteer, *NS* non-symptomatic patients, *TIA* patients presenting TIA without MR finding of cortical infarction, *I/TIA* patients presenting TIA with MR finding of cortical infarction, *PD* Patients presenting infarction with remaining severe permanent deficit, *H* patients with hemorrhagic onset. The figure was used with permission from an article by Nariai et al. [12]

that reduction of CPP is not as great when patients present with ischemic symptoms. This hypothesis might explain why indirect bypass surgery is effective for MMD with ischemic symptoms but not for atherosclerotic occlusive disease.

As a previous article indicated [12], the decrease of CPP is not uniform even among patients with moyamoya disease. As indicated in Fig. 24.2, the asymptomatic subtype and hemorrhagic subtype of this disease do not have as severe a decrease in CPP as the symptomatic ischemic subtypes. Therefore, indirect direct bypass surgery may not induce good arteriogenesis in such subtypes. Also, the region of the decreased CPP varies even among individuals with ischemic subtypes. Therefore, pre-operative neuroimaging to detect the degree and region of decreased CPP is tremendously important for the determination of whether and how to use indirect bypass surgery appropriately.

24.4 Pre-Operative Neuroimaging for Precise Application of Indirect-Bypass Surgery

Our group has been examining how pre-operative neuroimaging can predict the degree of post-operative arteriogenesis in the operative field [15, 16]. These works have proven that quantitated or semi-quantitated parameters of a cortex that is subject to surgery can predict the degree of collateral development. These parameters are as follows: cerebrovascular reactivity (CVR) by acetazolamide challenge measured by xenon CT (Fig. 24.3B) or ^{123}I isopropyl iodoamphetamine (IMP)

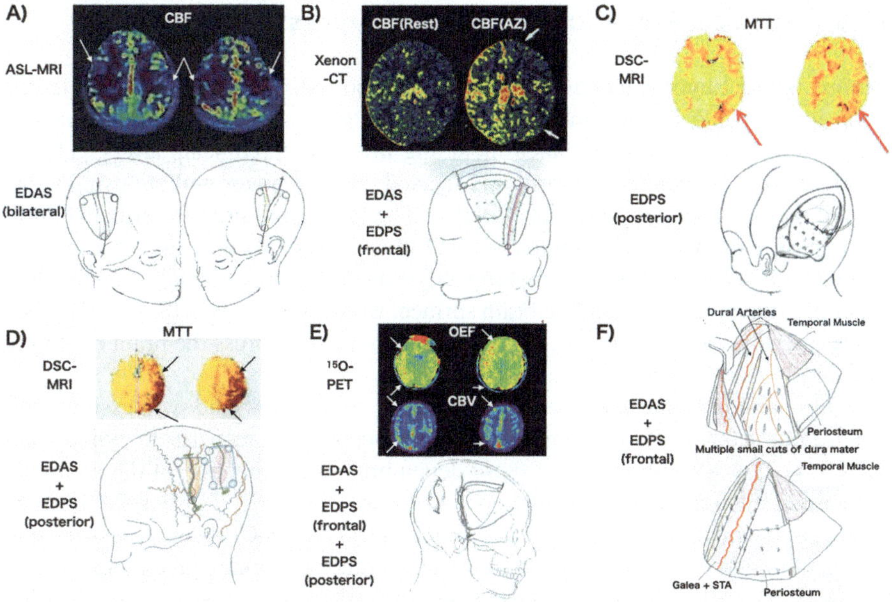

Fig. 24.3 (**A–E**) Various types of indirect bypass surgery for MMD performed at Tokyo Medical and Dental University are displayed. Various pre-operative neuroimaging modalities detecting a reduced area of CPP (indicated in each imaging by arrows). Surgical procedures were selected based on the spatial extent of hypoperfusion. (**F**) Principle of the operative procedure. We do not open dura mater widely; instead, many cuts are made, preserving all visible dural arteries (Fig. 24.3F), and flaps are sutured to the outside of the dura mater. *EDAS* encephalo-duro-arterio-synangiosis [1], *EDPS* encephalo-duro-periosto-synangiosis [17], *ASL-MRI*, arterial spin-labeling magnetic resonance imaging, *CBF* cerebral blood flow, *CBF (Rest)* cerebral blood flow in resting condition, *CBF (AZ)* cerebral blood flow after acetazolamide loading, *DSC-MRI* dynamic susceptibility contrast magnetic resonance imaging, *MTT* mean transit time, *PET* positron emission tomography, *OEF* oxygen extraction fraction, *CBV* cerebral blood volume

single-photon emission tomography (SPECT), CBV and oxygen extraction fraction (OEF) measured by PET (Fig. 24.3E), and mean transit time (MTT) measured by dynamic susceptibility contrast magnetic resonance imaging (DSC-MRI) (Fig. 24.3D and E).

Since the establishment of such neuroimaging techniques, potential adult or young-adult candidates for indirect bypass surgery have been screened to determine its suitability. Visualization of spatial distribution of the area with decreased CPP is also used to determine the operative procedure as will be described in the next chapter.

In the case of small children, all patients have been operated with an indirect bypass technique; therefore, pre-operative neuroimaging may not be necessary to determine the surgical indication. It is, however, still useful to visualize the extent of the hypo-perfused area and to determine the operative procedure. The recent development of arterial spin-labeling (ASL) MRI (Fig. 24.3A) has extended the use of brain perfusion imaging to children, due to its non-invasiveness [18].

24.5 Surgical Procedure of Indirect Bypass Surgery

Various indirect bypass techniques have been reported. Reported tissue implanted as an indirect flap include the temporal muscle [6], omentum [7], disconnected scalp artery [19], galea [20], galea including flow-preserved scalp artery [1], and pericranium [17]; another group simply incised the dura mater without using a flap [8]. All methods were reported as effective. The factors required for effective indirect bypass surgery may be summarized as follows: (1) performing the procedure in an area with decreased CPP, (2) making adhesion and granulation between the dura mater or implanted tissue and the brain surface, which will become the capillary bed where arteriogenesis will occur, (3) taking care not to compress the brain by flap or bleeding.

After gaining some experience with these procedures and witnessing their results, our team is now using EDAS [1], encephalo-duro-periosto-synangiosis (EDPS) [17] or a combination of these depending on the location of the area with decreased CPP. Examples of actual operations are summarized in Fig. 24.3. Many young patients with transient ischemic attack (TIA) have a CPP deficit restricted to the sensorimotor cortex; EDAS using a parietal branch of superficial temporal artery (STA) works well to ameliorate these symptoms (Fig. 24.3A). When the perfusion deficit exists in bilateral hemispheres, both sides can undergo surgery in a single anesthesia. When the CPP deficit extends more anteriorly to include the whole frontal lobe, frontal EDPS is often combined with EDAS (Fig. 24.3B). When the CPP deficit is located mainly among the area of posterior circulation, EDPS to the parieto-occipital area is performed (Fig. 24.3C). Such surgery is often performed on cases in whom occlusion of posterior cerebral artery (PCA) occurred several years after the initial treatment to the area of anterior circulation. When the area with the deficit extends further, these procedures are combined (Fig. 24.3D, E). Recently, we have refrained from opening the dura mater widely; instead, many small cuts are performed, preserving all visible dural arteries (Fig. 24.3F), and flaps are sutured to the outside of the dura mater [17].

Nakamura et al. [10] proved that arteriogenesis after an indirect bypass procedure starts after the formation of granulation tissue is completed during the wound healing process. One month after the operation, the arterial network was histologically observed in the operative field. Our recent neuro-imaging study examining the post-operative chronological changes of hemodynamics using DSC-MRI [21] indicated that statistically significant shortening of the MTT (=increase in CPP) was observed 15–30 days after surgery. In some individuals, shortening of MTT can be observed earlier, as in the representative case shown in Fig. 24.4. In this case, the MRI scan taken 12 days after surgery had a clearly shorter MTT than the preoperative scan. Because these recent experimental [10] and clinical [21] findings are so correspondent, amelioration of hemodynamics by indirect bypass surgery likely starts earlier than formerly thought.

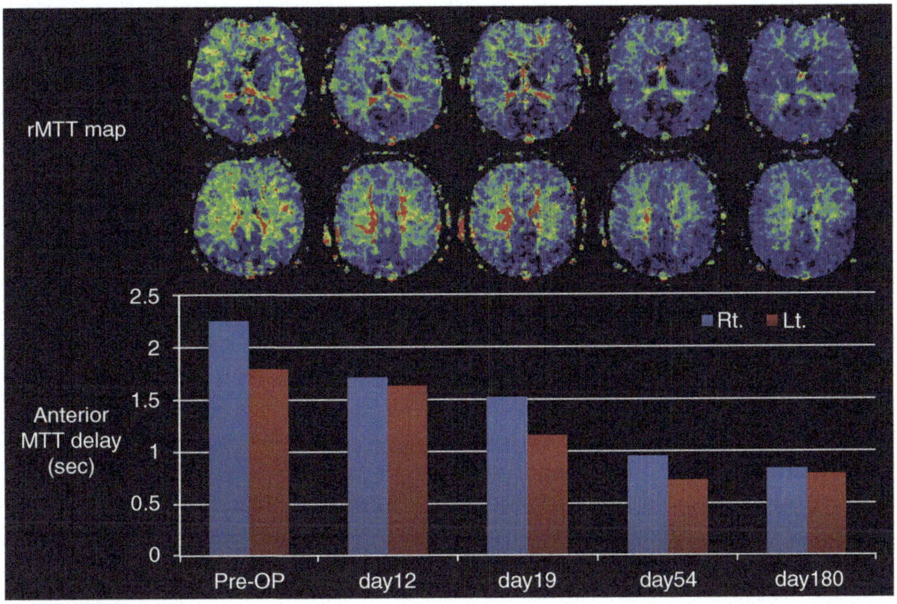

Fig. 24.4 A representative case of post-operative chronological follow-up using DSC-MRI. This is a 31-year-old woman who underwent bilateral indirect bypass surgery. Preoperative (Pre-OP) and postoperative relative mean transit time (rMTT) maps and the bar graph of anterior mean transit time (MTT) delay show that MTT had already begun to decrease 12 days after surgery and had almost stabilized at about 2 months after surgery. Anterior MTT delay: delay of the MTT compared with the control region (cerebellum) in the whole anterior circulation area. *Lt.* left, *Rt.* right, *sec* seconds. This figure was used with permission from an article by Ishii et al. [21]

24.6 Advantages and Limitations of Indirect Bypass Surgery

The advantage of indirect-bypass surgery lies in its non-invasiveness. As all procedures are epi-arachnoidal, and most of the procedures in our present surgical protocol are epi-dural, the indirect-bypass should be considered an operative procedure with no invasiveness to the brain. Therefore, no harmful events have occurred during operation. The only peri-operative complication is the possibility of a post-operative ischemic event within 1 week of the operation. During this week, close post-operative medical care and supervision are required to prevent the occurrence of a permanent deficit by cerebral infarction; this includes the use of antiplatelet and anticoagulation medication, sufficient fluid infusion, prevention of hypotension and anemia, etc. Post-operative management of indirect bypass surgery, however, is not overly complex because ischemia is the only potential complication. Post-operative management of direct bypass surgery is more complicated because complications deriving from either hypo-perfusion or hyper-perfusion are possible [22, 23].

By performing such peri-operative management, the recent perioperative infarction rate has been as low as 3% [24], with no focal neurological deficits remaining. Since peri-operative infarction, however, can cause cognitive decline after surgery [25], further efforts to reduce the rate of peri-operative infarction must be continued. Once the risk of peri-operative infarction is successfully averted, there is a greater chance of recovery of pre-operative cognitive decline by indirect bypass surgery [25]. This may be another advantage of indirect bypass surgery compared to direct bypass, as both the hypoperfusive and hyperperfusive peri-operative complications of the latter can cause cognitive decline [26].

The limitation of indirect bypass is that it is not effective for all types of MMD. As indicated in Fig. 24.2, the decrease in CPP (CBF/CBV) of hemorrhagic or non-symptomatic cases is not as large as that of symptomatic ischemic cases. Therefore, sufficient arteriogenesis by indirect bypass surgery may not be expected in those subtypes. Therefore, when we perform surgery to reduce the re-bleeding risk of hemorrhagic-onset cases, direct bypass surgery should be selected [27]. And, if evidence to support performing bypass surgery on asymptomatic cases is obtained by the ongoing multicenter study in Japan [28], only the direct bypass surgical method should be used.

24.7 Conclusions

Indirect bypass surgery is defined as a surgical technique to induce arteriogenesis in areas with highly reduced CPP among ischemic-type MMD cases. If such a condition is detected by the pre-operative neuro-imaging study, this technique is effective regardless of age. If ischemic conditions do not exist, this technique is not expected to be effective. Therefore, for the appropriate use of indirect bypass surgery, appropriate use of pre-operative neuroimaging to detect CPP deficit is mandatory. Also, peri-operative care is critical for reducing the rate of peri-operative infarction and thereby improving the chances of recovery from pre-operative cognitive decline.

References

1. Matsushima Y, Fukai N, Tanaka K, Tsuruoka S, Inaba Y, Aoyagi M, Ohno K. A new surgical treatment of moyamoya disease in children: a preliminary report. Surg Neurol. 1981;15:313–20.
2. Mukawa M, Nariai T, Matsushima Y, Tanaka Y, Inaji M, Maehara T, Aoyagi M, Ohno K. Long-term follow-up of surgically treated juvenile patients with moyamoya disease. J Neurosurg Pediatr. 2012;10:451–6.
3. Henschen C. [surgical revascularization of cerebral injury of circulatory origin by means of stratification of pedunculated muscle flaps]. Langenbecks Archiv fur klinische Chirurgie vereinigt mit deutsche Zeitschrift fur. Chirurgie. 1950;264:392–401.
4. Goldsmith HS, Chen WF, Duckett SW. Brain vascularization by intact omentum. Arch Surg. 1973;106:695–8.
5. Yonekawa Y, Yasargil MG. Brain vascularization by transplanted omentum: a possible treatment of cerebral ischemia. Neurosurgery. 1977;1:256–9.

6. Karasawa J, Kikuchi H, Furuse S, Sakaki T, Yoshida Y. A surgical treatment of "moyamoya" disease "encephalo-myo synangiosis". Neurol Med Chir. 1977;17:29–37.
7. Karasawa J, Kikuchi H, Kawamura J, Sakai T. Intracranial transplantation of the omentum for cerebrovascular moyamoya disease: a two-year follow-up study. Surg Neurol. 1980;14:444–9.
8. Endo M, Kawano N, Miyaska Y, Yada K. Cranial burr hole for revascularization in moyamoya disease. J Neurosurg. 1989;71:180–5.
9. Heil M, Eitenmuller I, Schmitz-Rixen T, Schaper W. Arteriogenesis versus angiogenesis: similarities and differences. J Cell Mol Med. 2006;10:45–55.
10. Nakamura M, Imai H, Konno K, Kubota C, Seki K, Puentes S, Faried A, Yokoo H, Hata H, Yoshimoto Y, Saito N. Experimental investigation of encephalomyosynangiosis using gyrencephalic brain of the miniature pig: histopathological evaluation of dynamic reconstruction of vessels for functional anastomosis. Laboratory investigation. J Neurosurg Pediatr. 2009;3:488–95.
11. Mukawa M, Nariai T, Inaji M, Tamada N, Maehara T, Matsushima Y, Ohno K, Negi M, Kobayashi D. First autopsy analysis of a neovascularized arterial network induced by indirect bypass surgery for moyamoya disease: case report. J Neurosurg. 2016;124:1211–4.
12. Nariai T, Matsushima Y, Imae S, Tanaka Y, Ishii K, Senda M, Ohno K. Severe haemodynamic stress in selected subtypes of patients with moyamoya disease: a positron emission tomography study. J Neurol Neurosurg Psychiatry. 2005;76:663–6.
13. Powers WJ. Cerebral hemodynamics in ischemic cerebrovascular disease. Ann Neurol. 1991;29:231–40.
14. Derdeyn CP, Videen TO, Yundt KD, Fritsch SM, Carpenter DA, Grubb RL, Powers WJ. Variability of cerebral blood volume and oxygen extraction: stages of cerebral haemodynamic impairment revisited. Brain: A Journal of Neurology. 2002;125:595–607.
15. Ishii Y, Nariai T, Tanaka Y, Mukawa M, Inaji M, Maehara T, Ohno K. Practical clinical use of dynamic susceptibility contrast magnetic resonance imaging (DSC-MRI) for the surgical treatment of Moyamoya disease. Neurosurgery. 2013;
16. Nariai T, Suzuki R, Matsushima Y, Ichimura K, Hirakawa K, Ishii K, Senda M. Surgically induced angiogenesis to compensate for hemodynamic cerebral ischemia. Stroke. 1994;25:1014–21.
17. Aoyagi M, Tanaka Y, Tamura K, Maehara T, Nariai T, Ohno K. Vascularized flap with multiple small dural opening for bypass surgery in moyamoya patients with occlusive lesioin in posterior circulation (in Japanese). Video J Japan Neurosurg. 2007:15.
18. Hara S, Tanaka Y, Ueda Y, Hayashi S, Inaji M, Ishiwata K, Ishii K, Maehara T, Nariai T. Noninvasive evaluation of CBF and perfusion delay of Moyamoya disease using arterial spin-labeling MRI with multiple Postlabeling delays: comparison with (15)O-gas PET and DSC-MRI. AJNR Am J Neuroradiol. 2017;38:696–702.
19. Adelson PD, Scott RM. Pial synangiosis for moyamoya syndrome in children. Pediatr Neurosurg. 1995;23:26–33.
20. Kim CY, Wang KC, Kim SK, Chung YN, Kim HS, Cho BK. Encephaloduroarteriosynangiosis with bifrontal encephalogaleo(periosteal)synangiosis in the pediatric moyamoya disease: the surgical technique and its outcomes. Child's Nervous System: ChNS: Official Journal of the International Society for Pediatric Neurosurgery. 2003;19:316–24.
21. Ishii Y, Tanaka Y, Momose T, Yamashina M, Sato A, Wakabayashi S, Maehara T, Nariai T. Chronologic evaluation of cerebral hemodynamics by dynamic susceptibility contrast magnetic resonance imaging after indirect bypass surgery for Moyamoya disease. World Neurosurg. 2017;108:427–35.
22. Hayashi T, Shirane R, Fujimura M, Tominaga T. Postoperative neurological deterioration in pediatric moyamoya disease: watershed shift and hyperperfusion. J Neurosurg Pediatr. 2010;6:73–81.
23. Fujimura M, Kaneta T, Mugikura S, Shimizu H, Tominaga T. Temporary neurologic deterioration due to cerebral hyperperfusion after superficial temporal artery-middle cerebral artery anastomosis in patients with adult-onset moyamoya disease. Surg Neurol. 2007;67:273–82.

24. Ishii Y, Nariai T, Tanaka Y, Mukawa M, Inaji M, Maehara T, Ohno K. Practical clinical use of dynamic susceptibility contrast magnetic resonance imaging for the surgical treatment of moyamoya disease. Neurosurgery. 2014;74:302–9.
25. Hara S, Kudo T, Hayashi S, Inaji M, Tanaka Y, Maehara T, Ishii K, Nariai T. Improvement in cognitive decline after indirect bypass surgery in adult moyamoya disease: implication of (15) O-gas positron emission tomography. Ann Nucl Med. 2020;34:467–75.
26. Yanagihara W, Chida K, Kobayashi M, Kubo Y, Yoshida K, Terasaki K, Ogasawara K. Impact of cerebral blood flow changes due to arterial bypass surgery on cognitive function in adult patients with symptomatic ischemic moyamoya disease. J Neurosurg. 2018;131:1716–24.
27. Miyamoto S, Yoshimoto T, Hashimoto N, Okada Y, Tsuji I, Tominaga T, Nakagawara J, Takahashi JC, Investigators JAMT. Effects of extracranial-intracranial bypass for patients with hemorrhagic moyamoya disease: results of the Japan adult Moyamoya trial. Stroke. 2014;45:1415–21.
28. Kuroda S, and Amore Study Group. Asymptomatic moyamoya disease: literature review and ongoing AMORE study. Neurol Med Chir. 2015;55:194–8.

Direct/Combined Bypass Surgery

25

Jun C. Takahashi

Abstract

Although numerous surgical techniques have been developed for moyamoya disease treatment, direct/combined bypass has recently been more popular than pure-indirect bypass due to its advantage of rapid increase of cerebral blood flow with less-frequent postoperative ischemic complications. This is especially true in adult cases, in which pure-indirect bypass is sometimes ineffective. In the Japan Adult Moyamoya Trial, a randomized controlled trial, which has proven the effectiveness of bypass surgery in preventing rebleeding attacks, surgical procedures are strictly confined to that including direct anastomosis. With all these benefits, however, surgeons should be alert to the adverse events after direct/combined bypass, such as postoperative hyperperfusion syndrome, and wound-related complications, especially when double procedures, which use both branches of the STA, are adopted.

Keywords

Direct bypass · Combined bypass · Hyperperfusion · Postoperative stroke

25.1 Direct/Combined Bypass Versus Indirect Bypass

Revascularization surgery for moyamoya disease can be classified into three types: direct anastomotic, indirect, and direct-indirect combined bypass. The advantage of direct bypass is reliability and immediate augmentation of cerebral blood flow in

J. C. Takahashi (✉)
Department of Neurosurgery, Kindai University Faculty of Medicine, Osaka, Japan
e-mail: juntak@med.kindai.ac.jp

S. Kuroda (ed.), *Moyamoya Disease: Current Knowledge and Future Perspectives*, https://doi.org/10.1007/978-981-33-6404-2_25

hemodynamically impaired cerebral hemispheres, which enables less-frequent postoperative ischemic complications [1–3]. However, the cortical arteries of patients with moyamoya disease are usually thin and fragile [4, 5], thus requiring substantially highly technical skills in accomplishing the vascular anastomosis, and the postoperative hyperperfusion syndrome has a relatively high rate compared to those of atherosclerotic arterial occlusion [6, 7].

Indirect bypass is grounded on a completely different concept. The collateral formation is expected to be derived by the spontaneous neovascularization from the pedicle vascularized tissue (i.e., temporal muscle) to the cortical surface. The biggest advantage of indirect bypass is its technical easiness, whereas the drawback is its delayed action. Indirect collateral formation requires several months to be established, which reportedly leads to a higher rate of ischemic complications in the early postoperative periods [3]. Another problem of the indirect bypass, which may be the most critical, is its insignificant effect in 30–40% of the adult patients [8]. Among pediatric patients, the benefit of indirect bypass has been widely known [2, 9]. However, even among them, failure of the indirect bypass, which requires reoperation with direct procedure, has still been reported [10].

Because a large randomized clinical trial has not been noted, the choice of surgical procedures largely depends on the preference and experience of each neurosurgeon. However, for the abovementioned reasons, the direct bypass seems to have become more frequent regardless of the patient age in recent years [11], whereas the pure-indirect bypass, such as encephalo-duro-arterio-synangiosis (EDAS), has not been preferred, especially in adult cases. Indirect bypass procedures with vascularized tissues, such as encephalo-myo-synangiosis (EMS), can be easily performed in addition to direct bypass. Consequently, various types of the direct-indirect combined bypass have emerged, achieving the benefits of both direct and indirect policies. Furthermore, the recent expanded indication of bypass surgery to the hemorrhagic moyamoya disease has made the direct anastomotic procedures more popular. The Japan Adult Moyamoya (JAM) Trial (conducted from 2001 to 2014) and its supplementary studies (2014–2020) have revealed that bypass surgery prevents rebleeding attacks in moyamoya disease with hemorrhagic presentation [12, 13]. In these studies, surgical procedures are strictly confined to the pure-direct or combined bypass.

25.2 Surgical Procedures of Direct/Combined Bypass

25.2.1 Superficial Temporal Artery (STA)-Middle Cerebral Artery (MCA) Anastomosis

STA-MCA anastomosis is the first reported revascularization surgery for moyamoya disease, which was performed in 1972 by Yasargil on a 4-year-old child [14, 15]. Although it is preferred to be performed together with the various indirect procedures, pure STA-MCA bypass is still popular especially among adult patients, whose temporal muscles are too thick to be used as donor tissues of the indirect procedures. The author, for example, uses direct bypass universally regardless of the patient's age and adds EMS in pediatric cases with thin temporal muscles. The choice of single- or double-barrel bypass depends on each neurosurgeon, both in the pure-direct and combined procedures.

Figure 25.1 shows the procedures for STA-MCA bypass. Following skin incision, subgaleal loose tissue is dissected, enabling reflection of skin flap. The temporal muscle is separated using a monopolar cutting device and reflected caudally. When the indirect bypass, such as EMS, is planned to be added, preservation of the deep temporal arteries, which run between the temporal muscle and pericranium, is important because it would serve as donor arteries. Frontotemporal craniotomy should be large enough for two reasons. First, cortical branches could be small in caliber and fragile, which often compels the surgeon to search for the good recipient artery all over the operative field. Second, when combined bypass is to be adopted, the pedicle vascularized tissue, such as the temporal muscle flap, should be contacted to as large area of the cortical surface as possible.

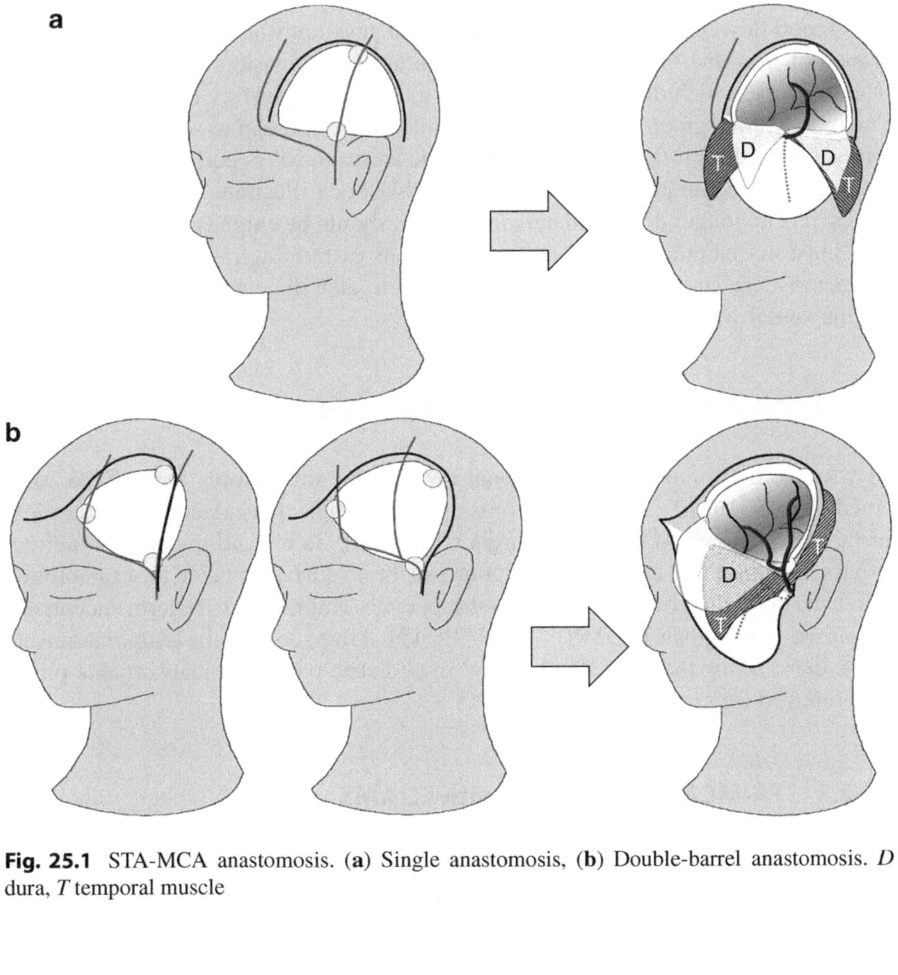

Fig. 25.1 STA-MCA anastomosis. (**a**) Single anastomosis, (**b**) Double-barrel anastomosis. *D* dura, *T* temporal muscle

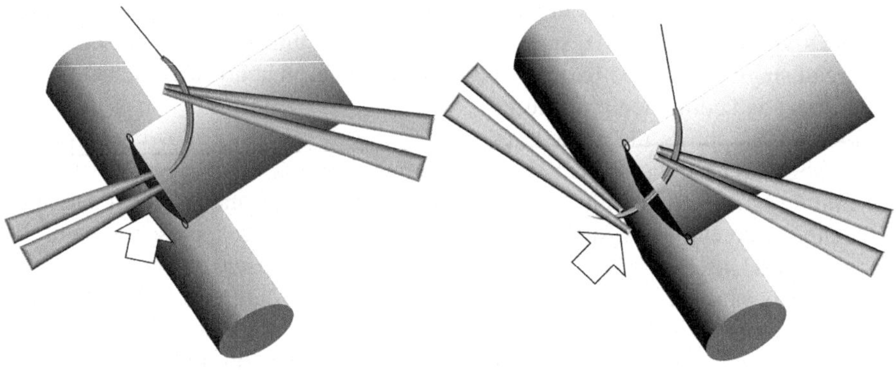

Fig. 25.2 Role of the forceps in direct bypass. The fragile MCA wall must not be pinched with forceps, the role of which is giving the counterforce by supporting the vessel walls (white arrows)

The STA is meticulously dissected under the operative microscope. The dura is opened while preserving the middle meningeal artery (MMA), especially if it supplies blood flow to the cortex via the transdural anastomosis. Typically, the anterior branch of the MMA ascends to the midline and then anastomoses to the anterior falcine artery, which finally supplies blood to the medial surface of the frontal lobe. The indocyanine green videoangiography allows the surgeon to select the recipient artery. Using the 11–0 suture, the end-to-side anastomosis is performed. Given that the operative technique of the direct bypass has been illustrated in numerous textbooks, it is no longer discussed here in detail. It should be emphasized that the MCA wall must not be pinched with forceps due to its extremely fragile and easy to tear characteristics. The main role of the forceps is to give the counterforce by supporting the vessel walls gently (Fig. 25.2).

25.2.2 STA-MCA Anastomosis with EMS/EDMS

STA-MCA anastomosis with additional EMS is the most simple form of the combined bypass [16, 17]. Pedicle flap of the temporal muscle is placed on the cortical surface and sutured to the dural margin (Fig. 25.3). To expand the area of indirect bypass, the dural flap can be reflected onto the brain surface outside the craniotomy. When the procedure of dural reflection is especially emphasized, the term encephalo-duro-myo-synangiosis (EDMS) is used [18, 19]. After suturing the temporal muscle to the dura, fixing the bone flap is done. In pediatric patients, bioabsorbable plates are preferred for cranial fixation.

25.2.3 STA-MCA Anastomosis with EDAMS

Houkin et al. proposed the method to expose as much of the brain surface as possible and to use the potential tissues as widely as possible as a source of indirect

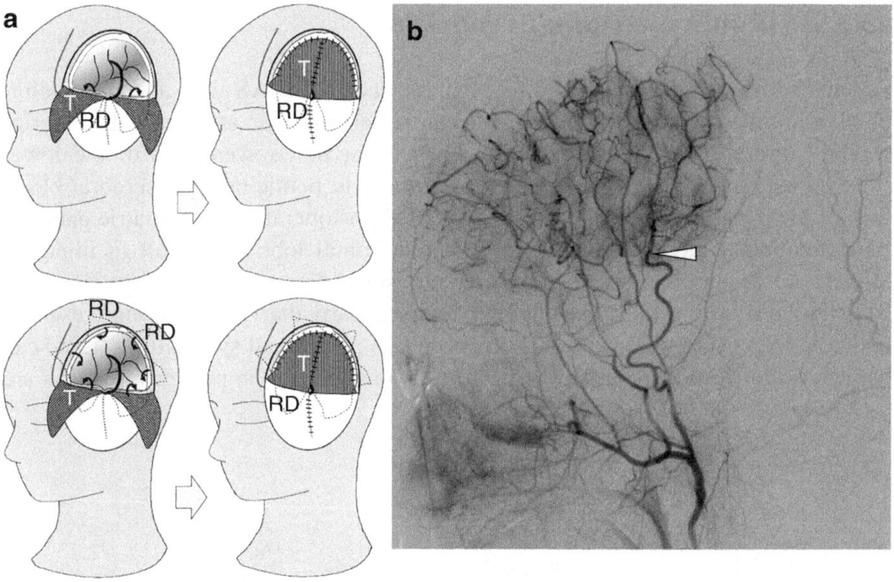

Fig. 25.3 STA-MCA anastomosis with EMS/EDMS. (**a**) EMS with dural reflection (2 types of the dural incision are illustrated), (**b**) The external carotid angiogram at 3 postoperative months showing sufficient revascularization from the STA parietal branch (white arrowhead) and the vascularized tissues (EDMS). *RD* reflected dura, *T* temporal muscle

revascularization (encephalo-duro-arterio-myo-synangiosis, EDAMS) [20, 21]. This method was derived from their inspection, as it was concluded that revascularization of the frontal lobe with severe hemodynamic failure cannot be fully achieved by the simple surgical technique. Using the STA frontal branch, single STA-MCA anastomosis is performed to the frontmost branch of the MCA to improve cerebral circulation of the frontal lobe. The dissected STA parietal branch is placed on the cortical surface while preserving the continuous flow to the distal side of the scalp, such as EDAS. Then the temporal muscle is placed on the brain surface and then sutured to the dural edge (EMS).

25.2.4 STA-MCA Anastomosis with EDMAPS

Kuroda et al. modified the EDAMS, proposing a more extensive combined bypass, which was called STA-MCA anastomosis with encephalo-duro-myo-arterio-pericranial synangiosis (EDMAPS) [22], with a larger craniotomy especially on the frontal side and using vascularized frontal pericranial flap to cover almost the whole frontal lobe. To date, this seems to be the most extensive combined bypass procedure.

25.2.5 STA-ACA Anastomosis with EPS

Patients who underwent only indirect bypass, such as EDAS with a small craniotomy, or simple direct/combined bypass can suffer ischemic attacks of the anterior cerebral artery (ACA) territory, such as transient motor weakness of the lower extremities, thereafter. Even in the cases without ischemic attacks, cerebral blood flow of the frontmost side can remain decreased postoperative. In pediatric patients, long-standing hemodynamic ischemia of the frontal lobe can result in impaired intellectual development [23]; therefore, persistent impaired hemodynamics of the frontal lobe warrants additional surgery, which is particularly true among preschool children. STA-ACA anastomosis with encephalo-pericranial synangiosis (EPS) can be the option (Fig. 25.4) [24]. Cortical ACA branches in the pediatric patients are

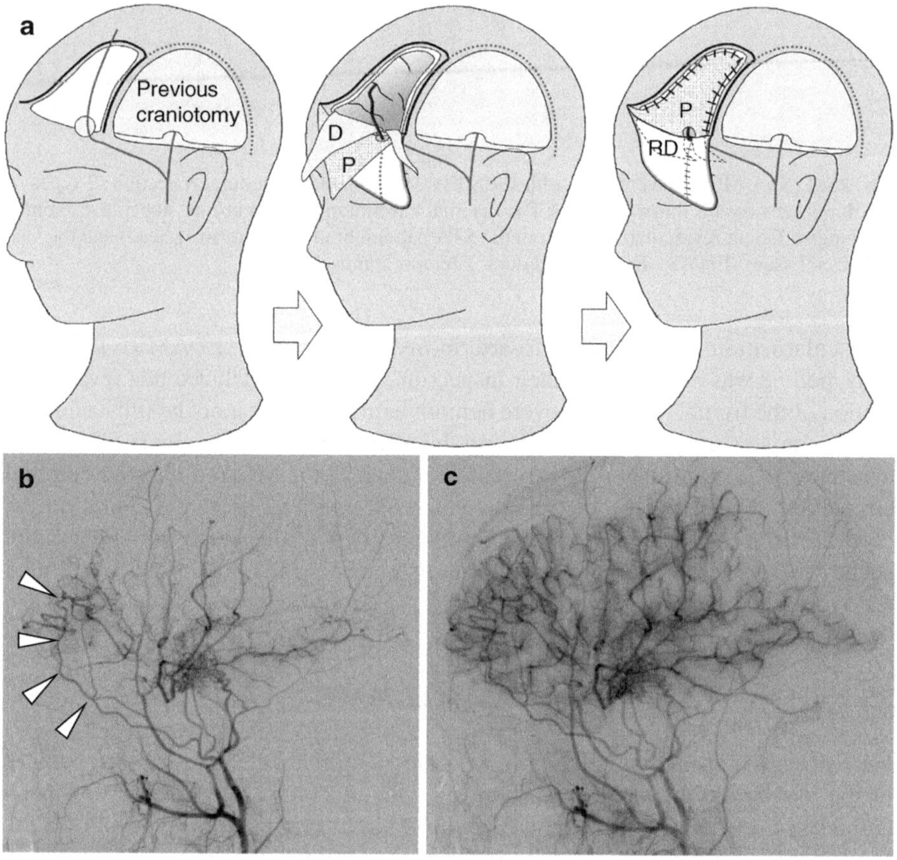

Fig. 25.4 STA-ACA anastomosis with EPS. (**a**) Surgical procedures of the additional STA-ACA anastomosis with EPS following the completion of the initial STA-MCA anastomosis with EMS. The frontal lobe is covered with the pericranium and the reflected dural flap. (**b** and **c**) The external carotid angiogram at 3 postoperative months (**b**: early phase, **c**: late arterial phase). *D* dura, *P* pericranium, *RD* reflected dura. White arrowheads: STA frontal branch

usually fragile and extremely small in caliber. Therefore, direct bypass for the ACA territory requires sufficient surgical training in vessel anastomosis. Skin incision should be designed to obtain as wide pericranial flap as possible.

Whether the extensive combined bypass covering the large area of the ACA as well as MCA territory is to be adopted in the initial surgery is controversial. Another option is considering the additional ACA bypass only for the selected patients following the completion of the initial simple combined bypass to the MCA territory. Both strategies have advantages and disadvantages in terms of effectiveness and invasiveness. The author performs STA-MCA bypass with EDMS routinely as the first operation for pediatric patients. Thereafter, the need for additional bypass for the ACA territory is considered individually according to the hemodynamic study and angiography at 3 postoperative months. In the author's retrospective analysis, the incidence of the additional ACA bypass was approximately 20% of the pediatric patients (data not published).

25.2.6 OA-PCA Anastomosis with EPS

The steno-occlusive change of the posterior cerebral artery (PCA) is observed in 25%–60% of patients with moyamoya disease. Therefore, in some, if not many, patients, the PCA lesion develops, causing ischemic attacks of the occipital lobe (i.e., transient visual field defect) after completing the bypass for the anterior circulation. In such cases, occipital artery (OA)-PCA anastomosis with EPS can be considered an additional surgery (Fig. 25.5) [25]. Cortical PCA branches are usually smaller in caliber than MCA branches, thus requiring the high-level skills of vascular anastomosis.

25.3 Surgical Complications of Direct/Combined Bypass

25.3.1 Postoperative Stroke

As the patients with a history of ischemic attacks naturally have an impaired cerebral hemodynamic state, they are susceptible to ischemic stroke in the early postoperative periods. The systematic review by Kazumata et al. revealed a less-frequent occurrence of postoperative stroke of the pediatric patients in direct/combined bypass than in pure-indirect bypass (2.5% vs 6.0%, $p < 0.001$), although no difference was observed in the adults [3]. They attributed this difference in pediatrics to the immediate increase in blood flow achieved by direct bypass. The immediate hemodynamic improvement can compensate postoperative adverse effects, such as hypocapnia induced by crying and circulation volume loss in pediatrics. When confined to the direct/combined bypass group, adult patients were significantly more susceptible to postoperative ischemic and hemorrhagic stroke than pediatric patients (7.6% vs 2.7%, $p < 0.001$), whereas such a difference was not observed in the indirect bypass group [3], which was partially attributed to less-developed collateral

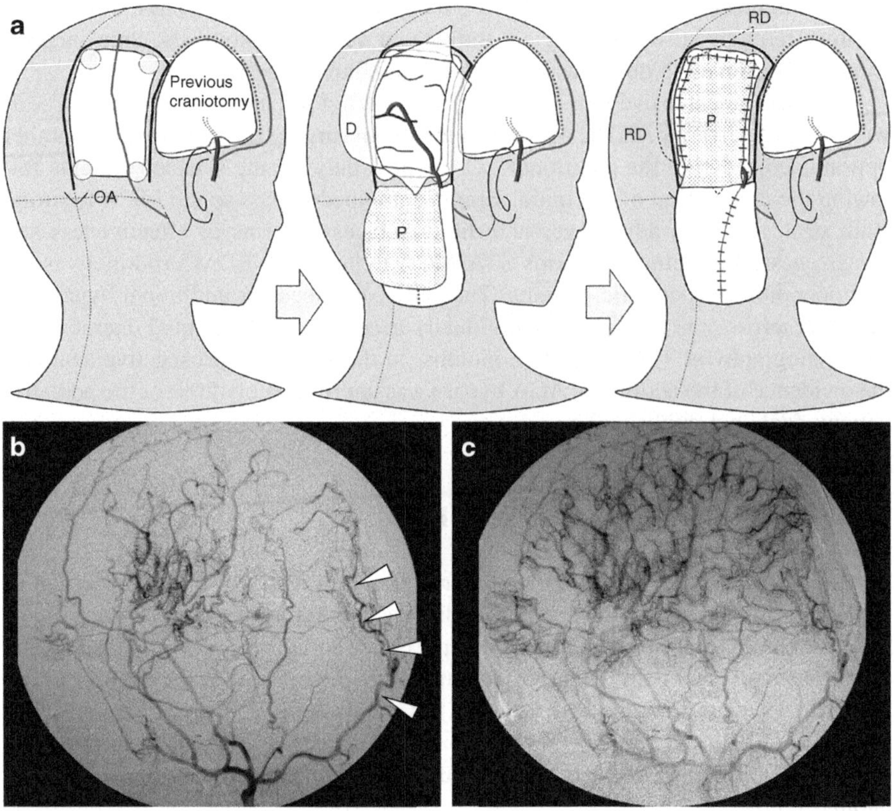

Fig. 25.5 OA-PCA anastomosis. (**a**) Surgical procedures of the additional OA-PCA anastomosis with EPS. The occipital lobe is covered with the pericranium and the reflected dural flap. (**b** and **c**) The external carotid angiogram at 3 postoperative months (B: early phase, C: late arterial phase). *D* dura, *P* pericranium, *RD* reflected dura. White arrowheads: OA

vessels in adults that failed to compensate for acute progressive occlusion in the main cerebral arteries after direct bypass [3]. Postoperative hyperperfusion, which is reportedly more common in adult patients, was hypothesized to have a more detrimental effect in adults than in pediatrics [3, 26].

25.3.2 Postoperative Hyperperfusion

Direct/combined bypass has a rapid and significant influence to the blood flow patterns, thus bringing about postoperative hyperperfusion in the operated hemispheres [7, 26, 27]. The incidence of both radiological and symptomatic hyperperfusions is reportedly much higher in adult patients than in pediatrics [26]. Uchino et al. demonstrated that radiological hyperperfusion was identified in 66% and 20% of the adults and pediatrics, respectively, by serial SPECT studies. Symptomatic hyperperfusion was found in 32% and 5% of the adults and pediatrics, respectively [26]. Clinical features of symptomatic hyperperfusion include transient motor weakness, aphasia, dysarthria, and seizure, most of which are transient and inadequate to be included in the category of surgical complications. The true complication, however, is intracerebral or subarachnoid hemorrhage, presumably caused by hyperperfusion. Postoperative intracranial hemorrhage is not rare and is found in 2.8% of the adult cases treated with combined bypass [3]. In the recent meta-analysis, the incidence of the hemorrhage accounted for 15% of the symptomatic hyperperfusion [28]. Although intracranial hemorrhage after bypass surgery seems to be less devastating than that after carotid endarterectomy [29], it can result in permanent deficits, such as hemiparesis, aphasia, and cognitive impairment. Adult patients with a cerebral blood volume increase have been reported to be the risk factors of both radiological and symptomatic hyperperfusions [26].

25.3.3 Operative Wound-Related Complications

Because of the well-developed vascular network in the scalp, wound-related complications are considered rare after the ordinary craniotomy surgery. However, bypass surgery, which requires harvesting the STAs, can compromise the blood supply and cause delayed wound healing or scalp necrosis [30]. Takanari et al. have reported that operative wound complications were found in 21.4% of the bypass surgeries [31], two-thirds of which are superficial necrosis in the epidermal level or poor adaptation, which could be treated with ointment or simple resuturing and thus classified as minor complications. One-third of the complication cases, on the other hand, had full-thickness skin necrosis, which consequently led to skin defects and required tissue transfer (major complications). Double procedures, which use both branches of the STA, and a history of diabetes have been found to be risk factors for wound-related complications [31]. Once infection is involved, the problem can be more serious. To reduce the wound-related complications, the skin incision, galeal incision, and vessel harvest line should be designed to compromise the blood supply as little as possible.

25.4 Special Considerations: Direct/Combined Bypass for Hemorrhagic Moyamoya Disease

Intracranial hemorrhage in moyamoya disease is assumed to be caused by the long-standing hemodynamic stress on the dilated collateral networks, which has been developed to compensate for the decrease in blood flow to the cerebral cortex. For years, these abnormal vessels have been ambiguously called "moyamoya vessels," but recent studies have clarified the precise anatomical features of these vessels and thus established the concept of "periventricular anastomosis [32–34]." The dilated lenticulostriate arteries, thalamic perforators, and anterior/posterior choroidal arteries extend to the periventricular area, forming the anastomoses to the medial end of the medullary or insular arteries, which finally supply the cortex [32–34]. Anastomoses can be classified into three subtypes, lenticulostriate, thalamic, and choroidal anastomoses, and the development of the periventricular anastomoses is associated with the hemorrhagic presentation of moyamoya disease [33].

The JAM Trial has revealed that direct/combined bypass suppresses the rate of rebleeding attacks from 7.6%/year to 2.7%/year in patients with hemorrhagic presentation [12]. In addition, choroidal anastomosis has been proven to be the significant risk factor for the rebleeding attacks (hazard ratio = 11.10), and this risk can be suppressed by direct/combined bypass surgery (hazard ratio = 0.33) [35]. Topographical analysis in the positive choroidal anastomosis cases has revealed good correspondence between bleeding points and the anatomical distribution of the choroidal arteries, including the posterior limb of the internal capsule, posterolateral part of the thalamus (pulvinar), and wall of the lateral ventricle atrium [34]. From these findings, reducing the hemodynamic burden of the periventricular anastomosis is critical, especially choroidal anastomosis, to prevent the rebleeding attacks.

Surgery should be designed as the bypass flow to cover the cortex, where the medullary arteries via the periventricular anastomosis are headed. If the targeted area becomes well-perfused from the bypass, periventricular anastomosis can be extremely diminished (Fig. 25.6).

25.5 Future Perspectives

Almost 50 years have passed since the first execution of bypass surgery in moyamoya disease. Numerous kinds of direct, indirect, and combined bypass procedures have been proposed, and there seems to be little room for an innovative surgical procedure anymore. However, some critical missions assigned to contemporary vascular neurosurgeons still exist. First, effective revascularization should be provided to the patients at the appropriate timing before devastating ischemic and hemorrhagic stroke occurs. Although the JAM Trial has demonstrated the effect of bypass surgery to prevent rebleeding attacks, the evidence is confined to the patients who have been already affected by hemorrhagic attacks, and the strategy to prevent "the first hemorrhagic event" in the patients' life remains to be established. Second, every effort should be made to suppress the rate of perioperative complications, such as intracerebral hemorrhage caused by hyperperfusion. Third, microvascular anastomosis skills should be properly handed down to the next generation. Since the effectiveness of STA-MCA anastomosis for atherosclerotic arterial occlusion has been denied in a randomized controlled trial in North America [36], the total numbers of direct bypass surgery seem to have been significantly declining, especially in the Western countries, where moyamoya disease, the major target of direct bypass, is rare. If no effective measures are taken, there could be a situation in which direct bypass surgery with minimum complication rate would not be available even in the advanced nations in the near future. Thus, we neurosurgeons must not allow such a scenario to occur.

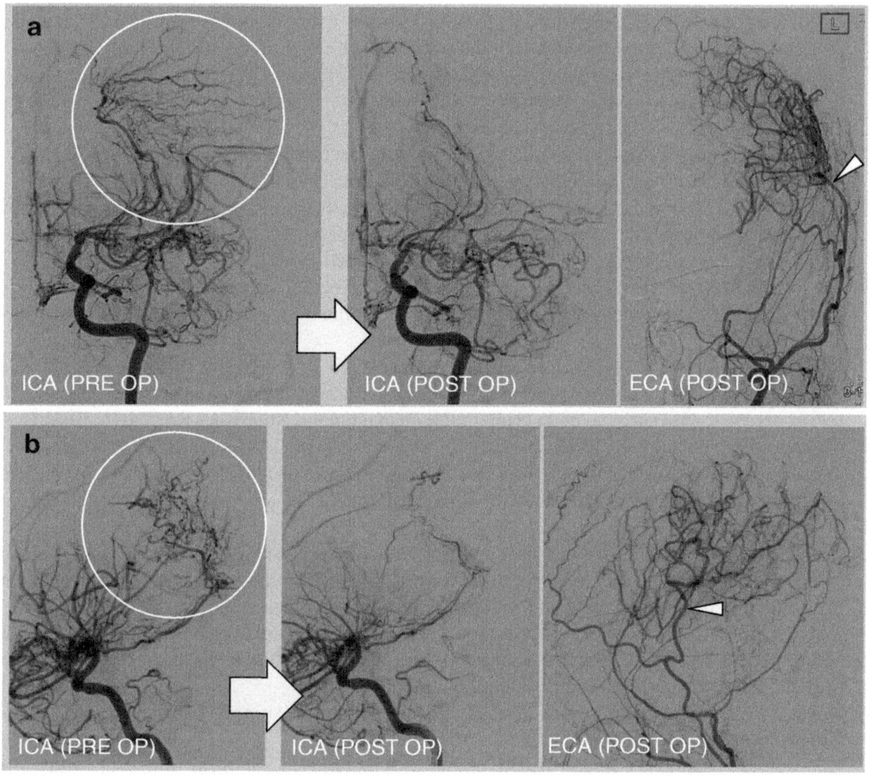

Fig. 25.6 Diminishment of the choroidal anastomosis after STA-MCA anastomosis. Preoperative angiograms show the well-developed choroidal anastomosis (white circles). Angiograms at 3 postoperative months reveal the sufficient bypass flow to the frontoparietal lobe and remarkable shrinkage of the choroidal anastomosis. (**a**) Anteroposterior view, (**b**) Lateral view. White arrowheads: STA parietal branch

References

1. Fung LW, Thompson D, Ganesan V. Revascularisation surgery for paediatric moyamoya: a review of the literature. Childs Nerv Syst. 2005;21:358–64.
2. Ishikawa T, Houkin K, Kamiyama H, et al. Effects of surgical revascularization on outcome of patients with pediatric moyamoya disease. Stroke. 1997;28:1170–3.
3. Kazumata K, Ito M, Tokairin K, Ito Y, Houkin K, Nakayama N, Kuroda S, Ishikawa T, Kamiyama H. The frequency of postoperative stroke in moyamoya disease following combined revascularization: a single-university series and systematic review. J Neurosurg. 2014;121:432–40.
4. Takagi Y, Kikuta K, Nozaki K, et al. Histological features of middle cerebral arteries from patients treated for Moyamoya disease. Neurol Med Chir(Tokyo). 2007;47:1–4.
5. Takagi Y, Kikuta K, Sadamasa N, et al. Caspase-3-dependent apoptosis in middle cerebral arteries in patients with moyamoya disease. Neurosurgery. 2006;59:894–900.
6. Fujimura M, Shimizu H, Inoue T, et al. Significance of focal cerebral hyperperfusion as a cause of transient neurologic deterioration after extracranial-intracranial bypass for moyamoya dis-

ease: comparative study with non-moyamoya patients using N-isopropyl-p-([123)I]iodoamphetamine singlephoton emission computed tomography. Neurosurgery. 2011;68:957–64.
7. Uno M, Nakajima N, Nishi K, et al. Hyperperfusion syndrome after extracranial-intracranial bypass in a patient with moyamoya disease—case report. Neurol Med Chir(Tokyo). 1998;38:420–4.
8. Mizoi K, Kayama T, Yoshimoto T, et al. Indirect revascularization for moyamoya disease: is there a beneficial effect for adult patients? Surg Neurol. 1996;45:541–8.
9. Matsushima T, Inoue T, Suzuki SO, Fujii K, Fukui M, Hasuo K. Surgical treatment of moyamoya disease in pediatric patients--comparison between the results of indirect and direct revascularization procedures. Neurosurgery. 1992;31:401–5.
10. Miyamoto S, Kikuchi H, Karasawa J, Nagata I, Yamazoe N, Akiyama Y. Pitfalls in the surgical treatment of moyamoya disease. Operative techniques for refractory cases. J Neurosurg. 1988;68:537–43.
11. Rashad S, Fujimura M, Niizuma K, Endo H, Tominaga T. Long-term follow-up of pediatric moyamoya disease treated by combined direct-indirect revascularization surgery: single institute experience with surgical and perioperative management. Neurosurg Rev. 2016;39:615–23.
12. Miyamoto S, Yoshimoto T, Hashimoto N, Okada Y, Tsuji I, Tominaga T, Nakagawara J, Takahashi JC. JAM trial investigators. Effects of extracranial-intracranial bypass for patients with hemorrhagic moyamoya disease: results of the Japan adult Moyamoya trial. Stroke. 2014;45:1415–21.
13. Takahashi JC, Funaki T, Houkin K, Inoue T, Ogasawara K, Nakagawara J, Kuroda S, Yamada K, Miyamoto S. JAM trial investigators. Significance of the hemorrhagic site for recurrent bleeding: Prespecified analysis in the Japan adult Moyamoya trial. Stroke. 2016;47:37–43.
14. Krayenbühl HA. The moyamoya syndrome and the neurosurgeon. Surg Neurol. 1975;4:353–60.
15. Vilela MD, Newell DW. Superficial temporal artery to middle cerebral artery bypass: past, present, and future. Neurosurg Focus. 2008;24(2):E2.
16. Nakagawa Y, Abe H, Sawamura Y, et al. Revascularization surgery for moyamoya disease. Neurol Res. 1988;10:32–9.
17. Karasawa J, Touho H, Ohnishi H, Miyamoto S, Kikuchi H. Long-term follow-up study after extracranial-intracranial bypass surgery for anterior circulation ischemia in childhood moyamoya disease. J Neurosurg. 1992;77:84–9.
18. Ishii K, Morishige M, Anan M, Sugita K, Abe E, Kubo T, Fujiki M, Kobayashi H. Superficial temporal artery-to-middle cerebral artery anastomosis with encephalo-duro-myo-synangiosis as a modified operative procedure for moyamoya disease. Acta Neurochir Suppl. 2010;107:95–9.
19. Zhao J, Liu H, Zou Y, Zhang W, He S. Clinical and angiographic outcomes after combined direct and indirect bypass in adult patients with moyamoya disease: a retrospective study of 76 procedures. Exp Ther Med. 2018;15:3570–6.
20. Houkin K, Kamiyama H, Abe H, et al. Surgical therapy for adult moyamoya disease. Can surgical revascularization prevent the recurrence of intracerebral hemorrhage? Stroke. 1996;27:1342–6.
21. Houkin K, Kamiyama H, Takahashi A, et al. Combined revascularization surgery for childhood moyamoya disease: STAMCA and encephalo-duro-arterio-myo-synangiosis. Childs Nerv Syst. 1997;13:24–9.
22. Kuroda S, Houkin K, Ishikawa T, et al. Novel bypass surgery for moyamoya disease using pericranial flap: its impacts on cerebral hemodynamics and long-term outcome. Neurosurgery. 2010;66:1093–101.
23. Kuroda S, Houkin K, Ishikawa T, et al. Determinants of intellectual outcome after surgical revascularization in pediatric moyamoya disease: a multivariate analysis. Childs Nerv Syst. 2004;20:302–8.
24. Iwama T, Hashimoto N, Tsukahara T, Miyake H. Superficial temporal artery to anterior cerebral artery direct anastomosis in patients with moyamoya disease. Clin Neurol Neurosurg. 1997;99(Suppl 2):S134–6.
25. Kazumata K, Kamiyama H, Saito H, Maruichi K, Ito M, Uchino H, Nakayama N, Kuroda S, Houkin K. Direct anastomosis using occipital artery for additional revascularization in

Moyamoya disease after combined superficial temporal artery-middle cerebral artery and indirect bypass. Oper Neurosurg (Hagerstown). 2017;13:213–23.
26. Uchino H, Kuroda S, Hirata K, Shiga T, Houkin K, Tamaki N. Predictors and clinical features of postoperative hyperperfusion after surgical revascularization for moyamoya disease: a serial single photon emission CT/positron emission tomography study. Stroke. 2012;43(10):2610–6.
27. Fujimura M, Kaneta T, Mugikura S, Shimizu H, Tominaga T. Temporary neurologic deterioration due to cerebral hyperperfusion after superficial temporal artery–middle cerebral artery anastomosis in patients with adult-onset moyamoya disease. Surg Neurol. 2007;67:273–82.
28. Yu J, Zhang J, Li J, Zhang J, Chen J. Cerebral Hyperperfusion syndrome after revascularization surgery in patients with Moyamoya disease. Syst Rev Meta-Analysis World Neurosurg. 2020;135:357–366.e4.
29. Piepgras DG, Morgan MK, Sundt TM Jr, Yanagihara T, Mussman LM. Intracerebral hemorrhage after carotid endarterectomy. J Neurosurg. 1988;68:532–6.
30. Kuroda S, Houkin K. Bypass surgery for moyamoya disease: concept and essence of surgical technique. Neurol Med Chir(Tokyo). 2012;52:287–94.
31. Takanari K, Araki Y, Okamoto S, Sato H, Yagi S, Toriyama K, Yokoyama K, Murotani K, Matsui S, Wakabayashi T, Kamei Y. Operative wound-related complications after cranial revascularization surgeries. J Neurosurg. 2015;123:1145–50.
32. Funaki T, Fushimi Y, Takahashi JC, Takagi Y, Araki Y, Yoshida K, Kikuchi T, Miyamoto S. Visualization of periventricular collaterals in moyamoya disease with flow-sensitive black-blood magnetic resonance angiography: preliminary experience. Neurol Med Chir (Tokyo). 2015;55:204–9.
33. Funaki T, Takahashi JC, Yoshida K, Takagi Y, Fushimi Y, Kikuchi T, Mineharu Y, Okada T, Morimoto T, Miyamoto S. Periventricular anastomosis in moyamoya disease: detecting fragile collateral vessels with MR angiography. J Neurosurg. 2016;124:1766–72.
34. Funaki T, Takahashi JC, Houkin K, Kuroda S, Takeuchi S, Fujimura M, Tomata Y, Miyamoto S. Angiographic features of hemorrhagic moyamoya disease with high recurrence risk: a supplementary analysis of the Japan adult Moyamoya trial. J Neurosurg. 2018;128:777–84.
35. Funaki T, Takahashi JC, Houkin K, Kuroda S, Takeuchi S, Fujimura M, Tomata Y, Miyamoto S. High rebleeding risk associated with choroidal collateral vessels in hemorrhagic moyamoya disease: analysis of a nonsurgical cohort in the Japan adult Moyamoya trial. J Neurosurg. 2019;130:337–673.
36. Powers WJ, Clarke WR, Grubb RL Jr, Videen TO, Adams HP Jr, Derdeyn CP. COSS investigators. Extracranial-intracranial bypass surgery for stroke prevention in hemodynamic cerebral ischemia: the carotid occlusion surgery study randomized trial. JAMA. 2011;306:1983–92.

Special Considerations: Infants

26

Satoshi Kuroda and Daina Kashiwazaki

Abstract

Infants and toddlers with moyamoya disease are known to usually have severely compromised cerebral hemodynamics and are to carry a higher risk for ischemic stroke than children 5 years or older. However, most clinical issues related to infants and toddlers with moyamoya disease are still unresolved, probably because their prevalence is extremely low in each institute and almost all of the previous studies have been conducted in a single center. In this chapter, therefore, we precisely review clinical features, surgical treatment, and outcome of infantile moyamoya disease by reviewing previous articles and also discuss future prospective to improve their functional and intellectual outcome even more.

Keywords

Moyamoya disease · Infants · Surgical treatment · Ischemic stroke · Prognosis

26.1 Introduction

Moyamoya disease is a very specific disease characterized by progressive stenosis of the terminal portion of the internal carotid artery and the formation of an abnormal network of dilated, fragile perforators around the basal ganglia and thalamus [1, 2]. Epidemiologically, there is a bimodal age distribution: one at 5–9 years and another lower peak at around 40 years. Young children with moyamoya disease have

S. Kuroda (✉) · D. Kashiwazaki
Department of Neurosurgery, Graduate School of Medicine and Pharmaceutical Science, University of Toyama, Toyama, Japan
e-mail: skuroda@med.u-toyama.ac.jp; dkashiwa@med.u-toyama.ac.jp

S. Kuroda (ed.), *Moyamoya Disease: Current Knowledge and Future Perspectives*, https://doi.org/10.1007/978-981-33-6404-2_26

historically been considered to be the most severely affected and the most challenging to surgically treat. Of these, infants and toddlers with moyamoya disease are known to usually have severely compromised cerebral hemodynamics and to carry a higher risk for ischemic stroke than children 5 years or older. However, these clinical issues related to infants and toddlers with moyamoya disease are still unresolved, as their sample size is relatively low in each institute and almost all of the previous studies have been conducted in a single center. In this chapter, therefore, we clarify unresolved issues on infantile moyamoya disease by reviewing previous articles and also discuss future prospective.

26.2 Epidemiology

As mentioned above, since the discovery of moyamoya disease in the 1950s, the number of infantile cases has not been consistently high. In a Korean cohort, the age-specific prevalence of patients with 0–4 years of age between 2007 and 2011 was reported less than 1.8 per 100,000 populations [3]. In a Taiwanese cohort, their annual incidence rate varied from 0.06 and 0.14 per 100,000 populations between 2000 and 2011 [4]. However, sporadic but infant patients have been reported from a variety of countries, so the number of patients is likely to be small but still occurring around the world [5–7].

It is not so easy to accurately evaluate the prevalence of infants and toddlers with moyamoya disease among total moyamoya disease patients because the awareness of the disease varies by country and time period and the age categories vary from report to report. We first discuss their proportion in the overall pediatric moyamoya disease population. In Korean case series, the incidence of infants with 0–2 years of age was 11.3% (23/204) [8]. The value was 14.5% (8/55) in our previous case series [8]. According to the report by Funaki et al. (2014), they performed surgical revascularization for 58 children with moyamoya disease. Of these, 19 (32.8%) were younger than 5 years [9]. In the case series at Harvard Medical School, infants aged 0–1 year accounted for only 7.9% (19/249) of pediatric patients [10]. In Japan, the incidence of infants and toddlers with 0–4 years of age was 15.3% in overall pediatric patients, based on a questionnaire survey in 2003 [11]. Next, we discuss their proportion in the total moyamoya patients. In Japan, the incidence of infants and toddlers with 0–4 years of age was 4.6% based on a questionnaire survey in 2003 [11]. The value in China and the USA was also very similar [12, 13]. There was no significant difference between Asian and non-Asian patients [13].

26.3 Clinical Presentations

It has long been known that the clinical manifestations are very different between infants/toddlers and school-age children. The formers more likely develop ischemic stroke than TIA, while the latter develop mostly TIAs and very rarely ischemic stroke [8, 10, 14–17]. Kuroda et al. (2003) reported that the incidence of ischemic stroke was 50% in children aged 0–5 years, but was 8.9% in school-age children [16]. Likewise, Kim et al. (2004) categorized 204 pediatric patients into Group A (n = 23, 0–2 years of age), Group B (n = 50, 3–6 years of age), and Group C (n = 131, 6 years of age). As a result, cerebral infarctions were more frequently observed in Group A (87%) and Group B (58%) than in Group C (46%) [8]. Mugikura et al. also divided pediatric patients into 4 categories: younger than 4 years (n = 14), 4–7 years (n = 29), 8–11 years (n = 21), and 12–15 years (n = 14). As a result, the prevalence of ischemic stroke was much higher in children younger than 4 years (85.7%) than the others (21–33%) [17]. According to the report from the USA, 17 (89.5%) of 19 infants with 0–2 years of age had clinical and radiological evidence of cerebral infarction [10]. Kim et al. (2013) found that ischemic stroke and seizure were most frequent in infants with 0–1 year of age and that infants and toddlers tended to suddenly develop TIA and/or ischemic stroke without any provoking events such as crying and eating hot foods [15]. These clinical profile differences may be related to the fact that metabolic demand in the developing brain is very high in children under 4 years of age followed by a gradual decrease in their growth (see also Chap. 7) [18, 19].

It is also known that clinical course is more aggressive in infants and toddlers than in school-age children. According to the report by Kim et al. (2004) cited above, ischemic stroke is more frequently repeated when waiting for surgery in Group A (39%) than in Group B (6%) and Group C (0.8%) [8]. Funaki et al. (2015) also reported that age younger than 3 years is an independent risk factor for unstable clinical course such as rapid disease progression or repeated ischemic stroke [20]. The finding correlates well with the fact that disease stage more likely advances in children aged 0–4 years than in older children. Representative case is shown in Fig. 26.1.

26.4 Radiological Findings

There are several studies that denote the findings on cerebral angiography in infantile moyamoya disease. Their disease stage is significantly earlier, but more aggressively progresses than school-age children [17]. In addition, the involvement of the posterior cerebral artery (PCA) is significantly more frequent in infants/toddlers than in school-age children, 50–66% and 20–30%, respectively [16, 17].

Children <4 or 5 years of age significantly more frequently have cerebral infarctions than older children [16, 17]. Thus, the prevalence of cerebral infarction was 65.6% (21/32) in children under 5 years of age, but was 17.4% (4/23) in school-age children. Especially, cerebral infarct was highly located in the cortical branch territories in those <5 years of age (Fig. 26.1) [16]. This finding seems inconsistent with the fact that their disease stage is significantly earlier than that of school-age children, but they have a significantly higher rate of PCA involvement, one of the important collateral circulation channels, and a significantly lower rate of transdural anastomosis [16, 17]. More importantly, normal cerebral blood flow is much higher

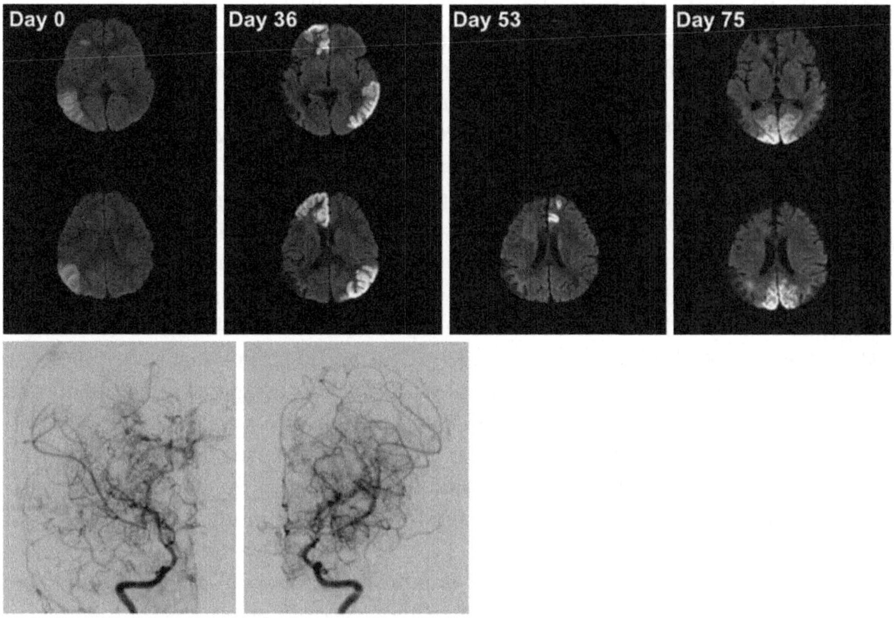

Fig. 26.1 Radiological findings of a 3-year-old boy who repeated ischemic stroke while waiting for surgical revascularization at prior hospital. Note that cerebral infarcts on diffusion-weighted MRI (*upper*) are distributed in the cortical area every time. The findings on cerebral angiography are very typical for moyamoya disease (lower)

in infants and toddlers than in school-age children, as described in Chap. 7. These facts would be directly related to a higher prevalence of cerebral infarct development in children <5 years of age.

26.5 Surgical Treatments

As described in Chap. 18, surgical revascularization is the only way to improve cerebral hemodynamics and reduce the further risk for ischemic/hemorrhagic stroke in moyamoya disease. Roughly, the procedures can be divided into three categories: indirect bypass, direct bypass, and combined bypass. This theory is also true in infants and toddlers with moyamoya disease. However, it should be noted that there are unique concerns when performing surgical revascularization for them, as follows:

Surgical revascularization is usually considered safe to perform when the brain condition has stabilized several weeks after the last ischemic or hemorrhagic stroke. In the cases of infants and toddlers, however, the timing of surgical revascularization may be frequently missed, as the patient repeats ischemic strokes one after another while waiting for several weeks (Fig. 26.1). Therefore, clinical factors to determine the optimal timing of surgical revascularization for them should be determined in near future.

As aforementioned, surgical procedures do not largely differ from those of the school-age children just because the patient is an infant or toddler. Direct bypass, typically represented by superficial temporal artery to middle cerebral artery (STA-MCA) anastomosis, is also technically feasible. We usually use 11–0 nylon threads for STA-MCA anastomosis for them (Fig. 26.2) [20].

It is still controversial whether children younger than 3–4 years of age are at higher risk for perioperative complications than school-age children. Kuroda et al. (2003) reported that the incidence of perioperative stroke was 6.3% (2/32) and 8.7% (2/23) after indirect or combined bypass procedures in infants/toddlers and school-age children, respectively [16]. Kim et al. found no significant differences in the incidence of perioperative complications after encephalo-duro-arterio-synangiosis (EDAS) among Group A (<3 years of age), Group B (3–6 years of age), and Group C (>6 years of age) [8]. However, the same group subsequently reported that the incidence of newly developed cerebral infarcts was about 11% in children younger than 6 years after indirect bypass procedures, being three-fold higher than school-age children [21]. Another Korean group performed EDAS for 170 hemispheres in 90 children with moyamoya disease and found postoperative ischemic complications in 12 hemispheres (7.1%). The prevalence of children younger than 3 years was higher in children with postoperative ischemic complications (41.7%) than

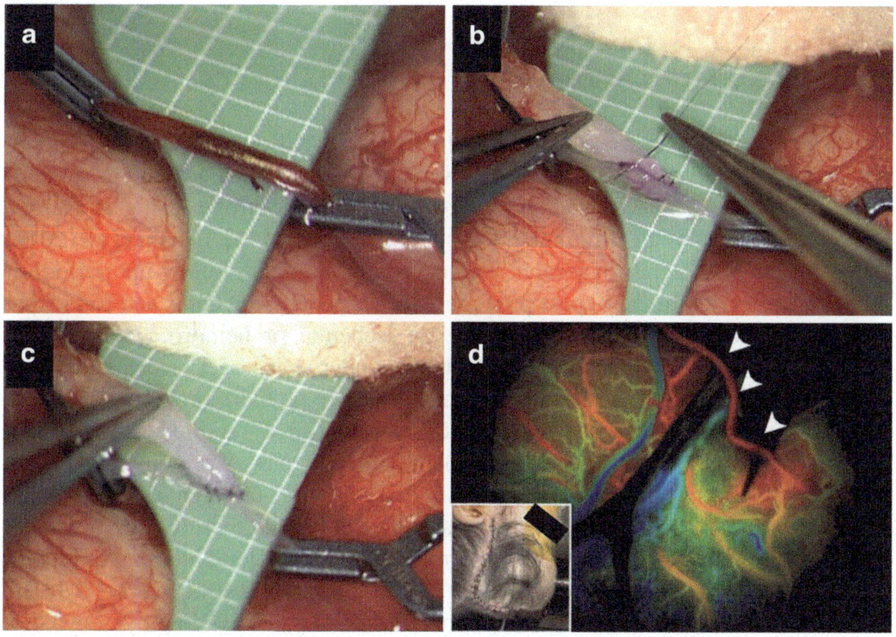

Fig. 26.2 Intraoperative findings of STA-MCA anastomosis combined with indirect bypass for a 11-month-old boy with moyamoya disease. (**a**) Clamping of the cortical branch of MCA with a diameter of 0.6 mm. (**b**) Suturing with a 11–0 nylon thread for STA-MCA anastomosis. (**c**) Completion of STA-MCA anastomosis. (**d**) Intra-operative indocyanine (ICG) videoangiography shows a good patency of STA-MCA anastomosis (arrowheads). Small picture demonstrates the surgical wound. Note that the procedure can be performed with partial shaving of the hair

those without (8.2%) [22]. Jackson et al. (2014) performed pial synangiosis for 19 patients younger than 2 years of age and experienced unanticipated staged operations due to persistent EEG changes during the initial surgery in two patients and due to intraoperative brain swelling requiring ventriculostomy in another. The other two cases developed postoperative seizures due to a newly developed cerebral infarct. Therefore, the incidence of perioperative complications was 26.3% (5/19) [10]. More recently, Bot et al. (2019) performed 11 combined bypass procedures for 6 children ≤3 years of age and reported that perioperative stroke occurred in one (9.1%) [23]. As is widely known in moyamoya disease in general, therefore, direct bypass may contribute to reduce perioperative ischemic stroke even in infants and toddlers.

In addition to surgical procedures, perioperative managements may influence the occurrence of perioperative complications. Matsushima et al. (1991) reported 6 pediatric patients, including 3 cases younger than 3 years, developed cerebral infarcts as the result of crying-associated hyperventilation [24]. Sato et al. (1997) also indicated that intraoperative blood loss and excessive urinary output were potential contributors to ischemic complications in pediatric patients and presented a 1-year-old case that suffered a postoperative ischemic stroke due to these two factors [25]. Smaller circulating blood volume in infants would be responsible for such ischemic complications after surgery.

26.6 Long-Term Outcome

The risk of recurrent stroke during the follow-up period after surgical revascularization does by no means seem to differ between infants/toddlers and school-age children. Kuroda et al. (2003) found no recurrence of ischemic stroke during an average of 7.5 years of follow-up after indirect or combined bypass [16]. Funaki et al. (2014) analyzed the late cerebrovascular events during a mean follow-up period of 18.1 years after combined bypass procedure for 58 pediatric patients and found that 4 of 56 followed patients experienced late ischemic or hemorrhagic stroke at 8–33 years post-surgery. The ages at which they underwent surgery were 3, 4, 6, and 7 years old, respectively, and infants do not appear to be more prone to suffer late cerebrovascular events [9]. Conversely, Jackson et al. (2014) reported that new cerebral infarcts developed in 2 cases (10.5%) and repeat bypass was required for frontal lobe ischemic symptoms in other 2 cases (10.5%) in 19 children <2 years of age after pial synangiosis [10]. Kimiwada et al. (2018) reported that PCA involvement during follow-up periods after surgical revascularization for anterior circulation more likely occurs in younger children (5.1 ± 2.5 years vs. 8.2 ± 4.0 years) [26]. The PCA is known as one of the most important collateral pathways in moyamoya disease, thus PCA involvement would carry the risk of late cerebrovascular events in infants and toddlers.

In addition, infantile patients are known to have worse functional outcome compared to school-age children. Kim et al. (2004) found lower rate of favorable outcome in Group A (58%, <3 years of age) than in Group B (84%, 3–6 years of age) and Group C (86%, >6 years of age) [8]. Based on recent multivariate analysis, however, ischemic stroke that occurred between the time of onset and surgical revascularization, but not the onset age itself, is considered as its primary cause (odds ratio, 4.9) [27]. In addition, postoperative ischemic complications would contribute to poor functional outcome [22].

Furthermore, intellectual outcome is known worse in children who developed moyamoya disease before school age. Thus, Matsushima et al. (1990) studied cognitive outcomes following EDAS in children with the onset of the disease before the age of 5 years. As a result, 7 of 8 cases that presented moyamoya disease at <2 years of age had an IQ lower than 61 [28]. Kuroda et al. (2003) also reported that a mean full-scale IQ value was 85 in infants and toddlers, being significantly lower than 98 in school-age children [16]. Most of other earlier reports have also shown that the onset of the disease in infants adversely affects higher brain function probably because most of them more likely suffer ischemic stroke due to single or multiple cortical infarcts [29–33].

26.7 Conclusion

In summary, a number of studies have gradually revealed the clinical picture and long-term prognosis of moyamoya disease in infancy. However, many issues, including the timing of surgical revascularization after an ischemic stroke and the clinical factors that predispose to perioperative complications, remain unclear. This is partly due to their small sample size in single institute and the lack of a comprehensive and precise survey. Therefore, we are conducting a multi-center observational cohort study, "*M*oyamoya Disease with *A*ggressive *C*linical Course in The *In*fan*t*s f*o*r *S*afety and *H*ealthy Growth [MACINTOSH] study in Japan now. It is our great hope that the functional and intellectual outcomes of infants affected by moyamoya disease will improve even more through these studies in near future.

References

1. Kuroda S, Houkin K. Moyamoya disease: current concepts and future perspectives. Lancet Neurol. 2008;7:1056–66.
2. Suzuki J, Takaku A. Cerebrovascular "moyamoya" disease. Disease showing abnormal net-like vessels in base of brain. Arch Neurol. 1969;20:288–99.
3. Ahn IM, Park DH, Hann HJ, Kim KH, Kim HJ, Ahn HS. Incidence, prevalence, and survival of moyamoya disease in Korea: a nationwide, population-based study. Stroke. 2014;45:1090–5.
4. Chen PC, Yang SH, Chien KL, Tsai IJ, Kuo MF. Epidemiology of moyamoya disease in Taiwan: a nationwide population-based study. Stroke. 2014;45:1258–63.
5. Amlie-Lefond C, Zaidat OO, Lew SM. Moyamoya disease in early infancy: case report and literature review. Pediatr Neurol. 2011;44:299–302.
6. Law-Ye B, Saliou G, Toulgoat F, Tardieu M, Deiva K, Adamsbaum C, Husson B. Early-onset stroke with moyamoya-like syndrome and extraneurological signs: a first reported paediatric series. Eur Radiol. 2016;26:2853–62.

7. Lee S, Rivkin MJ, Kirton A, deVeber G, Elbers J, International Pediatric Stroke S. Moyamoya disease in children: results from the international pediatric stroke study. J Child Neurol. 2017;32:924–9.
8. Kim SK, Seol HJ, Cho BK, Hwang YS, Lee DS, Wang KC. Moyamoya disease among young patients: its aggressive clinical course and the role of active surgical treatment. Neurosurgery. 2004;54:840–4. discussion 844–846
9. Funaki T, Takahashi JC, Takagi Y, Yoshida K, Araki Y, Kikuchi T, Kataoka H, Iihara K, Sano N, Miyamoto S. Incidence of late cerebrovascular events after direct bypass among children with moyamoya disease: a descriptive longitudinal study at a single center. Acta Neurochir. 2014;156:551–9. discussion 559
10. Jackson EM, Lin N, Manjila S, Scott RM, Smith ER. Pial synangiosis in patients with moyamoya younger than 2 years of age. J Neurosurg Pediatr. 2014;13:420–5.
11. Kuriyama S, Kusaka Y, Fujimura M, Wakai K, Tamakoshi A, Hashimoto S, Tsuji I, Inaba Y, Yoshimoto T. Prevalence and clinicoepidemiological features of moyamoya disease in Japan: findings from a nationwide epidemiological survey. Stroke. 2008;39:42–7.
12. Duan L, Bao XY, Yang WZ, Shi WC, Li DS, Zhang ZS, Zong R, Han C, Zhao F, Feng J. Moyamoya disease in China: its clinical features and outcomes. Stroke. 2012;43:56–60.
13. Starke RM, Crowley RW, Maltenfort M, Jabbour PM, Gonzalez LF, Tjoumakaris SI, Randazzo CG, Rosenwasser RH, Dumont AS. Moyamoya disorder in the United States. Neurosurgery. 2012;71:93–9.
14. Hoshino H, Izawa Y, Suzuki N, Research Committee on Moyamoya D. Epidemiological features of moyamoya disease in Japan. Neurol Med Chir (Tokyo). 2012;52:295–8.
15. Kim YO, Joo SP, Seo BR, Rho YI, Yoon W, Woo YJ. Early clinical characteristics according to developmental stage in children with definite moyamoya disease. Brain and Development. 2013;35:569–74.
16. Kuroda S, Nanba R, Ishikawa T, Houkin K, Kamiyama H, Iwasaki Y. Clinical manifestations of infantile moyamoya disease. No Shinkei Geka. 2003;31:1073–8.
17. Mugikura S, Higano S, Shirane R, Fujimura M, Shimanuki Y, Takahashi S. Posterior circulation and high prevalence of ischemic stroke among young pediatric patients with Moyamoya disease: evidence of angiography-based differences by age at diagnosis. AJNR Am J Neuroradiol. 2011;32:192–8.
18. Epstein HT. Stages of increased cerebral blood flow accompany stages of rapid brain growth. Brain and Development. 1999;21:535–9.
19. Kuroda S, Kamiyama H, Abe H, Yamauchi T, Kohama Y, Houkin K, Mitsumori K. Cerebral blood flow in children with spontaneous occlusion of the circle of Willis (moyamoya disease): comparison with healthy children and evaluation of annual changes. Neurol Med Chir (Tokyo). 1993;33:434–8.
20. Funaki T, Takahashi JC, Takagi Y, Kikuchi T, Yoshida K, Mitsuhara T, Kataoka H, Okada T, Fushimi Y, Miyamoto S. Unstable moyamoya disease: clinical features and impact on perioperative ischemic complications. J Neurosurg. 2015;122(2):400–7.
20. Kuroda S, Houkin K. Bypass surgery for moyamoya disease - concept and essence of surgical technique. Neurol Med Chir (Tokyo). 2012;52:287–94.
21. Choi JW, Chong S, Phi JH, Lee JY, Kim HS, Chae JH, Lee J, Kim SK. Postoperative symptomatic cerebral infarction in pediatric Moyamoya disease: risk factors and clinical outcome. World Neurosurg. 2020;136:e158–64.
22. Kim SH, Choi JU, Yang KH, Kim TG, Kim DS. Risk factors for postoperative ischemic complications in patients with moyamoya disease. J Neurosurg. 2005;103:433–8.
23. Bot GM, Burkhardt JK, Gupta N, Lawton MT. Superficial temporal artery-to-middle cerebral artery bypass in combination with indirect revascularization in moyamoya patients </= 3 years of age. J Neurosurg Pediatr. 2018;23:198–203.
24. Matsushima Y, Aoyagi M, Suzuki R, Tabata H, Ohno K. Perioperative complications of encephalo-duro-arterio-synangiosis: prevention and treatment. Surg Neurol. 1991;36:343–53.
25. Sato K, Shirane R, Yoshimoto T. Perioperative factors related to the development of ischemic complications in patients with moyamoya disease. Childs Nerv Syst. 1997;13:68–72.

26. Kimiwada T, Hayashi T, Shirane R, Tominaga T. Posterior cerebral artery stenosis and posterior circulation revascularization surgery in pediatric patients with moyamoya disease. J Neurosurg Pediatr. 2018;21:632–8.
27. Ha EJ, Kim KH, Wang KC, Phi JH, Lee JY, Choi JW, Cho BK, Yang J, Byun YH, Kim SK. Long-term outcomes of indirect bypass for 629 children with Moyamoya disease: longitudinal and cross-sectional analysis. Stroke. 2019;50:3177–83.
28. Matsushima Y, Aoyagi M, Masaoka H, Suzuki R, Ohno K. Mental outcome following encephaloduroarteriosynangiosis in children with moyamoya disease with the onset earlier than 5 years of age. Childs Nerv Syst. 1990;6:440–3.
29. Karasawa J, Touho H, Ohnishi H, Miyamoto S, Kikuchi H. Long-term follow-up study after extracranial-intracranial bypass surgery for anterior circulation ischemia in childhood moyamoya disease. J Neurosurg. 1992;77:84–9.
30. Kuroda S, Houkin K, Ishikawa T, Nakayama N, Ikeda J, Ishii N, Kamiyama H, Iwasaki Y. Determinants of intellectual outcome after surgical revascularization in pediatric moyamoya disease: a multivariate analysis. Childs Nerv Syst. 2004;20:302–8.
31. Matsushima T, Inoue T, Suzuki SO, Fujii K, Fukui M, Hasuo K. Surgical treatment of moyamoya disease in pediatric patients--comparison between the results of indirect and direct revascularization procedures. Neurosurgery. 1992;31:401–5.
32. Matsushima Y, Aoyagi M, Nariai T, Takada Y, Hirakawa K. Long-term intelligence outcome of post-encephalo-duro-arterio-synangiosis childhood moyamoya patients. Clin Neurol Neurosurg. 1997;99(Suppl 2):S147–50.
33. Miyamoto S, Akiyama Y, Nagata I, Karasawa J, Nozaki K, Hashimoto N, Kikuchi H. Long-term outcome after STA-MCA anastomosis for moyamoya disease. Neurosurg Focus. 1998;5:e5.

Special Considerations: Elderly

27

Miki Fujimura and Teiji Tominaga

Abstract

Moyamoya disease (MMD) is a chronic, occlusive cerebrovascular disease with unknown etiology characterized by progressive stenosis/occlusion at the terminal portion of the internal carotid artery and an abnormal vascular network formation at the base of the brain. MMD was known to have bimodal age distribution with a peak each in childhood and young adulthood, and presentation in the elderly has been considered to be relatively rare. Recently, there is an increasing number of the elderly patients being diagnosed as having MMD and undergoing management under the modern diagnostic criteria, which also includes patients with atherosclerosis and/or with unilateral involvement as the definitive MMD. The aim of this chapter is to summarize the current status of revascularization surgery for elderly MMD patients. We also introduce the tips and pitfall of the diagnosis and the management of elderly MMD patients.

Keywords

Moyamoya vasculopathy · Moyamoya disease · Elderly · Revascularization surgery · Cerebral hyperperfusion

M. Fujimura (✉)
Department of Neurosurgery, Kohnan Hospital, Sendai, Japan

Division of Advanced Cerebrovascular Surgery, Tohoku University Graduate School of Medicine, Sendai, Japan
e-mail: fujimur@nsg.med.tohoku.ac.jp

T. Tominaga
Department of Neurosurgery, Tohoku University Graduate School of Medicine, Sendai, Japan
e-mail: tomi@nsg.med.tohoku.ac.jp

S. Kuroda (ed.), *Moyamoya Disease: Current Knowledge and Future Perspectives*, https://doi.org/10.1007/978-981-33-6404-2_27

27.1 Introduction

Moyamoya disease (MMD) is characterized by progressive stenosis/occlusion at the terminal portion of the internal carotid artery (ICA) and an abnormal vascular network formation at the base of the brain [1, 2]. MMD has been known to have bimodal age distribution with a peak each in childhood and young adulthood [3, 4], but there is an increasing number of elderly patients being diagnosed as having MMD and undergoing management under the modern diagnostic criteria [5]. In this chapter, we sought to summarize the current status of revascularization surgery for elderly MMD patients, while introducing the tips and pitfall of their diagnosis and the management.

27.2 Current Diagnostic Criteria of MMD

Original diagnostic criteria of definitive MMD in the 1960s included stenosis/occlusion at the bilateral ICA terminus, associated with abnormal vascular network formation at the base of the brain [1]. In light of the increasing number of the MMD patients with unilateral involvement and the similarity of the genetic background between patients with bilateral and unilateral involvement, diagnostic criteria of MMD in Japan were updated in 2015 to include patients having both bilateral and unilateral involvement of terminal ICA stenosis/occlusion, in association with the abnormal vascular network formation at the surrounding area [5]. Regarding moyamoya vasculopathy associated with atherosclerosis, the previous diagnostic criteria had categorized them into moyamoya syndrome (akin/quasi MMD), but the modern diagnostic criteria allow it to be diagnoses as definitive (idiopathic) MMD [5]. Based on these backgrounds, the number of the elderly MMD patients could be markedly increasing more recently.

27.3 Significance of the Supportive Diagnostic Tools

Definitive diagnosis of MMD is not always easy, especially in the elderly patients, because the current diagnostic criteria might lead to the misdiagnosis of atherosclerotic patients with unilateral involvement to the definitive MMD. To resolve this critical issue, it is essential to understand the diagnostic value of high-resolution magnetic resonance (MR) vessel wall imaging (VWI) focusing on the intracranial major arteries. Ryoo and colleagues reported the characteristic VWI finding of MMD, such as the concentric moderate enhancement on distal ICA and shrinkage of middle cerebral artery (MCA), which is distinct from atherosclerosis representing focal eccentric enhancement at the symptomatic segment of intracranial arteries [6]. Similar observation was reported by Yuan et al. that the vascular wall-thinning and the arterial outer diameter narrowing shown by high-resolution MR VWI could be the characteristic finding of MMD [7]. Taken together, MR VWI provides important information for the accurate diagnosis of MMD, especially in the elderly patients. Alternatively, genetic analysis of a MMD susceptibility gene, ring finger protein 213 (RNF213), would also provide supportive information for the accurate diagnosis of MMD among East Asian population [8].

27.4 Surgical Indication and Management Procedure for Elderly MMD Patients

Concept of the revascularization surgery for adult MMD includes both the microsurgical reconstruction by superficial temporal artery (STA)-MCA bypass and the consolidation for the extracranial–intracranial neovascularization by indirect pial synangiosis such as encephalo-myo-synangiosis, encephalo-duro-arterio-synangiosis (EDAS), and encephalo-duro-myo-synangiosis (EDMS) [9]. For the adult MMD patients, including the elderly, STA-MCA bypass with or without indirect pial synangiosis is a preferred management not only to prevent recurrent stroke by improving cerebral hemodynamics in ischemic-onset patients, but also to ameliorate the hemodynamic stress to the vulnerable collateral anastomosis at the base of the brain, thus reducing the risk of re-bleeding from the affected vessels in hemorrhagic-onset patients [5, 10]. This 72-year-old woman had undergone left STA-MCA bypass with EDMS at the age of 60 years (Fig. 27.1), which relieved her ischemic symptom on the left hemisphere. Twelve years later, external carotid angiogram indicated patent STA-MCA bypass (arrow in Fig. 27.1f) and marked pial synangiosis via middle meningeal artery and deep temporal artery, indicating the efficacy of combined revascularization in the elderly MMD patient (Fig. 27.1e and f). In light of her newly-developed ischemic symptom of the right hemisphere as confirmed by N-isopropyl-p-[^{123}I] iodoamphetamine SPECT (^{123}I-IMP SPECT), we diagnosed her as having surgical indication also for the right hemisphere twelve years after the initial management (Fig. 27.1g).

Since March 2004, the single surgeon (M.F.) performed over 530 consecutive procedures of STA-MCA (M4) single bypass with EDMS at Kohnan Hospital, Tohoku University Hospital, and Sendai Medical Center according to the previously described procedure [11]. Intra-operative finding of the representative case of this 72-year-old woman is shown (Fig. 27.2). Craniotomy is performed around the Sylvian fissure end, approximately 8 cm in diameter, and the stump of the STA, either frontal or parietal branch, is prepared as semi-fish mouth shape with the stump of 1.6 ~ 2.0 mm (Fig. 27.2a and b). Then the stump of STA is anastomosed by 10–0 nylon monofilament suture to the M4 segment of the MCA, approximately 0.8 ~ 1.2 mm in diameter (Fig. 27.2c and d). After reperfusion, the patency of STA-MCA bypasss is confirmed by intra-operative indocyanine green (ICG) video angiography and Doppler ultrasonography (Fig. 27.2e and f). The direct anastomosis procedure is followed by indirect pial synangiosis such as EDMS. Postoperative course of this patient was uneventful, and MR angiography demonstrated apparently patent STA-MCA bypass as shown by thick high signal intensity (asterisk in Fig. 27.3d). T2-weighted MR imaging showed the absence of parenchymal lesion after surgery (Fig. 27.3e). Efficacy of STA-MCA bypass for elderly patients with

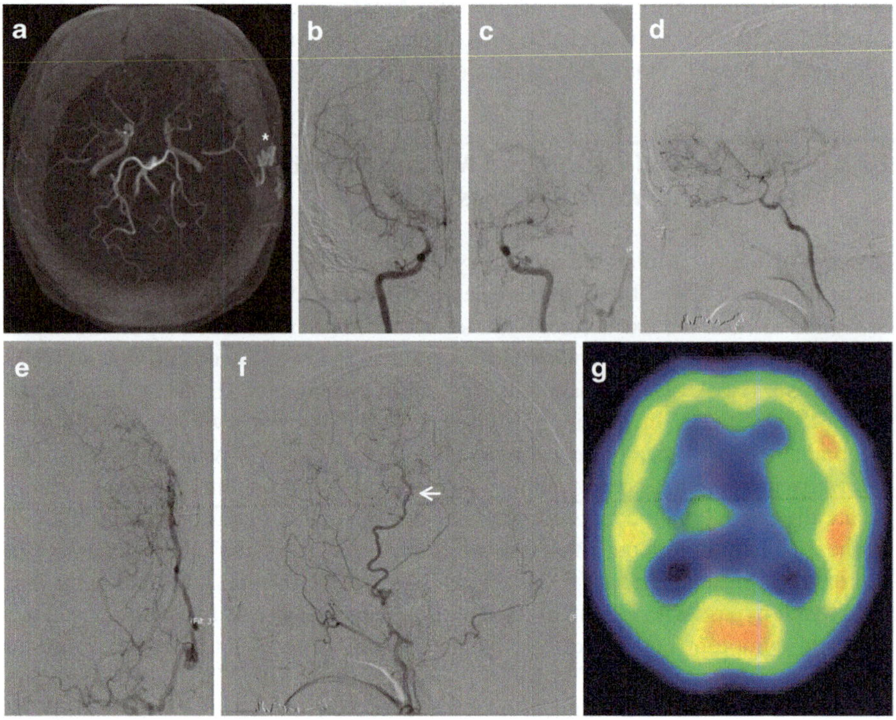

Fig. 27.1 (**a**) Representative case of a 72-year-old woman with moyamoya disease (MMD). MR angiography demonstrated an apparently patent bypass, undergone at the age of 60 years (**a**). Bilateral internal carotid angiograms indicated the definitive MMD (**b–d**). Left external carotid angiogram demonstrated patent STA-MCA bypass (arrow) and pial synangiosis via middle meningeal artery and deep temporal artery (**e** and **f**). ^{123}I-IMP SPECT indicated favorable hemodynamics on the hemisphere operated on, while apparent hemodynamic compromise on the right hemisphere (**g**)

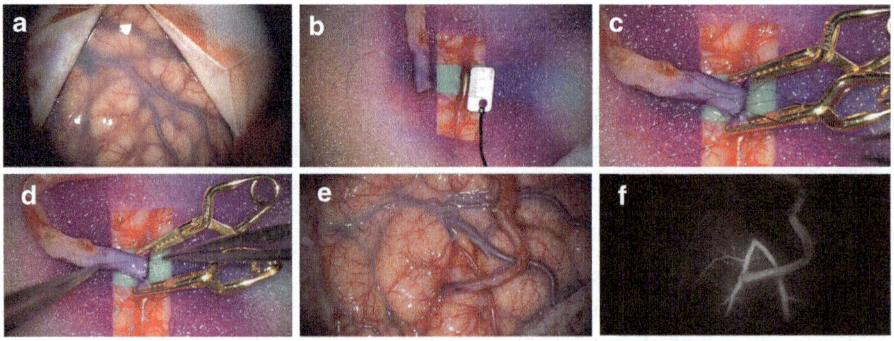

Fig. 27.2 Intra-operative view of right combined revascularization. Surgical view before (**a**, **b**), during (**c**, **d**), and after right STA-MCA bypass (**e**, **f**). Vascular wall structure was very thin and fragile, compatible with the characteristic finding of MMD (**c**, **d**). Indocyanine green video angiography demonstrated patent bypass (**f**)

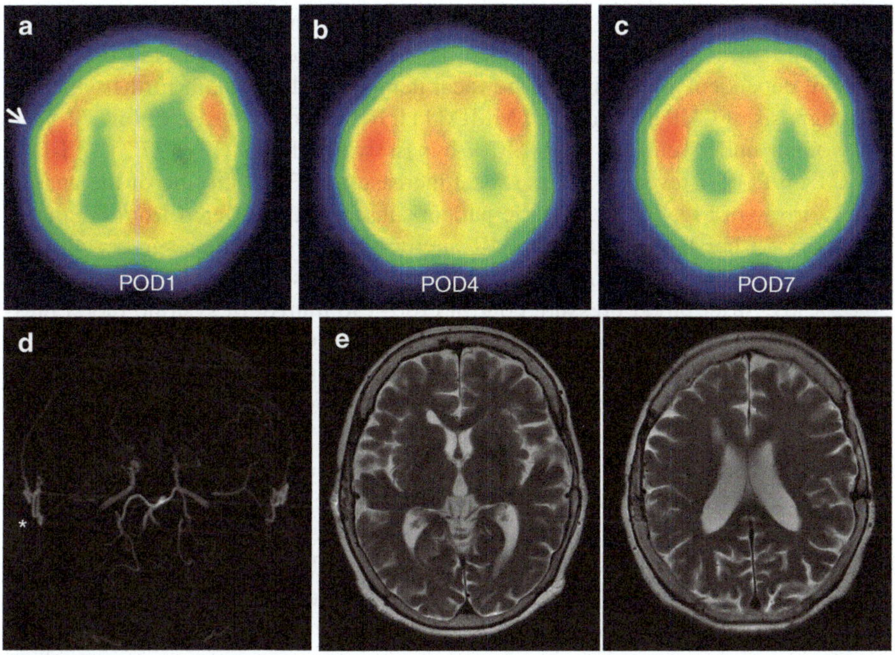

Fig. 27.3 ^{123}I-IMP SPECT after STA-MCA bypass (**a**, **b**, **c**) indicated temporary local hyperperfusion (arrow in **a**). Postoperative MR angiography showing patent bypass (asterisks in **d**), and the absence of brain damage by T2-weighted MR imaging (**e**). *POD* postoperative day(s)

MMD was reported from multiple institutes [12–14], indicating revascularization surgery could be beneficial for the elderly MMD patients as well as for the younger adult patients.

27.5 Potential Complications of the Revascularization Surgery for Elderly MMD Patients

Surgical complications of the combined revascularization procedure for adult MMD include perioperative ischemic stroke and cerebral hyperperfusion (CHP) syndrome [11, 15–17]. Perioperative cerebral ischemia could be caused by a variety of factors including intra-operative hypotension, anemia, inadequate general anesthesia (hypocapnia, etc.), and surgical procedure. While considering the association of atherosclerosis in the elderly MMD patients, ischemic complication should be carefully avoided by prompt perioperative management [14]. Besides perioperative ischemic stroke, CHP syndrome is one of the most deleterious complications after STA-MCA bypass for MMD, especially in the elderly [14]. Excessive focal increase in cerebral blood flow (CBF) at the site of the STA-MCA bypass could result in focal hyperemia associated with vasogenic edema and/or hemorrhagic conversion in adult MMD, and elderly patients are known to have higher risk for CHP syndrome [16, 17]. Clinical presentation of local CHP includes transient neurological deteriorations, seizure, and delayed intracerebral hemorrhage [11, 16]. Blood pressure dependent worsening of the focal neurological symptom further supports the diagnosis of CHP syndrome in MMD [11]. Representative case of this 72-year-old woman underwent left STA-MCA bypass with EDMS (Fig. 27.2). ^{123}I-IMP SPECT on POD 1 revealed intense focal increase in CBF at the site of the anastomosis (arrow in Fig. 27.3a), and the patient subsequently suffered from fluctuated numbness on her left extremities. MR angiography 2 days after surgery showed apparently patent STA-MCA bypass with thick high signal intensity (asterisk in Fig. 27.3d). Strict blood pressure control (100–130 mmHg of systolic blood pressure) improved her symptom, and serial ^{123}I-IMP SPECT indicated the gradual distribution of local hyperperfusion to the wider vascular territory on the affected hemisphere (Fig. 27.3b and c). As shown in this case, blood pressure lowering is generally an effective management of CHP in adult MMD patients, but the concomitant ischemic complication at remote area should be carefully avoided by prompt blood pressure control, such as the avoidance of the excessive hypotension [11, 14]. Besides the blood pressure control, protective role of minocycline hydrochloride and edaravone was reported to ameliorate CHP after revascularization surgery for adult MMD, based on their pharmacological effects of blood–brain barrier maintenance and anti-oxidant/anti-inflammatory roles [18, 19].

Acknowledgement This study was supported by JSPS KAKENHI grant number 20 K09362 (Miki Fujimura). The ethical committee of Kohnan Hospital approved the clinical study of postoperative CBF analysis. The authors have no conflict of interest regarding this study.

References

1. Suzuki J, Takaku A. Cerebrovascular 'moyamoya' disease. Disease showing abnormal net-like vessels in base of brain. Arch Neurol. 1969;20:288–99.
2. Fujimura M, Bang OY, Kim JS. Moyamoya disease. Front Neurol Neurosci. 2016;40:204–20.
3. Kuriyama S, Kusaka Y, Fujimura M, Wakai K, Tamakoshi A, Hashimoto S. Prevalence and clinico-pathological features of moyamoya disease in Japan: findings from a nationwide epidemiological survey. Stroke. 2008;39:42–7.
4. Kim JS. Moyamoya disease: epidemiology, clinical features, and diagnosis. J Stroke. 2016;18:2–11.
5. Tominaga T, Suzuki N, Miyamoto S, Koizumi A, Kuroda S, Takahashi JC, et al. Recommendations for the management of Moyamoya disease: a statement from research committee on spontaneous occlusion of the circle of Willis (Moyamoya disease) [2nd edition]. Surg Cereb Stroke. 2018;46:136–40. (in Japanese)
6. Ryoo S, Cha J, Kim SJ, Choi JW, Ki CS, Kim KH, et al. High- resolution magnetic resonance wall imaging findings of Moyamoya disease. Stroke. 2014;45:2457–60.
7. Yuan M, Liu ZQ, Wang ZQ, Li B, Xu LJ, Xiao XL. High-resolution MR imaging of the arterial wall in moyamoya disease. Neurosci Lett. 2015;584:77–82.
8. Fujimura M, Sonobe S, Nishijima Y, Niizuma K, Sakata H, Kure S, et al. Genetics and biomarkers of moyamoya disease: significance of RNF213 as a susceptibility gene. J Stroke. 2014;16:65–72.

9. Fujimura M, Tominaga T. Current status of revascularization surgery for moyamoya disease: special consideration for its 'internal carotid-external carotid (IC-EC) conversion' as the physiological reorganization system. Tohoku J Exp Med. 2015;236:45–53.
10. Jeon JP, Kim JE, Cho WS, Bang JS, Son YJ, Oh CW. Meta-analysis of the surgical outcomes of symptomatic moyamoya disease in adults. J Neurosurg. 2018;128:793–9.
11. Fujimura M, Shimizu H, Inoue T, Mugikura S, Saito A, Tominaga T. Significance of focal cerebral hyperperfusion as a cause of transient neurologic deterioration after EC-IC bypass for moyamoya disease: comparative study with non-moyamoya patients using n-isopropyl-p-[(123)i]iodoamphetamine single-photon emission computed tomography. Neurosurgery. 2011;68:957–65.
12. Gupta R, Moore JM, Adeeb N, Griessenauer CJ, Patel AS, Chua MH, et al. Clinical presentation, progression, and treatment outcomes of moyamoya disease in the elderly. Acta Neurochir. 2016;158:2409–14.
13. Williamson RW, Abla AA, Zabramski JM, Nakaji P, Spetzler RF, Wanebo JE. Revascularization of Moyamoya Angiopathy in older adults. World Neurosurg. 2017;99:37–40.
14. Fujimura M, Shimizu H, Inoue T, Niizuma K, Tominaga T. Issues in revascularization surgery for elderly patients with moyamoya disease. Surg Cereb Stroke. 2014;42:37–41. (in Japanese)
15. Kim JE, Oh CW, Kwon OK, Park SQ, Kim SE, Kim YK. Transient hyperperfusion after superficial temporal artery/middle cerebral artery bypass surgery as a possible cause of postoperative transient neurological deterioration. Cerebrovasc Dis. 2008;25:580–6.
16. Fujimura M, Mugikura S, Kaneta T, Shimizu H, Tominaga T. Incidence and risk factors for symptomatic cerebral hyperperfusion after superficial temporal artery-middle cerebral artery anastomosis in patients with moyamoya disease. Surg Neurol. 2009;71:442–7.
17. Uchino H, Kuroda S, Hirata K, Shiga T, Houkin K, Tamaki N. Predictors and clinical features of postoperative hyperperfusion after surgical revascularization for moyamoya disease: a serial single photon emission CT/positron emission tomography study. Stroke. 2012;43:2610–6.
18. Fujimura M, Niizuma K, Inoue T, Sato K, Endo H, Shimizu H, et al. Minocycline prevents focal neurologic deterioration due to cerebral hyperperfusion after extracranial-intracranial bypass for moyamoya disease. Neurosurgery. 2014;74:163–70.
19. Uchino H, Nakayama N, Kazumata K, Kuroda S, Houkin K. Edaravone reduces hyperperfusion-related neurological deficits in adult moyamoya disease: historical control study. Stroke. 2016;47:1930–2.

GPSR Compliance

The European Union's (EU) General Product Safety Regulation (GPSR) is a set of rules that requires consumer products to be safe and our obligations to ensure this.

If you have any concerns about our products, you can contact us on ProductSafety@springernature.com

In case Publisher is established outside the EU, the EU authorized representative is:

Springer Nature Customer Service Center GmbH
Europaplatz 3
69115 Heidelberg, Germany

Batch number: 10738115

Printed by Printforce, the Netherlands